AF798938

Colonic Diverticular Disease

Foreword

The detection of diverticula in the colon is frequent and on a continuous rise which is due to a series of factors that include the increasing number of colonoscopies for colon cancer screening purpose and the demographic evolution with an increase of the elderly population. Although often detected in the complete absence of symptoms, colon diverticuli may present with a broad spectrum of clinical manifestations that range from mild abdominal symptoms and mild inflammation to severe inflammation with complications and life-threatening conditions. In the context of symptomatic colonic diverticular disease, among the many challenges posed is also the question whether diverticuli are the cause of irritable bowel syndrome or simply an innocuous bystander.

The pathophysiology underlying the various phenotypes of diverticular disease is multifactorial and complex. Basic and translational research has advanced our knowledge and led to a change in paradigm which is reflected by a significant progress in the clinical management of colon diverticular disease in all its facets.

The clinician and clinical scientist will find all the relevant questions answered in this most comprehensive book on colon diverticular disease presented by Tursi, Bafutto, Brandimarte, and Oliveira. With the contribution of authoritative colleagues, all critical aspects and novel areas around colonic diverticular diseases are presented in an impressive didactic manner and in excellent style.

This book provides an up-to-date and comprehensive overview on diverticular disease of the colon including all the recent innovations in the management, from modifiable risk factors to medical and surgical therapies.

This book should be delivered to the desk of all clinicians who demand for a comprehensive update on Colonic Diverticular Disease.

My compliments to the editors and all the authors who contributed to the edition of this book.

September 2nd, 2021

Peter Malfertheiner
Department of Gastroenterology,
Hepatology and Infectious Diseases,
Otto-von-Guericke, University Hospital,
Magdeburg, Germany

Antonio Tursi • Mauro Bafutto
Giovanni Brandimarte • Enio Chaves de Oliveira
Editors

Colonic Diverticular Disease

Springer

Editors
Antonio Tursi
Territorial Gastroenterology Service
Local Sanitary Agency
Barletta-Andria-Trani
Barletta, Italy

Mauro Bafutto
Department of Internal Medicine
Division of Gastroenterology
Universidade Federal de Goiás
Goiânia, Brazil

Giovanni Brandimarte
Division of Internal Medicine and
Gastroenterology
"Cristo Re" Hospital
Roma, Italy

Enio Chaves de Oliveira
Department of Surgery
Universidade Federal de Goiás
School of Medicine
Goiânia, Brazil

ISBN 978-3-030-93760-7 ISBN 978-3-030-93761-4 (eBook)
https://doi.org/10.1007/978-3-030-93761-4

© The Editor(s) (if applicable) and The Author(s), under exclusive license to Springer Nature Switzerland AG 2022
This work is subject to copyright. All rights are solely and exclusively licensed by the Publisher, whether the whole or part of the material is concerned, specifically the rights of translation, reprinting, reuse of illustrations, recitation, broadcasting, reproduction on microfilms or in any other physical way, and transmission or information storage and retrieval, electronic adaptation, computer software, or by similar or dissimilar methodology now known or hereafter developed.
The use of general descriptive names, registered names, trademarks, service marks, etc. in this publication does not imply, even in the absence of a specific statement, that such names are exempt from the relevant protective laws and regulations and therefore free for general use.
The publisher, the authors and the editors are safe to assume that the advice and information in this book are believed to be true and accurate at the date of publication. Neither the publisher nor the authors or the editors give a warranty, expressed or implied, with respect to the material contained herein or for any errors or omissions that may have been made. The publisher remains neutral with regard to jurisdictional claims in published maps and institutional affiliations.

This Springer imprint is published by the registered company Springer Nature Switzerland AG
The registered company address is: Gewerbestrasse 11, 6330 Cham, Switzerland

Preface

Although diverticular disease seems to be a neglected disease yet, in the past few years several fine papers have been published on this topic and help us to understand better the pathogenesis and the natural history of the disease. This book represents the state of the art of this disease, but much needs to be studied and understood, in particular what is the best treatment for patients suffering from symptomatic uncomplicated diverticular disease, how to prevent acute diverticulitis occurrence, and how to prevent its recurrence. Further studies are therefore warranted in the next few years.

The editors are very grateful to all the contributors for their high-quality manuscripts, which made the publication of this book possible.

The editors are also very grateful to Springer Nature for its support in publishing this volume. Furthermore, the authors wish to thank Catherine Mazars, publishing editor, and Karthik Rajasekar, project coordinator for Springer Nature, for their help and cooperation in preparing this book.

Barletta, Italy — Antonio Tursi
Goiânia, Brazil — Mauro Bafutto
Roma, Italy — Giovanni Brandimarte
Goiânia, Brazil — Enio Chaves de Oliveira

Contents

Part VII Surgical Treatment

Contributors

Antonio Amato Department of Surgery, Imperia Hospital, Imperia, Italy

Department of General Surgery, S. Agata Hospital, Imperia, Italy

Alexandre Ferreira Bafutto Department of Surgery, Hospital da Santa Casa de Misericórdia de São Paulo, São Paulo, Brazil

Eduardo Ferreira Bafutto Department of Internal Medicine, Division of Gastroenterology and Endoscopy, Hospital Estadual Geral de Goiânia Dr. Alberto Rassi, Goiânia, Brazil

Mauro Bafutto Department of Internal Medicine, Division of Gastroenterology, Universidade Federal de Goiás, Goiânia, Brazil

Gabrio Bassotti Department of Clinical and Experimental Medicine, Gastroenterology and Hepatology Section, "Santa Maria della Misericordia" Hospital, University of Perugia, Perugia, Italy

Nunzia Bernardini Department of Clinical and Experimental Medicine, University of Pisa, Pisa, Italy

Department of Pharmacy, University of Pisa, Pisa, Italy

Gian Andrea Binda General Surgery, BioMedical Institute, Genoa, Italy

Sebastiano Biondo Department of General and Digestive Surgery, Colorectal Unit, Bellvitge University Hospital and IDIBELL, University of Barcelona, Barcelona, Spain

Ingvar Bjarnason Department of Gastroenterology, King's College Hospital, London, UK

Dmitry Bordin Healthcare Institution of Moscow, Moscow Clinical Scientific Center, Moscow, Russia

Department of Pancreatic, Biliary and Upper Digestive Tract Disorders, A. S. Loginov Moscow Clinical Scientific Center, Moscow, Russia

Department of Outpatient Therapy and Family Medicine, Tver State Medical University, Tver, Russian Federation

Department of Propaedeutic of Internal Diseases and Gastroenterology, A.I. Yevdokimov Moscow State University of Medicine and Dentistry, Moscow, Russia

Giovanni Brandimarte Division of Internal Medicine and Gastroenterology, "Cristo Re" Hospital, Rome, Italy

Maria Alessandra Brandimarte Department of Hygiene and Public Health, ASL RM1, Rome, Italy

Department of Prevention, ASL Roma 1, Rome, Italy

Leonardo Bustamante-Lopez Department of Diverticular Disease, "Clinica da Cidade Saõ Paulo" Hospital, Saõ Paulo, Brazil

Valeria Clemente Division of Nutritional and Digestive Endoscopy, "S. Eugenio" Hospital, Rome, Italy

Debora Compare Department of Clinical and Experimental Medicine, University "Federico II", Naples, Italy

Pellegrino Crafa Department of Pathology, "Ospedale Maggiore" University Hospital, University of Parma, Parma, Italy

Silvio Danese Gastroenterology and Endoscopy, IRCCS Ospedale "San Raffaele", "Vita-Salute San Raffaele" University, Milan, Italy

Silvio De Melo Oregon Health and Science University, Portland, OR, USA

Salvador J. Diaz-Cano Queen Elizabeth Hospital, Birmingham, UK

Department of Pathology and Molecular Pathology, King's Health Partners, University of London, London, UK

Francesco Di Mario Gastroenterology Unit, "Ospedale Maggiore" University Hospital, University of Parma, Parma, Italy

Carolina Di Paolo Department of Hygiene and Public Health, ASL RM1, Rome, Italy

Department of Prevention, ASL Roma 1, Rome, Italy

Enrico Di Rosa Department of Hygiene and Public Health, ASL RM1, Rome, Italy

Department of Prevention, ASL Roma 1, Rome, Italy

Dan L. Dumitrascu 2nd Medical Department, Iuliu Hațieganu University of Medicine and Pharmacy Cluj Napoca, Napoca, Romania

Walter Elisei Division of Gastroenterology, "S. Camillo" Hospital, Rome, Italy

Annarita Eramo Division of Nutritional and Digestive Endoscopy, "S. Eugenio" Hospital, Rome, Italy

Ricardo Escalante Universidad Central de Venezuela, Loira Medical Center, Caracas, Venezuela

Nicola Flor Division of Radiology, "L. Sacco" University Hospital, ASST "Fatebenefratelli-Sacco", Milan, Italy

Gian Marco Giorgetti Division of Nutritional and Digestive Endoscopy, "S. Eugenio" Hospital, Rome, Italy

Thomas Golda Colorectal Unit—Department of General and Digestive Surgery, Bellvitge University Hospital, University of Barcelona, Barcelona, Spain

Kok-Ann Gwee National University of Singapore and Gleneagles Hospital, Singapore, Singapore

László Herszènyi 2 Department of Medicine, Semmelweis University, Budapest, Hungary

Alois Hollerweger Department of Radiology, Hospital Barmherzige Brüder, Salzburg, Austria

David Humes Nottingham Digestive Diseases Centre and National Institute for Health Research (NIHR), Nottingham Biomedical Research Centre, Nottingham University Hospitals NHS Trust, University of Nottingham, Nottingham, UK

Silvia Innamorati Postgraduation School in Radiodiagnostic, Facoltà di Medicina e Chirurgia, Università degli Studi di Milano, Milan, Italy

Maria Ellionore Jarbrink-Sehgal Department of Gastroenterology, Veterans Affairs Medical Center, Baylor College of Medicine, Houston, TX, USA

Keiji Koda Department of Surgery, Teikyo University Chiba Medical Center, Ichihara City, Chiba, Japan

Chihiro Kosugi Department of Surgery, Teikyo University Chiba Medical Center, Ichihara City, Chiba, Japan

Wolfgang Kruis Innere Medizin, Evangelische Krankenhaus Kalk, Cologne, Germany

Juozas Kupcinskas Institute for Digestive Research, Lithuanian University of Health Sciences, Kaunas, Lithuania

Gastroenterology, Lithuanian University of Health Sciences, Kaunas, Lithuania

Adi Lahat Department of Gastroenterology, Chaim Sheba Medical Center, Tel Hashomer, Ramat Gan, Tel Aviv, Israel

Angel Lanas Service of Digestive Diseases, University Clinic Hospital Lozano Blesa, University of Zaragoza, IIS Aragón, Zaragoza, Spain

Giovanni Latella Gastroenterology Unit, "San Salvatore" Hospital, University of L'Aquila, L'Aquila, Italy

Gastroenterology, Hepatology and Nutrition Division, Department of Life, Health and Environmental Sciences, University of L'Aquila, L'Aquila, Italy

Loris R. Lopetuso CEMAD Digestive Disease Center, Dipartimento di Scienze Mediche e Chirurgiche, Fondazione Policlinico Universitario "A. Gemelli" IRCCS, Università Cattolica del Sacro Cuore, Rome, Italy

Department of Medicine and Ageing Sciences, "G. d'Annunzio" University of Chieti-Pescara, Chieti, Italy

Center for Advanced Studies and Technology (CAST), "G. d'Annunzio" University of Chieti-Pescara, Chieti, Italy

Jaune Ieva Lukosiene Department of Gastroenterology and Institute for Digestive Research, Lithuanian University of Health Sciences, Kaunas, Lithuania

Giovanni Maconi Department of Clinical Sciences, Gastrointestinal Unit, "L. Sacco" University Hospital, Milan, Italy

Peter Malfertheiner Department of Gastroenterology, Hepatology and Infectious Diseases, Otto-von-Guericke, University Hospital, Magdeburg, Germany

Cristina Marmorale Department of Experimental and Clinical Medicine, School of Medicine and Surgery, Politechnical University of Marche, Ancona, Italy

Paola Mastromarino Department of Public Health and Infectious Diseases, "Sapienza" University, Rome, Italy

Tomica Milosavljević Clinical Centre of Serbia, University of Belgrade, Belgrade, Serbia

Akira Mizuki Department of Internal Medicine, Keiyu Hospital, Yokohama, Japan

Department of Internal Medicine, Tokyo Sea Fort Square Clinic, Tokyo, Japan

Atsushi Nakajima Department of Gastroenterology and Hepatology, Yokohama City University School of Medicine, Yokohama, Kanagawa, Japan

Gerardo Nardone Department of Clinical and Experimental Medicine, University "Federico II", Naples, Italy

Veronica Ojetti Department of Emergency Medicine, "A. Gemelli" IRCCS Foundation, School of Medicine, Catholic University of the Sacred Heart, Rome, Italy

Enio Chaves de Oliveira Department of Surgery, Universidade Federal de Goiás, School of Medicine, Goiânia, Brazil

Lorenzo Paglione Department of Hygiene and Public Health, ASL RM1, Rome, Italy

Department of Prevention, ASL Roma 1, Rome, Italy

Alfredo Papa Centro Malattie Apparato Digerente (CEMAD), Fondazione Policlinico A. Gemelli, IRCCS, Università Cattolica del S. Cuore, Rome, Italy

Savvas Papagrigoriadis Department of Colorectal Surgery, King's College Hospital, London, UK

Valerio Papa Department of Digestive Surgery, "A. Gemelli" IRCCS Foundation, School of Medicine, Catholic University of the Sacred Heart, Rome, Italy

Carolina Pellegrini Department of Clinical and Experimental Medicine, University of Pisa, Pisa, Italy

Department of Pharmacy, University of Pisa, Pisa, Italy

Roberto Persiani Department of Surgical Sciences, First General Surgery Unit, "A. Gemelli" IRCCS Foundation, School of Medicine, Catholic University of the Sacred Heart, Rome, Italy

Roberto Pezzuto Department of Surgical Sciences, First General Surgery Unit, "A. Gemelli" IRCCS Foundation, School of Medicine, Catholic University of the Sacred Heart, Rome, Italy

Marcello Picchio Division of General Surgery, "P. Colombo" Hospital, ASL Roma 6, Velletri (Roma), Italy

Perry Pickhardt University of Wisconsin School of Medicine & Public Health, Madison, WI, USA

Guilherme Piovezani Ramos Division of Gastroenterology and Hepatology, Mayo Clinic, Rochester, MN, USA

Odery Ramos Department of Internal Medicine, Division of Gastroenterology, Hispital del Clinical, Universidade, federal do Paranà, Rua general Cameiro, Curitiba, Brazil

Jaroslaw Regula Department of Oncological Gastroenterology, Maria Sklodowska-Curie National Research Institute of Oncology and Department of Gastroenterology, Hepatology and Clinical Oncology, Centre of Postgraduate Medical Education, Warsaw, Poland

Cristina Maria Sabo 2nd Medical Department, Iuliu Haţieganu University of Medicine and Pharmacy Cluj Napoca, Napoca, Romania

Narimantas Evaldas Samalavicius Department of Surgery, Klaipėda University Hospital, Klaipėda, Lithuania

Edoardo Savarino Division of Gastroenterology, Department of Surgery, Oncology and Gastroenterology, University of Padua, Padua, Italy

Angela Saviano Emergency Department, Fondazione Policlinico Universitario A. Gemelli IRCCS, Università Cattolica del Sacro Cuore, Rome, Italy

Carmelo Scarpignato Faculty of Medical Sciences, LUdeS University, United Campus of Malta, Msida, Malta

Department of Health Sciences, United Campus of Malta, Msida, Malta

Faculty of Medicine, Chinese University of Hong Kong, Shatin, Hong Kong, China

Johannes Schultz Department of Gastrointestinal Surgery, Akershus University Hospital, Lørenskog, Norway

Neil Stollman Division of Gastroenterology, Alta Bates Summit Medical Center, East Bay Center for Digestive Health, Oakland, CA, USA

School of Medicine, University of California San Francisco (UCSF), San Francisco, CA, USA

Antonio Tursi Territorial Gastroenterology Service, Local Sanitary Agency Barletta-Andria-Trani, Barletta, Italy

Department of Medical and Surgical Sciences, Post-graduate School of Digestive Diseases, Catholic University, Rome, Italy

Lorenzo Maria Vetrone Centro Malattie Apparato Digerente (CEMAD), Fondazione Policlinico A. Gemelli, IRCCS, Università Cattolica del S. Cuore, Rome, Italy

Eiji Yamada Department of Gastroenterology and Hepatology, Yokohama City University School of Medicine, Yokohama, Kanagawa, Japan

Gastroenterology Division, National Hospital Organization Yokohama Medical Center, Yokohama-shi, Kanagawa, Japan

Part I

Epidemiology

Prevalence of Diverticulosis and Diverticular Disease

1

Alfredo Papa, Lorenzo Maria Vetrone, Atsushi Nakajima, and Eiji Yamada

1.1 Introduction

The most frequent anatomical alteration of the colon is diverticulosis, constituted by multiple outpockets with herniation of the mucosa and the submucosa. Diverticulosis is generally an age-related alteration and in most of the cases remains asymptomatic [1]. It is generally expected that about one-fourth/one-fifth of patients may develop symptoms linked to the presence of diverticula, and these patients are generally considered to be suffering from 'diverticular disease' (DD) [1]. It includes both diverticulitis with or without complications and symptomatic uncomplicated diverticular disease (SUDD). The latter is the most frequent form of DD affecting about 80% of all patients with symptoms attributable to diverticula [2].

A. Papa (✉) · L. M. Vetrone
Centro Malattie Apparato Digerente (CEMAD), Fondazione Policlinico A. Gemelli, IRCCS, Università Cattolica del S. Cuore, Rome, Italy
e-mail: alfredo.papa@unicatt.it

A. Nakajima · E. Yamada
Department of Gastroenterology and Hepatology, Yokohama City University School of Medicine, Yokohama, Kanagawa, Japan
e-mail: nakajima-tky@umin.ac.jp

© The Author(s), under exclusive license to Springer Nature Switzerland AG 2022
A. Tursi et al. (eds.), *Colonic Diverticular Disease*,
https://doi.org/10.1007/978-3-030-93761-4_1

The prevalence of diverticulosis and DD has been widely investigated. However, available data are not homogeneous and are often difficult to analyze since the diagnosis of diverticulosis and DD could be obtained with different diagnostic modalities and in cohorts of patients not comparable for age, symptoms, and ethnicity, only for citing the most important confounding factors.

In this chapter, we report the results of the most important studies regarding the prevalence of diverticulosis and DD, analyzing data from Western and Eastern countries separately.

1.2 Prevalence of Diverticulosis in Western Countries

The actual prevalence of colonic diverticulosis is difficult to determine because most individuals with diverticula are asymptomatic. In addition, several epidemiological studies report remarkable variations of prevalence rates and predominant location of diverticula depending on ethnicity. It is generally accepted that diverticula in Western countries are predominantly located in the left colon, whereas in Asian countries they occur predominantly in the right colon.

Colonoscopy remains the main tool used for the diagnosis of diverticulosis and DD; in fact, diverticulosis is the most reported finding on routine colonoscopy, although endoscopic diagnosis of diverticulosis is generally incidental. However, other diagnostic techniques could be used to pose the diagnosis of diverticulosis. For example, Carabotti et al., during their analysis of an Italian registry, found that diagnosis of colonic diverticula was obtained by colonoscopy in 77.1% of cases, whereas in the other 22.9% of cases it was posed by abdominal CT (10.6% of cases), barium enema (5.1% of cases), ultrasound (4% of cases), and CT colonography (3.2% of cases) [3]. This means that a colonoscopy-based study could lose about 23% of cases and therefore underestimated the prevalence. Epidemiological studies report that the prevalence of diverticulosis in Europe and North America ranges from 20 to 42% [4–6], whereas it is lower in Africa (usually under 10%), reflecting not only different dietary habits and lifestyle but also genetic background [7, 8]. Further data are obtained from a French cohort of 796 consecutive patients referred for total colonoscopy; 40% of these showed uncomplicated diverticulosis [9]. In this population, the prevalence of colonic diverticula increased from <10% in adults under 40 years of age to about 75% in those over 75 years of age, and nearly one-third presented with right-sided involvement [9]. Pooled data from the endoscopy database of the Clinical Outcomes Research Initiative (CORI) showed a prevalence of diverticulosis of 32.6% in patients aged 50–59 years [10]. This percentage steadily increased to around 71.4% of all examinations in patients aged ≥80 years [10]. To conclude, we can affirm that the prevalence of diverticulosis in Western countries has been increasing in the last few decades due to both the increasing spread of colonoscopy, especially for colorectal cancer screening reasons, and the growing age of the population.

1.3 Prevalence of DD and Diverticulitis in Western Countries

DD and its complications represent a burden for health-care systems all over the world. Data obtained from ambulatory surveys (National Ambulatory Medical Care Survey and National Hospital Ambulatory Medical Care Survey) in 2010 in the United States showed that DD is the eighth most frequent outpatient gastrointestinal diagnosis with 2.7 million clinic visits [11]. In addition, the 2012 Nationwide Inpatients Sample (NIS) reported that cases with diverticulitis without hemorrhage admissions were more than 200,000 with an increase of 21% when compared to the 2003 data [11]. Diverticular hemorrhage (included in gastrointestinal hemorrhage diagnosis) had an adjunctive burden of admissions and costs. In 2003, Delvaux et al. reported an estimation of the prevalence of DD in the European Union (EU), which included at that time 15 countries with a total population of 376,481,775 inhabitants [12]. About 27.3% of the EU population, corresponding to more than one hundred million people, had colonic diverticula. According to the authors' assumptions, the number of perforation cases/year was 60,237 and the annual rate of hospital admission for DD was nearly 800,000 [12].

The Scottish Morbidity Records, a cohort study including all patients with a hospital admission for DD as the primary diagnosis, reported data on 90,990 admissions from 2000 to 2010 [13]. It showed that the increase in admissions for DD during the study period was higher than the admission rate for all digestive diseases or for all kinds of admissions in the same period of time, with an average annual increase of 4.5% [13]. This finding confirms the increasing prevalence of DD in the last few decades. In the same study, the standardized mortality ratio (SMR) among patients having a first admission for DD was also assessed. Data were divided according to the primary management of DD, surgical or medical, and according to the admission route, in election or in emergency. The highest SMR of 4.95 was observed among patients having an operative primary management in the group of age $\leq$ 55 years in case of an emergency admission route compared to an SMR of 2.80 for patients with the same age but with an elective admission route [13]. As expected, mortality rates were lower in the case of nonoperative management. Binda et al. reported Italian data regarding 174,436 hospitalizations for DD with an increasing rate in the 2008–2015 period from 39 to 48 per 100,000 inhabitants ($p < 0.001$) [14]. The rate of hospitalization was higher for women, but the increasing trend over time was even more pronounced among men (mean increase per year 3.9 and 2.1% among men and women, respectively) ($p < 0.001$) [14]. Putting these data together, we can observe that the incidence of diverticulitis has increased over time and increases with patient age. In particular, in recent decades, the relative increase in diverticulitis has been the highest in young patients as reported by Bharucha et al. who found that, from 1980 through 2007, the incidence of diverticulitis in individuals aged 40–49 years increased by 132% [15].

With regard to the prevalence of acute diverticulitis in patients with diverticulosis, it has been suggested that the lifetime risk of acute diverticulitis is 10–25%

[16]. However, these risk estimates were based on older literature without accurate studies on the true prevalence. A recent retrospective observational cohort study including 2222 patients with baseline diverticulosis identified at colonoscopy has addressed this issue, providing information on the long-term risk of complications of colonic diverticulosis [17]. Over an 11-year follow-up period, 95 patients developed diverticulitis (4.3%; 6 per 1000 patient years); of these, 23 met the rigorous definition of diverticulitis (1%; 1.5 per 1000 patient years) [17]. Further data were reported by Loffeld in a cohort of 433 patients with diverticulosis undergoing colonoscopy [18]. The sum of follow-up years was 6191, with a mean follow-up of 14.1 years per patient [18]. A total of 30 cases of diverticulitis (7%) were identified corresponding to 4.8 cases per 1000 years [18]. Based on these population-based colonoscopy studies, the natural history of colonic diverticulosis seems favorable with a far lower incidence of complications, thus contradicting the common belief that diverticulosis has a high rate of progression.

1.4 Prevalence of Complicated Diverticulitis in Western Countries

Complicated diverticulitis, as defined by the presence of any of the manifestations, such as abscess, peritonitis, obstruction, or fistula, is burdened with considerable morbidity and mortality [1, 2]. Complications of acute diverticulitis occur in approximately 12% of patients [15], and mortality after complicated diverticulitis is the highest among individuals with perforation or abscesses [19]. In fact, in a population-based cohort study performed in the United Kingdom, mortality at 1 year was 20% in patients with perforated diverticulitis compared to 4% in age- and sex-matched controls [19].

A population-based cohort study based on computerized records from the General Practice Research Database linked to Hospital Episode Statistics data from the UK found that increasing episodes of acute diverticulitis were associated with an increased risk of developing a fistula (two or more prior episodes; OR 1.54, 95% CI 1.08–2.19), but there was no clear relationship with stricture or perforation/abscess [20]. In addition, diverticular bleeding is a common cause of lower gastrointestinal hemorrhage in adults, sometimes requiring surgery or arterial embolization after the failure of endoscopic hemostasis [21]. Wheat and Strate analyzed data from the Nationwide Inpatient Sample from 2000 through 2010 and identified adult patients with a discharge diagnosis of diverticular bleeding or diverticulitis [22]. They reported that the prevalence of hospitalizations per 100,000 persons for diverticular bleeding decreased over the 10-year period from 32.5 to 27.1 (−5.4; 95% confidence interval − 5.1 to −5.7) and that the prevalence of diverticular bleeding was the highest in Blacks (34.4/100,000 in 2010), whereas the prevalence of diverticulitis was the highest in whites (75.5/100,000 in 2010) [22].

1.5 Prevalence of SUDD and Progression from SUDD to Diverticulitis

As previously reported, most DD patients suffer from SUDD; they have a low quality of life, requiring frequent therapeutic courses [1, 2]. Tursi et al. found that SUDD was recorded in about 7% of the patients having diverticulosis [23]. Furthermore, they showed that a small but not irrelevant percentage of patients suffering from SUDD occurred after an episode of acute diverticulitis. This clinical entity, defined as post-diverticulitis (PD)-SUDD, was found in about 2% of the patients having diverticulosis [23]. Overall, considering the prevalence of 'primary' SUDD and PD-SUDD, it affected about 10% of patients having diverticulosis. Four studies investigated the outcomes of SUDD in terms of occurrence of acute diverticulitis and its complications [24–27]. The first study performed by Salem et al. in 2007 included 167 SUDD patients during a 5-year follow-up [24]. Acute uncomplicated diverticulitis occurred in only 1.7% of cases, and only a single patient underwent a sigmoid colectomy for recurrent symptoms [24]. The second study was a prospective, open-label study that compared SUDD patients taking either 800 mg of mesalamine b.i.d. for 10 days every month or no mesalamine [25]. Gatta et al. reported acute diverticulitis occurrence in eight SUDD patients (10.4%) not taking mesalamine during a 5-year follow-up [25]. The third was a double-blind placebo-controlled study assessing the role of mesalamine, with or without probiotics, in maintaining remission in SUDD patients during a 1-year follow-up [26]. The authors found that acute diverticulitis occurred in 3.5% of patients [26]. Recently, Tursi et al. performed a 13-year analysis on an SUDD population and found that acute diverticulitis occurred in a significant percentage of patients. Indeed, during the follow-up, about 8% of patients developed acute diverticulitis and 1.1% died from diverticulitis complications [27]. Taking all the data together, the risk of acute diverticulitis occurrence in SUDD seems to be significantly higher than the risk in people who have simple diverticulosis, in whom acute diverticulitis occurs in 4.3% of cases [17].

1.6 Prevalence and Characteristics of Diverticulosis and DD in Eastern Countries

The most important feature of diverticulosis in the Eastern countries is that it is predominant in the right-sided colon. The prevalence of diverticulosis in the Eastern countries is reported to be 13–25%, and right-sided diverticula are common. Colonoscopy-based studies have shown that the prevalence of diverticulosis was 12% in Korea (mean age: 51 years) and 14% in Taiwan (mean age: 53 years). Barium-based studies in Japan have shown a significant increase in the prevalence of diverticulosis from 2.1% in 1967 and 7.8% in 1983 to 28% in 1997. In Korea, 15% of patients with colonic diverticulosis had left-sided diverticula, whereas half of the Japanese and Taiwanese populations with colonic diverticulosis had left-sided diverticula. It is interesting that the prevalence of diverticulosis in Lebanon was 33% (mean age: 61 years), and most subjects had left-sided diverticulosis. However, other studies from the Middle East suggest a much lower prevalence with predominantly right-sided diverticulosis [28]. Very recently, a colonoscopy-based study in Singapore has shown that the prevalence of diverticulosis progressively increased from 2006 to 2016 (14.9 vs 23.9%, adjusted trend <0.001), with an overall prevalence of 19.6%. Patients with diverticulosis were older and had higher body mass index, and diverticulosis was significantly more prevalent in Chinese than in Malay and Indian races (20.5 vs 18.9 vs 15.5%, $P < 0.05$). Right-sided diverticulosis was more common than left-sided or pan diverticulosis (16.2 vs 8.3 vs 4.8%, $P < 0.05$). As Singapore is a multiethnic country with rapid recent westernization, this report is of great interest for understanding the recent situation of diverticulosis in Eastern countries [29].

A recent Japanese colonoscopy-based study has shown that diverticulosis was detected in 11,771 (18.8%; 10,023 men and 1748 women) out of 62,503 subjects (47,325 men and 15,178 women; age: 52.1 ± 9.2 years). The incidences of diverticulosis in 1990–2000 and 2001–2010 were 13.0% (3771 of 29,071) and 23.9% (8000 of 33,432) respectively: the latter was much higher than the former in all age groups and for both genders. According to the analysis of the location of diverticular disease, left-sided ones significantly increased with age but did not significantly change with time [30]. In studies analyzing the risk factors for the development of diverticulosis in Asian countries, a colonoscopy-based study in Singapore has shown that age (odds ratio (OR) 1.060, 95% confidence interval (CI) 1.052–1.068), BMI (OR 1.051, 95% CI 1.028–1.075), male gender (OR 1.317, 95% CI 1.084–1.600), and abdominal pain (OR 1.409, 95% CI 1.168–1.699) were positively associated with diverticulosis, whereas constipation (OR 0.566, 95% CI 0.452–0.709) was negatively associated with diverticulosis [29]. In Japan, it has been demonstrated that age (β = 0.217–0.674, OR = 1.24–1.96), male gender (β = 0.185, OR = 1.20), smoking (β = 0.142–0.200, OR = 1.15–1.22), severe weight increase in adulthood (β = 0.153, OR = 1.17), HbA1c (β = 0.136, OR = 1.15), drinking (β = 0.109, OR = 1.11), and serum triglyceride (β = 0.098, OR = 1.10) showed significantly positive association with diverticulosis, whereas body mass index and blood pressure did not by utilizing the multiple logistic analysis calculating standardized coefficients (β) and odds ratio (OR) [30]. In the past, the association between constipation and colonic diverticulosis has been pointed out, but, in recent years, reports of an inverse correlation have been seen from Asia [29, 31, 32]. In conclusion, colonic diverticulosis is increasing in Asian countries and is predominantly present on the right side of the colon in Asian countries. This increase may be associated with the adoption of a Western lifestyle, and the incidence of left-sided diverticulosis has markedly increased with age. Although it is difficult to make a pure comparison of the incidence of diverticulosis between Western and Eastern populations because of differences in patient background and evaluation methods of diverticulosis, the incidence of diverticulosis seems to be slightly lower in Asia than in Europe and the United States.

1.7 Prevalence of DD and Diverticulitis in Eastern Countries

There are few reports showing the incidence rate of colonic diverticulitis in Asia. Different from Western countries, right-sided diverticulitis shows a higher incidence in Asian countries [33–36]. It is reported that 38% of diverticulitis was on the right side and 49% was on the left side of the colon in Singapore [33] and also that 76% of diverticulitis was on the right side and 24% on the left side in Korea [34]. Patients with right-sided diverticulitis are significantly younger, but the incidence of overall complications is higher on the left side. A Japanese multicenter study showed that diverticulitis of the left side was significantly more frequent (61.0%) in elderly patients although significantly more eligible patients presented with right-sided diverticulitis (70.1%) [36]. Another Japanese multicenter study showed that the mortality rate of colonic diverticulitis was significantly higher in patients with complications than in those without complications (2.8 vs. 0.2%) [37]. It is also reported that the mortality rate was significantly higher in patients with left-sided diverticulitis than in patients with the right-sided one (10.8 vs. 0%) [34].

Reports from Asia indicate that patients with colonic diverticula have a high incidence of abdominal pain, especially irritable bowel syndrome-like symptoms. The frequency is particularly high in patients with left-sided diverticulosis [37, 38]. This result suggests that the right side and the left side may both have different pathologies. There are no reports of SUDD in Asia. A report from Japan on diverticular bleeding showed that the cumulative incidence of bleeding from diverticulosis was approximately 2% in 5 years and 10% in 10 years and that the overall incidence was 0.46 per 1000 patient years, and an age of more than 70 years and both-sided diverticulosis increased the risk of bleeding [39]. Another report in Japan also showed that the incidence of diverticular bleeding was 1.5%, the mean age was 69.7 years with a higher incidence in men (66.3%), and the bleeding was predominantly of the both-sided type (47.0%) [40]. The proportion of diverticular bleeding increased significantly from 1.02% (22 of 2157 subjects) in 2003 to 1.67% (69 of 4159 subjects) in 2011. Using a national database in Japan, it is estimated that the in-hospital mortality rate in patients with diverticular bleeding was 0.7% [41]. To conclude, although the prevalence of diverticulitis is unknown in Asia, it is more common on the right side, but left-sided diverticulitis increases with age, and complications and mortality are higher on the left side. Diverticular bleeding is increasing in Asia and occurs bilaterally. SUDD has not yet been reported in Asia, but diverticulosis with IBS symptoms is more common on the left side than on the right.

1.8 Conclusions

The prevalence of diverticulosis and DD, which includes both diverticulitis with its complications and SUDD, has been increasing in the last few decades. This is attributable to both the increase in the average age of the population and the increasing diffusion of diagnostic methods, especially colonoscopy, mainly for colorectal cancer screening. It is not easy to compare the prevalence data of diverticulosis between populations of Western and Eastern countries due to the nonhomogeneity of the different studies; however, it seems to be slightly lower in Asia than in Europe and the United States. Although the prevalence of diverticulitis is unknown in Asia, it is more common on the right side unlike in Western countries where it is found mostly in the left colon. Finally, diverticular bleeding prevalence is on the rise in both Asia and the United States; however, in Asia, it can occur bilaterally, whereas in the West it is more common in the left colon.

References

1. Tursi A, Scarpignato C, Strate LL, Lanas A, Kruis W, Lahat A, Danese S. Colonic diverticular disease. Nat Rev Dis Primers. 2020;6:20.
2. Tursi A, Papa A, Danese S. Review article: the pathophysiology and medical management of diverticulosis and diverticular disease of the colon. Aliment Pharmacol Ther. 2015;42(6):664–84. https://doi.org/10.1111/apt.13322. Epub 2015 Jul 22
3. Carabotti M, Cuomo R, Barbara G, Pace F, Andreozzi P, Cremon C, Annibale B. Demographic and clinical features distinguish subgroups of diverticular disease patients: results from an Italian nationwide registry. United European Gastroenterol J. 2018;6:926–34.
4. Manousos ON, Truelove SC, Lumsden K. Prevalence of colonic diverticulosis in general population of Oxford area. BMJ. 1967;3:762–3.
5. Loffeld RJ, Van der Putten AB. Diverticular disease of the colon and concomitant abnormalities in patients undergoing endoscopic evaluation of the large bowel. Color Dis. 2002;4:189–92.
6. Peery AF, Keku TO, Martin CF, Eluri S, Runge T, Galanko JA, Sandler RS. Distribution and characteristics of colonic diverticula in a United States screening population. Clin Gastroenterol Hepatol. 2016;14(7):980–5.
7. Reichert MC, Lammert F. The genetic epidemiology of diverticulosis and diverticular disease: emerging evidence. United European Gastroenterol J. 2015;3(5):409–18. https://doi.org/10.1177/2050640615576676. PMID: 26535118; PMCID: PMC4625748
8. Tănase I, Păun S, Stoica B, Negoi I, Gaspar B, Beuran M. Epidemiology of diverticular disease—systematic review of the literature. Chirurgia. 2015;110(1):9–14.
9. Faucheron JL, Roblin X, Bichard P, Heluwaert F. The prevalence of right-sided colonic diverticulosis and diverticular haemorrhage. Color Dis. 2013;15(5):e266–70.
10. Everhart JE, Ruhl CE. Burden of digestive diseases in the United States part II: lower gastrointestinal diseases. Gastroenterology. 2009;136:741–54.
11. Peery AF, Crockett SD, Barritt AS, Dellon ES, Eluri S, Gangarosa LM, Jensen ET, Lund JL, Pasricha S, Runge T, Schmidt M, Shaheen NJ, Sandler RS. Burden of gastrointestinal, liver, and pancreatic diseases in the United States. Gastroenterology. 2015;149(7):1731–1741.e3.
12. Delvaux M. Diverticular disease of the colon in Europe: epidemiology, impact on citizen health and prevention. Aliment Pharmacol Ther. 2003;18(Suppl 3):71–4.
13. Paterson HM, Arnott ID, Nicholls RJ, Clark D, Bauer J, Bridger PC, Crowe AM, Knight AD, Hodgkins P, Solomon D, Dunlop MG. Diverticular disease in Scotland: 2000-2010. Color Dis. 2015;17(4):329–34.
14. Binda GA, Mataloni F, Bruzzone M, Carabotti M, Cirocchi R, Nascimbeni R, Gambassi G, Amato A, Vettoretto N, Pinnarelli L, Cuomo R, Annibale B. Trends in hospital admission for acute diverticulitis in Italy from 2008 to 2015. Tech Coloproctol. 2018;22(8):597–604.
15. Bharucha AE, Parthasarathy G, Ditah I, Fletcher JG, Ewelukwa O, Pendlimari R, Yawn BP, Melton LJ, Schleck C, Zinsmeister AR. Temporal trends in the incidence and natural history of diverticulitis: a population-based study. Am J Gastroenterol. 2015;110(11):1589–96.
16. Hughes LE. Postmortem survey of diverticular disease of the colon. II. The muscular abnormality of the sigmoid colon. Gut. 1969;10:344–51.

17. Shahedi K, Fuller G, Bolus R, Cohen E, Vu M, Shah R, et al. Longterm risk of acute diverticulitis among patients with incidental diverticulosis found during colonoscopy. Clin Gastroenterol Hepatol. 2013;11:1609–13.
18. Loffeld RJ. Long-term follow-up and development of diverticulitis in patients diagnosed with diverticulosis of the colon. Int J Color Dis. 2016;31(1):15–7. https://doi.org/10.1007/s00384-015-2397-1. Epub 2015 Sep 26
19. Humes DJ, Solaymani-Dodaran M, Fleming KM, Simpson J, Spiller RC, West J. A population-based study of perforated diverticular disease incidence and associated mortality. Gastroenterology. 2009;136(4):1198–205. https://doi.org/10.1053/j.gastro.2008.12.054. Epub 2008
20. Humes DJ, West J. Role of acute diverticulitis in the development of complicated colonic diverticular disease and 1-year mortality after diagnosis in the UK: population-based cohort study. Gut. 2012;61(1):95–100.
21. Jensen DM, Machicado GA, Jutabha R, Kovacs TOG. Urgent colonoscopy for the diagnosis and treatment of severe diverticular hemorrhage. N Engl J Med. 2000;342:78–82.
22. Wheat CL, Strate LL. Trends in hospitalization for diverticulitis and diverticular bleeding in the United States from 2000 to 2010. Clin Gastroenterol Hepatol. 2016;14(1):96–103.
23. Tursi A, Elisei W, Franceschi M, Picchio M, Di Mario F, Brandimarte G. The prevalence of symptomatic uncomplicated diverticular disease could be lower than expected: a single-center colonoscopy-based cohort study. Eur J Gastroenterol Hepatol. 2021;33(1S Suppl 1):e478–83.
24. Salem TA, Molloy RG, O'Dwyer PJ. Prospective, five-year follow-up study of patients with symptomatic uncomplicated diverticular disease. Dis Colon Rectum. 2007;50:1460–4.
25. Gatta L, Di Mario F, Curlo M, et al. Long-term treatment with mesalazine in patients with symptomatic uncomplicated diverticular disease. Intern Emerg Med. 2012;7:133–7.
26. Tursi A, Brandimarte G, Elisei W, Picchio M, Forti G, Pianese G, Rodino S, D'Amico T, Sacca N, Portincasa P, Capezzuto E, Lattanzio R, Spadaccini A, Fiorella S, Polimeni F, Polimeni N, Stoppino V, Stoppino G, Giorgetti GM, Aiello F, Danese S. Randomised clinical trial: mesalazine and/or probiotics in maintaining remission of symptomatic uncomplicated diverticular disease—a double-blind, randomised, placebo-controlled study. Aliment Pharmacol Ther. 2013;38(7):741–51.
27. Tursi A, Franceschi M, Elisei W, Picchio M, Mario FD, Brandimarte G. The natural history of symptomatic uncomplicated diverticular disease: a long-term follow-up study. Ann Gastroenterol. 2021;34(2):208–13. https://doi.org/10.20524/aog.2020.0560. Epub 2020 Dec 7. PMID: 33654361; PMCID: PMC7903564
28. Imaeda H, Hibi T. The burden of diverticular disease and its complications: West versus East. Inflamm Intest Dis. 2018;3(2):61–8. https://doi.org/10.1159/000492178.
29. Soh YSA, Ooi SQD, Chan YH, Siah TK, Lee SE, Lee WJJ, Zhu F, Yeoh KG, Gwee KA. Rising prevalence of colonic diverticulosis in a westernized multi-ethnic Asian community. J Gastroenterol Hepatol. 2021;36(2):413–20. https://doi.org/10.1111/jgh.15165.
30. Yamamichi N, Shimamoto T, Takahashi Y, et al. Trend and risk factors of diverticulosis in Japan: age, gender, and lifestyle/metabolic-related factors may cooperatively affect on the colorectal diverticula formation. PLoS One. 2015;10(4):e0123688.
31. Yamada E, Nakajima A, et al. Constipation is not associated with colonic diverticula: a multicenter study in Japan. Neurogastroenterol Motil. 2015;27(3):333–8. 32
32. Yamada E, Kuriyama H, Uchida E, Murata Y, Hata Y, Tagri M, Isozaki Y, Oyamada H, Ozawa Y, Ito T, Mizuki A, Inamori M, Manabe N, Haruma K, Nakajima A. Association between endoscopic findings related to colonic diverticula and bowel habits: a multicenter study in Japan. J Gastroenterol Hepatol. 2017;32(12):1938–42.
33. Wong SK, Ho YH, Leong AP, Seow-Choen F. Clinical behavior of complicated right-sided and left-sided diverticulosis. Dis Colon Rectum. 1997;40:344–8.
34. Kim JH, Cheon JH, Park S, Kim BC, Lee SK, Kim TI, Kim WH. Relationship between disease location and age, obesity, and complications in Korean patients with acute diverticulitis: a comparison of clinical patterns with those of Western populations. Hepato-Gastroenterology. 2008;55:983–6.

35. Oh HK, Han EC, Ha HK, Choe EK, Moon SH, Ryoo SB, Jeong SY, Park KJ. Surgical management of colonic diverticular disease: discrepancy between right- and left-sided diseases. World J Gastroenterol. 2014;20:10115–20.
36. Manabe N, Haruma K, Nakajima A, Yamada M, Maruyama Y, Gushimiyagi M, Yamamoto T. Characteristics of colonic diverticulitis and factors associated with complications: a Japanese multicenter, retrospective, cross-sectional study. Dis Colon Rectum. 2015;58:1174–81.
37. Jung H-k, Choung RS, Richard Locke G III, et al. Diarrhea-predominant irritable bowel syndrome is associated with diverticular disease: a population-based study. Am J Gastroenterol. 2010;105(3):652–61.
38. Yamada E, Nakajima A, et al. Association between the location of diverticular disease and the irritable bowel syndrome: a multicenter study in Japan. Am J Gastroenterol. 2014;109(12):1900–5.
39. Niikura R, Nagata N, Shimbo T, Aoki T, Yamada A, Hirata Y, Sekine K, Okubo H, Watanabe K, Sakurai T, Yokoi C, Mizokami M, Yanase M, Akiyama J, Koike K, Uemura N. Natural history of bleeding risk in colonic diverticulosis patients: a long-term colonoscopy-based cohort study. Aliment Pharmacol Ther. 2015;41(9):888–94.
40. Nagata N, Niikura R, Aoki T, Shimbo T, Itoh T, Goda Y, Suda R, Yano H, Akiyama J, Yanase M, Mizokami M, Uemura N. Increase in colonic diverticulosis and diverticular hemorrhage in an aging society: lessons from a 9-year colonoscopic study of 28,192 patients in Japan. Int J Color Dis. 2014;29:379–85.
41. Niikura R, Yasunaga H, Yamaji Y, Horiguchi H, Fushimi K, Yamada A, Hirata Y, Koike K. Factors affecting in-hospital mortality in patients with lower gastrointestinal tract bleeding: a retrospective study using a national database in Japan. J Gastroenterol. 2015;50:533–40.

Burden of Diverticulosis and Diverticular Disease

2

Maria Alessandra Brandimarte, Enrico Di Rosa, Lorenzo Paglione, and Carolina Di Paolo

2.1 Diverticulosis and Diverticular Disease: A Neglected Condition?

The term "diverticular disease" (DD) covers a variety of conditions associated with the presence of colonic diverticula, herniations of the colonic mucosa through the muscular membrane and the clinical manifestations associated with their inflammation [1]. DD represents one of the most common gastrointestinal diseases in the Western industrialized countries, and the prevalence tends to increase with increasing age, thus showing an increasing incidence in younger patients [2]. Diverticulosis remains clinically asymptomatic in most patients during their lifetime, but up to 25% of them develop symptoms and up to a quarter experience at least one episode of acute diverticulitis (AD), an acute inflammatory process of diverticula with various complications (e.g., perforation, obstruction, fistula, etc.) described in 15–20% of cases [3–6]. AD incidence has been increasing in the last few decades, representing one of the main reasons for hospitalization for DD patients and consequently one of the factors that most impact the disease burden [3, 7]. The Global Burden of Disease in 2019 assessed DD as the leading cause of death in the group "other digestive diseases", which includes various codes of International Statistical Classification of Diseases and Related Health Problems, tenth Revision (ICD-10) [8].

Despite the significant epidemiological burden and the consequent impact on health services of this condition, there are no major studies in European countries that evaluate its impact.

M. A. Brandimarte (✉) · E. Di Rosa · L. Paglione · C. Di Paolo
Department of Prevention, ASL Roma 1, Rome, Italy
e-mail: ale.brandimarte@aslroma1.it; enrico.dirosa@aslroma1.it; lorenzo.paglione@aslroma1.it; carolina.dipaolo@aslroma1.it

© The Author(s), under exclusive license to Springer Nature Switzerland AG 2022
A. Tursi et al. (eds.), *Colonic Diverticular Disease*,
https://doi.org/10.1007/978-3-030-93761-4_2

2.1.1 An Overview

The complexity of this multifactorial condition has so far not been accompanied by guidelines that explain causal pathways and management paths.

Different aspects of management and treatment of DD patients are still controversial. Some studies with the aim of summarizing the most recent evidence show that it is crucial to determine a patient's optimal stratification level according to the severity of the disease to guarantee therapeutic success [9–12]. For this reason, it seems essential to deepen and implement the most recent radiological and endoscopic classifications to guide the management of this condition.

At present, this condition is ranked as the fifth most important gastrointestinal disease in terms of direct and indirect costs [13]. In Italy, some studies tried to estimate the burden of DD on health-care expenditure using hospitalization data [3, 7, 14]. As already pointed out, in most patients, DD occurs in an asymptomatic or a paucisymptomatic manner, and so, the use of hospital data does not seem to be exhaustive for an assessment of the impact of this disease on health services. It was also assessed that only a small percentage of hospitalized patients are admitted specifically for DD [5].

Therefore, both to evaluate and to contain the economic impact of this condition, and to optimize the management of patients at different levels, it seems crucial to implement the systematization of a tool for taking charge through territorial primary care structures up to acute hospitals, in which the most complex situations can be managed.

2.1.2 Integrating Data for a Better Healthcare

Particularly in the Italian context, there is a lack of updated and usable information flows that can allow a valid exploration of the disease burden of diverticular disease in terms of public health. Beyond evaluations, which are necessarily partial, such as those from real-world data epidemiology [3] or from databases obtainable from groups of general practitioners [5], for example, there are no dedicated national or regional information flows. In this regard, the SDO flow [14] represents a precious ally for defining the burden attributable to diverticular disease not only in terms of hospital budget but also in terms of workload with regard to days of hospitalization. It therefore becomes important, starting from evaluations conducted by scientific societies [13], to carry out an overall advocacy work with competent administrative bodies to stimulate a national discussion on the subject.

Attention to the territorial management of diverticular disease is almost completely lacking in both the national and international panoramas. Moreover, in this case, there would be the possibility of collecting and evaluating data from outpatient specialist flows, which are unfortunately still extremely fragile in terms of reliability. The availability of such data could lead to, for example, the improvement of risk stratification capacity, appropriately directing patients toward the most appropriate diagnostic and therapeutic paths, thus improving the outcome and quality of life.

Evaluation epidemiology, once again a public health tool for assessing the burden of diseases, could thus actively contribute to the definition of needs and to an appropriate global care of the patient.

2.2 Risk Factors, Time to Act

The prevalence of diverticular disease is increasing [1, 2]. In addition to biomedical causal pathways, it is important, in view of the sustainability of health services, to act on risk factors related to habits and lifestyles. These are defined as partially modifiable health determinants although they are dependent in turn on other factors, as evidenced by the literature on social health inequalities [15]. Like all causal pathways in epidemiology, it is therefore necessary to frame the field from a broad point of view to be able to evaluate the actions to be taken in the fight against noncommunicable diseases [16].

The importance of lifestyle, mediated by economic and cultural contexts, in the epidemiology of DD is well known. Evidence from ecological studies shows that DD is more prevalent in the so-called Western countries and also shows how the prevalence of this disease in the migrant population increases with the length of time spent in emigration countries [17]. This shows how the disease, and its burden in terms of public health, indeed has a strong sociocultural component, identified in some individual lifestyles typical of advanced capitalist countries.

There are two main areas of intervention in promoting individual healthy lifestyle [18]: sedentary lifestyle [19, 20] and nutrition [21, 22], which are distinguishable by two specific risk factors, namely, the excessive consumption of meat [20] and the reduced intake of fibers, fruit, and vegetables [23, 24], while being aware that individual behaviors are attributable to what are defined as root causes or the social determinants of health [15], such as the degree of urbanization of the population [25]. Public health professionals must frame the issue starting from the specificity of their discipline and the possibility of intervention given by the tools available. The prevalence of these risk factors within the population is also unequal among social classes [26].

With regard to the Italian population, from the data available from the information and surveillance flows[1] we found interesting results, which represent as many possibilities as possible for public health intervention.

[1] Tables are extracted from a national database, COESDI, from the Italian Contributo all'Esposizione delle Disuguaglianze, literally "contribution of inequalities to exposure" [https://www.dors.it/tool-dis/]. Data are from the Italian surveillance system, PASSI, Progressi delle Aziende Sanitarie per la Salute in Italia, literally "Progress by local health units towards a healthier Italy".

2.2.1 Physical Activity

Physical activity is one of the main public health problems [27] and is one of the main risk factors for chronic diseases, cardiovascular and metabolic [18, 27, 28]. It is a risk factor that is unequally distributed among social classes [29], strongly linked to the urban issue [30].

Physical activity, in terms of a sedentary lifestyle, is also one of the main risk factors for diverticular disease [31]. Promoting physical activity to reduce sedentary lifestyle and the prevalence of overweight and obese populations is one of the objectives of the National Prevention Plan [32]. The declination of this theme in the context of diverticular disease poses a challenge to the public health sector, as it requires a differentiated intervention, for example, with respect to age groups. In fact, action on the school population, for example, is configured as a primary prevention activity, whereas acting on the most advanced age groups, considering the growing prevalence of the disease [1], configures an intervention that is characterized more as secondary prevention (early detection of disease) if not tertiary (prevention of adverse outcome).

A sedentary lifestyle represents one of the main priorities for public health intervention in the Italian population, as it is highly prevalent in all age groups—more than 50% of the population in all age groups under analysis, male and female, is sedentary—and, above all, is strongly dependent on social inequalities (Table 2.1).

2.2.2 Healthy Eating

With regard to nutrition, the health promotion intervention can be declined in terms of primary or secondary prevention, by acting on the population in different age groups and with different health objectives. This aim can be achieved through campaigns aimed at not only training subjects on the advantages of a healthy diet but also by acting on obstacles, regarding the accessibility of healthy foods throughout the year, with particular attention to the most disadvantaged sections of the population. It is interesting to see how, based on the information available today on the Italian population, there is an inverse gradient regarding the consumption of meat, evidently a cultural heritage fueled by the ease of availability of fresh meats and sausages (Table 2.1). With regard to the consumption of fruit and vegetables, interventions should be promoted in the school environment, since, despite the lower impact of inequalities regarding the difference in prevalence in the Italian population, younger age groups are those with the highest prevalence of low consumption of fruit and vegetables, indicating a possible trend in increased risk and also in diverticular disease.

Inequalities in food quality and accessibility are therefore one of the possible areas of action of public health and health promotion policies and practices, as they have a considerable impact on the health of the population. The action, therefore, must once again be targeted on a specific population, as there is a need to act not only on the individual person but also on the general cultural and social conditions [33].

Table 2.1 Prevalence and population-attributable fraction of inequalities of the main risk factors, men and women by age group (extracted from COESDI)

Men	Age classes	Prevalence	Population-attributable fraction of inequalities
Low consumption of fruit and vegetables			
	30–44	25.2%	19.8%
	45–54	19.8%	26.1%
	55–64	14.9%	15.9%
	65–74	10.7%	29.2%
Excessive consumption of meat			
	30–44	49.1%	5.2%
	45–54	49.3%	−1.6%
	55–64	50.5%	−2.4%
	65–74	53.7%	−3.6%
Sedentary lifestyle			
	30–44	43.6%	41.8%
	45–54	51.3%	37.3%
	55–64	52.1%	31.5%
	65–74	52.3%	29.5%
Women	Age classes	Prevalence	Population-attributable fraction of inequalities
Low consumption of fruit and vegetables			
	30–44	17%	11.8%
	45–54	12.5%	21%
	55–64	9.6%	28.6%
	65–74	8.9%	32.8%
Excessive consumption of meat			
	30–44	54.4%	−0.8%
	45–54	55.8%	−4.8%
	55–64	58.2%	−5.3%
	65–74	60%	−2%
Sedentary lifestyle			
	30–44	52.5%	22.6%
	45–54	55.1%	26.8%
	55–64	57.6%	27.9%
	65–74	64.3%	29.4%

2.2.3 Public Health Intervention on Reducing the Burden of Disease

Interventions of the preventive area generally fall within the national or local prevention plans. These plans aim to reduce the burden of preventable diseases, with a view to promoting health.

Therefore, regarding the burden of disease, it is necessary to be able to identify not only the individual risk factors, an area of preeminence in biomedicine, but also to act on the social determinants of health that underlie them.

These types of health promotion interventions can be carried out by creating alliances between clinicians, public health doctors, and institutions. Public health interventions should be aimed at younger age groups, working in concert with schools to promote physical activity and a healthier diet, to train the population and preserve their state of health. Valuable work can also be done through local administrations [34], favoring, from the point of view of spatial accessibility and temporal availability, the purchase of fresh products from local markets [35], with a view to co-benefit both environment and health [36].

Therefore, the assessment of social vulnerability, regarding diverticular disease, thus becomes a useful public health tool to reduce the burden on local and national hospital services, thus guaranteeing an overall empowerment of the population regarding the management of the disease.

2.3 A Public Health Approach

2.3.1 Management

The burden of disease of a pathology with a multifactorial etiology and a chronic degenerative course, with phases of exacerbation and the need for management in complex structures, is always rather complex to evaluate [37]. As previously described, real-world data or hospital information flows do not exhaust the necessary epidemiological evaluation of the incidences, costs, complications, appropriateness of care, and effectiveness of management. However, all these problems can become useful public health tools, especially if an effective integration of assistance tools and pathways between the territory, in its various forms, and acute-care hospitals is achieved [38, 39].

The goal must be to act as secondary prevention, with respect to early management to avoid complications, and as tertiary prevention, to reduce the overall burden of residual disability, especially after invasive interventions.

2.3.2 Risk Factors

Public health policies have the possibility of acting in three directions: reducing the incidence (and therefore the prevalence); reducing the burden of disease, improving the state of health of the population; reducing the growing commitment of hospitals with respect to diverticular disease, also with a view to an overall reduction in economic and social costs.

Primary prevention and health promotion action can be practiced using a community- and population-based approach, through action mainly on the determinants of the disease, such as individual lifestyles. However, in this regard, it must be remembered that without an action on the social determinants of health, education, degree of urbanization, and income, it is difficult to reduce the burden of disease.

2.4 Conclusions: A Proposal

The integration of disciplines can be a useful approach for combating the growing burden of diverticular disease. In fact, when comparing the disciplines, it is possible to define priorities in terms of areas of intervention to develop integrated methodologies concerning prevention, management, and evaluation of pathways.

Nowadays biomedicine has made possible an effective resolution of diverticular disease, thanks to continuous technological development. Today it is more than ever a priority to address, starting from the experience gained in the development of diagnostic and assistance paths, to integrate this knowledge and skills with further possible actions in the field of public health, with a population view and an evaluation approach.

In a perspective of sustainability and equity of health services, it is fundamental to create a synergy between disciplines to manage pathologies with multifactorial etiopathogenesis, especially in the European context where the constant process of aging of the population leads to a growth in health needs.

References

1. Tursi A. Current and evolving concepts on the pathogenesis of diverticular disease. J Gastrointestin Liver Dis. 2019;28:225–35.
2. Nalamati S, Munie S. Epidemiology and pathophysiology of diverticular disease. Clin Colon Rectal Surg. 2018;31(04):209–13.
3. Cammarota S, Cargiolli M, Andreozzi P, Toraldo B, Citarella A, Flacco M, et al. Increasing trend in admission rates and costs for acute diverticulitis during 2005–2015: real-life data from the Abruzzo Region. Ther Adv Gastroenterol. 2018;11:175628481879150.
4. Shahedi K, Fuller G, Bolus R, Cohen E, Vu M, Shah R, et al. Long-term risk of acute diverticulitis among patients with incidental diverticulosis found during colonoscopy. Clin Gastroenterol Hepatol. 2013;11(12):1609–13.
5. Ubaldi E, Grattagliano I, Lapi F, Pecchioli S, Cricelli C. Overview on the management of diverticular disease by Italian General Practitioners. Dig Liver Dis. 2019;51(1):63–7.
6. Binda G, Arezzo A, Serventi A, Bonelli L. Multicentre observational study of the natural history of left-sided acute diverticulitis. Br J Surg. 2011;99(2):276–85.
7. Mennini F, Sciattella P, Marcellusi A, Toraldo B, Koch M. Economic burden of diverticular disease: an observational analysis based on real world data from an Italian region. Dig Liver Dis. 2017;49(9):1003–8.
8. Global Burden of Disease 2019. Other digestive diseases—level 3 cause [Internet]. Institute for Health Metrics and Evaluation. 2021 [cited 1 May 2021]. Available from: http://www.healthdata.org/results/gbd_summaries/2019/other-digestive-diseases-level-3-cause
9. Tursi A, Brandimarte G, Di Mario F, Andreoli A, Annunziata M, Astegiano M, et al. Development and validation of an endoscopic classification of diverticular disease of the colon: the DICA classification. Dig Dis. 2014;33(1):68–76.
10. Tursi A, Brandimarte G, Di Mario F, Annunziata M, Bafutto M, Bianco M, et al. Predictive value of the Diverticular Inflammation and Complication Assessment (DICA) endoscopic classification on the outcome of diverticular disease of the colon: an international study. United European Gastroenterol J. 2016;4(4):604–13.

11. Tursi A, Papa A, Danese S. Review article: the pathophysiology and medical management of diverticulosis and diverticular disease of the colon. Aliment Pharmacol Ther. 2015;42(6):664–84.
12. Tursi A, Elisei W, Picchio M, Nasi G, Mastromatteo A, Di Mario F, et al. Impact of diverticular inflammation and complication assessment classification on the burden of medical therapies in preventing diverticular disease complications in Italy. Ann Transl Med. 2017;5(16):320.
13. Cuomo R, Barbara G, Pace F, Annese V, Bassotti G, Binda G, et al. Italian consensus conference for colonic diverticulosis and diverticular disease. United European Gastroenterol J. 2014;2(5):413–42.
14. Aprea G, Giugliano A, Canfora A, Cardin F, Ferronetti A, Guida F, et al. Diverticular disease hospital cost impact analysis: evaluation of testings and surgical procedures in inpatient and outpatient admissions. BMC Surg. 2012;12(Suppl 1):S3.
15. Marmot M. Social determinants of health inequalities. Lancet. 2005;365(9464):1099–104.
16. Davey SG. Post–modern epidemiology: when methods meet matter. Am J Epidemiol. 2019;188:1410–9.
17. Hjern F, Johansson C, Mellgren A, Baxter N, Hjern A. Diverticular disease and migration—the influence of acculturation to a Western lifestyle on diverticular disease. Aliment Pharmacol Ther. 2006;23:797–805.
18. Lanier JB, Bury DC, Richardson SW. Diet and physical activity for cardiovascular disease prevention. Am Fam Physician. 2016;93(11):919–24.
19. Violi A, Cambiè G, Miraglia C, Barchi A, Nouvenne A, Capasso M, Leandro G, Meschi T, De' Angelis GL, Di Mario F. Epidemiology and risk factors for diverticular disease. Acta Biomed. 2018;89(9-S):107–12.
20. Strate LL. Lifestyle factors and the course of diverticular disease. Dig Dis. 2012;30(1):35–45.
21. Järbrink-Sehgal M, Schmidt P, Sköldberg F, Hemmingsson T, Hagström H, Andreasson A. Lifestyle factors in late adolescence associate with later development of diverticular disease requiring hospitalization. Clin Gastroenterol Hepatol. 2018;16:1474–1480.e1.
22. Böhm SK, Kruis W. Lifestyle and other risk factors for diverticulitis. Minerva Gastroenterol Dietol. 2017 Jun;63(2):110–8.
23. Korzenik JR. Case closed? Diverticulitis: epidemiology and fiber. J Clin Gastroenterol. 2006;40(Suppl 3):S112–6.
24. Crowe F, Appleby P, Allen N, Key T. Diet and risk of diverticular disease in Oxford cohort of European Prospective Investigation into Cancer and Nutrition (EPIC): prospective study of British vegetarians and non-vegetarians. BMJ. 2011;343:d4131.
25. Capolongo S, Rebecchi A, Dettori M, et al. Healthy design and urban planning strategies, actions, and policy to achieve salutogenic cities. Int J Environ Res Public Health. 2018;15:2698.
26. Marmot M. Social justice, epidemiology and health inequalities. Eur J Epidemiol. 2017;32:537–46.
27. Warburton D, Bredin S. Health benefits of physical activity. Curr Opin Cardiol. 2017;32:541–56.
28. Lavie C, Ozemek C, Carbone S, Katzmarzyk P, Blair S. Sedentary behavior, exercise, and cardiovascular health. Circ Res. 2019;124:799–815.
29. Althoff T, Sosič R, Hicks J, King A, Delp S, Leskovec J. Large-scale physical activity data reveal worldwide activity inequality. Nature. 2017;547:336–9.
30. Appolloni L, Corazza MV, D'Alessandro D. The pleasure of walking: an innovative methodology to assess appropriate walkable performance in urban areas to support transport planning. Sustainability. 2019;11:3467.
31. Hjern F, Wolk A, Håkansson N. Obesity, physical inactivity, and colonic diverticular disease requiring hospitalization in women: a prospective cohort study. Am J Gastroenterol. 2021;107(2):296–302. Accessed 15 May 2021
32. Italian Ministry of Health. National Prevention Plan 2020–2025. https://www.salute.gov.it/portale/documentazione/p6_2_2_1.jsp?lingua=italiano&id=2955.
33. Mayén A, de Mestral C, Zamora G, Paccaud F, Marques-Vidal P, Bovet P, Stringhini S. Interventions promoting healthy eating as a tool for reducing social inequalities in diet in low- and middle-income countries: a systematic review. Int J Equity Health. 2016;15(1):205.

34. Lange S, Moore L, Galuska D. Local government retail incentives for healthier food retailers in the USA, 2014. Public Health Nutr. 2019;22:2521–9.
35. Noy S, Patrick R, Henderson-Wilson C, Nuttman S, Ryan I. New frontiers in community initiatives to increase vegetable consumption. Health Promot J Austr. 2018;30:52–61.
36. Vineis P, Beagley J, Bisceglia L, Carra L, Cingolani R, Forastiere F, et al. Strategy for primary prevention of non-communicable diseases (NCD) and mitigation of climate change in Italy. J Epidemiol Community Health. 2021;75(9):917–24.
37. Weizman A, Nguyen G. Diverticular disease: epidemiology and management. Can J Gastroenterol. 2011;25:385–9.
38. König HH, Leicht H, Bickel H, Fuchs A, Gensichen J, Maier W, et al. MultiCare study group. Effects of multiple chronic conditions on health care costs: an analysis based on an advanced tree-based regression model. BMC Health Serv Res. 2013;13:219.
39. Reddy VB, Longo WE. The burden of diverticular disease on patients and healthcare systems. Gastroenterol Hepatol. 2013;9(1):21–7.

Part II

Pathogenesis

Genetics

3

Jaune Ieva Lukosiene and Juozas Kupcinskas

The etiology of colonic diverticular disease (DD) is considered to be a multifactorial process, involving environmental and dietary factors, structural and functional changes of the colonic wall and enteric nervous system, and genetic predisposition [1]; however, to this day, the exact pathogenesis of this disease is incompletely understood. Compiled data from recent decades have indicated that genetic factors undoubtedly contribute to the development of the disease and to its complications [2]. This chapter provides an overview of the most significant findings in this field of research.

Prior to this time, the role of inherited factors in the development of DD seems to have been overlooked. The existing transethnic differences in prevalence rates and the predominant location of diverticula between Western and Asian populations (*Asians are more likely to have acquired pseudodiverticula in the ascending colon, whereas Westerners tend to have acquired pseudodiverticula in the descending and sigmoid colon* [3, 4]) were pointing toward the potential role of heritability in DD occurrence. An attempt to investigate the significance of genetics in the development of the disease was made in two European epidemiological twin studies [5, 6]. Granlund et al. linked the Swedish Twin Registry to the Swedish Inpatient Registry

J. I. Lukosiene
Department of Gastroenterology and Institute for Digestive Research, Lithuanian University of Health Sciences, Kaunas, Lithuania
e-mail: jaune.lukosiene@lsmuni.lt

J. Kupcinskas (✉)
Department of Gastroenterology, Lithuanian University of Health Sciences, Kaunas, Lithuania

Institute for Digestive Research, Lithuanian University of Health Sciences, Kaunas, Lithuania
e-mail: juozas.kupcinskas@lsmuni.lt

© The Author(s), under exclusive license to Springer Nature Switzerland AG 2022

A. Tursi et al. (eds.), *Colonic Diverticular Disease*,
https://doi.org/10.1007/978-3-030-93761-4_3

[5]. With the use of mathematical models, the heritability was estimated to be 40% in a cohort of twins with (2296 people) or without (102,156 people) DD, and the nonshared environmental effects were calculated to account for 60% of the trait variability [5]. A comparable result was evidenced by a Danish twin study. Using the Danish National Registry of Patients linked to the Danish Twin Registry, the heritability of DD was estimated to be 53% in a twin cohort comprising twins with (923 people) and without (29,399 people) DD [6].

The evidence described above suggests an important role of genetic predisposition in the development of DD. However, possible genetic variants involved in the pathogenesis of this common disease remain widely unknown.

One classical pathogenetic concept suggests that DD might develop due to weakening of the colonic wall musculature, caused by structural alterations of the connective tissue [7–9]. Two major extracellular matrix components, collagen and elastin, have been found to be altered in diverticular disease [8, 9]. In addition, studies have shown that matrix metalloproteinases or their inhibitors responsible for collagen metabolism are also altered in patients with DD [10, 11]. The hypothesis that these changes may be genetically predisposed is further supported by the fact that in some hereditary disorders of the connective tissue, including autosomal dominant polycystic kidney disease (ADPKD), Coffin–Lowry syndrome, Ehler–Danlos syndrome (EDS) type IV, and Williams–Beuren syndrome, colonic diverticula are observed in increased frequency and at an extremely early age [4, 12].

ADPKD is the most frequent hereditary renal cystic disease and one of the most common causes of end-stage kidney disease. Mutations in different genes, such as PKD1, PKD2, and PKD3, cause a similar phenotype. Diverticulosis is a common finding in ADPKD, with one research showing a prevalence of 83% [13] and another 75% [14]. The diverticula are most commonly located in the right colon. Due to the higher prevalence and severity of diverticulitis in patients with ADPKD [15], a prophylactic colectomy before kidney transplantation is recommended in some individual cases. Although larger case series are needed, diverticulosis seems to be a plausible extrarenal manifestation of ADPKD.

The Coffin–Lowry syndrome is an X-chromosomal semidominant genetic disease that is caused by mutations in RPS6KA3, which encodes for ribosomal S6 kinase 2. This kinase plays a role in skeletal and neural development. Mental retardation is a defining feature of the syndrome, which is frequently associated with auditory and visual impairments as well as kyphoscoliosis. Despite the lack of larger case series, an autopsy case in siblings suggests that these patients might be prone to the development of diverticula [16].

EDS is an inherited heterogeneous group of connective tissue disorders characterized by defects in collagen synthesis that affect the skin, ligaments, joints, blood vessels and gastrointestinal tract. Hyperelasticity of the skin and hypermobility of the joints are two major symptoms. EDS type IV is an autosomal dominant defect of type III collagen synthesis due to COL3A1 mutations. The phenotype is characterized by a distinct facial appearance and spontaneous rupture of the bowel and large arteries. Small case series finding diverticulosis at an early age (two cases each) [17, 18], two larger studies finding 28% colonic complications [19], and various intestinal complications in an older study [20] all suggest an increased prevalence of DD in EDS type IV.

The Williams–Beuren syndrome is a rare genetic disorder that is characterized by distinctive facial features, a varying degree of mental deficiency, growth delays, and cardiovascular malformations. It is caused by a deletion on chromosome 7q11.23. The deleted region includes more than 25 genes (CLIP2, ELN, GTF2I, and LIMK1 are among the genes that are typically deleted). Gastrointestinal symptoms, such as gastroesophageal reflux, constipation, rectal prolapse, and hernias, are among the most common manifestations of the syndrome, as well as the occurrence of DD at an early age in one series (prevalence of 10.9% at a mean age of 26.9 years) [21] and a case report of diverticulitis in a 9-year-old boy [22].

Moreover, genetic loci and polymorphisms associated with maintenance of the connective tissue and degradation of collagen were identified in other pathologies, which, traditionally, are linked to connective tissue malfunction: *rs2236479* located in the collagen XVIII (*COL18A1*) gene was identified as a candidate variant for pelvic organ prolapse in genome-wide association studies (GWASs) [23]. A whole-genome linkage analysis revealed that *COL3A1* is linked to gastroesophageal reflux disease and identified AA homozygotes in *rs3134646* as a risk factor for hiatal hernia in men [24]. In a Dutch study, the probability of pelvic organ prolapse was higher in women carrying the *COL3A1* 2209G > A allele [25]. A recent GWAS in patients with inguinal hernia has identified four single nucleotide polymorphisms (SNPs) in genes involved in the regulation of the connective tissue [26].

Thus far, only two small case–control studies using the candidate gene approach have attempted to identify certain SNPs in DD; however, they were underpowered to provide conclusive results [27, 28].

More recently, new data on genetic loci and polymorphisms involved in the occurrence of DD have become available. In 2018, a case–control study including 422 patients with diverticulosis and 285 controls found an SNP (rs3134646) in collagen type III alpha 1 chain (COL3A1) to be associated with the risk of developing colonic diverticulosis in white men [29].

The most important data supporting the role of genetic predisposition in DD have been obtained from three extremely recent genome-wide association studies (GWASs). The first genome-wide association study in DD and diverticulitis was performed in 2017 in Iceland and The Netherlands [30]. The study showed that intronic variants rs4662344 and rs7609897, established within the DNase hypersensitivity sites located in Rho-GTPase-activating protein 15 (ARHGAP15) and the collagen-like tail subunit of asymmetric acetylcholinesterase (COLQ) genes, were linked to uncomplicated DD [30]. rs67153654 within an intron of FAM155A (family with sequence similarity 155A) was also significantly associated with diverticulitis occurrence [30]. These were the first loci shown to associate with diverticular disease in a genome-wide study.

Additionally, one of the two largest to date GWASs was conducted in 2018 in the United States [31]. Maguire et al. analyzed 27,444 cases and 382,284 controls from the UK Biobank and tested for replication in the Michigan Genomics Initiative (2572 cases; 28,649 controls) [31]. The study identified 42 loci associated with DD

(39 of them novel), genes that are significantly enriched for expression in the mesenchymal stem cells and multiple connective tissue cell types and are coexpressed with genes that have a role in vascular and mesenchymal biology [31].

The largest GWAS to date employed the UK Biobank and imputed genotypes using 31,964 cases and 419,135 controls [32]. These associations were then replicated in a European sample of 3893 cases and 2829 diverticula-free controls and evaluated for risk contribution to diverticulitis and uncomplicated diverticulosis, and they identified 48 genetic risk loci. The most significant novel risk variant rs9960286 was located near CTAGE1 (cutaneous T-cell lymphoma-associated antigen 1), and the most significant novel replicated risk variant rs60869342 was located in NOV (nephroblastoma overexpressed) [32]. Based on 95% confidence intervals (CIs), the authors found four loci having stronger effects for diverticulitis, namely, variants at PHGR1 (proline, histidine, and glycine-rich 1), FAM155A-2, calcitonin-related polypeptide beta (CALCB), and the S100A10 locus [32].

The functional link between DD and many of the genes identified by the aforementioned GWAS is unknown. To confirm gene-variant associations, functional characterizations should yet be established. However, it is noteworthy that among genes in the newly determined risk loci associated with DD, many have a role in immunity, extracellular matrix biology, cell adhesion, membrane transport, and intestinal motility, thus contributing to the pathophysiology of the disease [31] (Fig. 3.1).

The genetic data from all three GWASs clearly show that DD is primarily a disorder of intestinal neuromuscular function and impaired connective fiber support,

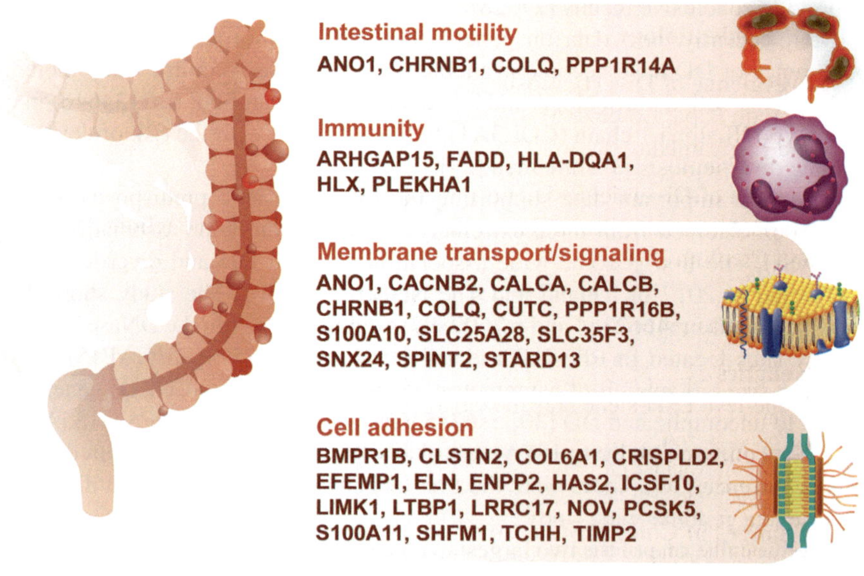

Fig. 3.1 Plausible functional characteristics of GWAS identified risk loci associated with diverticular disease

while an additional diverticulitis risk might be conferred by epithelial dysfunction-related genes. To date, there are no studies evaluating how identified genetic risk factors could serve for clinical decision-making in DD prevention or management, and these subjects are topics for future research.

References

1. Von Rahden BHA, Germer CT. Pathogenesis of colonic diverticular disease. Langenbeck's Arch Surg. 2012;397(7):1025–33. https://doi.org/10.1007/s00423-012-0961-5.
2. Tursi A. Current and evolving concepts on the pathogenesis of diverticular disease. J Gastrointest Liver Dis. 2019;28:225–35. https://doi.org/10.15403/jgld-184.
3. Tursi A, Scarpignato C, Strate LL, Lanas A, Kruis W, Lahat A, Danese S. Colonic diverticular disease. Nat Rev Dis Prim. 2020;6:20.
4. Reichert MC, Lammert F. The genetic epidemiology of diverticulosis and diverticular disease: emerging evidence. United Eur Gastroenterol J. 2015;3(5):409–18. https://doi.org/10.1177/2050640615576676.
5. Granlund J, Svensson T, Olén O, Hjern F, Pedersen NL, Magnusson PKE, Thelin Schmidt P. The genetic influence on diverticular disease—a twin study. Aliment Pharmacol Ther. 2012;35:1103–7.
6. Strate LL, Erichsen R, Baron JA, Mortensen J, Pedersen JK, Riis AH, Christensen K, Sørensen HT. Heritability and familial aggregation of diverticular disease: a population-based study of twins and siblings. Gastroenterology. 2013;144:736–742.e1.
7. Böttner M, Wedel T. Abnormalities of neuromuscular anatomy in diverticular disease. Dig Dis. 2012;30:19–23.
8. Wess L, Eastwood MA, Wess TJ, Busuttil A, Miller A. Cross linking of collagen is increased in colonic diverticulosis. Gut. 1995;37:91–4.
9. Whiteway J, Morson BC. Elastosis in diverticular disease of the sigmoid colon. Gut. 1985;26:258–66.
10. Stumpf M, Cao W, Klinge U, Klosterhalfen B, Kasperk R, Schumpelick V. Increased distribution of collagen type III and reduced expression of matrix metalloproteinase 1 in patients with diverticular disease. Int J Color Dis. 2001;16:271–5.
11. Mimura T, Bateman AC, Lee RL, Johnson PA, McDonald PJ, Talbot IC, Kamm MA, MacDonald TT, Pender SLF, Koltun W. Up-regulation of collagen and tissue inhibitors of matrix metalloproteinase in colonic diverticular disease. Dis Colon Rectum. 2004;47:371–9.
12. Leganger J, Søborg MLK, Mortensen LQ, Gregersen R, Rosenberg J, Burcharth J. Association between diverticular disease and Ehlers-Danlos syndrome: a 13-year nationwide population-based cohort study. Int J Color Dis. 2016;31:1863–7.
13. Scheff RT, Zuckerman G, Harter H, Delmez J, Koehler R. Diverticular disease in patients with chronic renal failure due to polycystic kidney disease. Ann Intern Med. 1980;92:202–4.
14. Pourfarziani V, Mousavi-Nayeeni SM, Ghaheri H, Assari S, Saadat SH, Panahi F, Noorbala MH, Vasei A, Norouzi AR, Simforoosh N. The outcome of diverticulosis in kidney recipients with polycystic kidney disease. Transplant Proc. 2007;39:1054–6.
15. Lederman ED, McCoy G, Conti DJ, Lee EC. Diverticulitis and polycystic kidney disease. Am Surg. 2000;66:200–3.
16. Machin GA, Walther GL, Fraser VM. Autopsy findings in two adult siblings with Coffin-Lowry syndrome. Am J Med Genet Suppl. 1987;3:303–9.
17. Bläker H, Funke B, Hausser I, Hackert T, Schirmacher P, Autschbach F. Pathology of the large intestine in patients with vascular type Ehlers-Danlos syndrome. Virchows Arch. 2007;450:713–7.
18. Lindor NM, Bristow J. Tenascin-X deficiency in autosomal recessive Ehlers-Danlos syndrome. Am J Med Genet A. 2005;135:75–80.

19. Pepin M, Schwarze U, Superti-Furga A, Byers PH. Clinical and genetic features of Ehlers–Danlos syndrome type IV, the vascular type. N Engl J Med. 2000;342:673–80.
20. Beighton PH, Murdoch JL, Votteler T. Gastrointestinal complications of the Ehlers-Danlos syndrome. Gut. 1969;10:1004–8.
21. Partsch CJ, Siebert R, Caliebe A, Gosch A, Wessel A, Pankau R. Sigmoid diverticulitis in patients with Williams-Beuren syndrome: relatively high prevalence and high complication rate in young adults with the syndrome. Am J Med Genet A. 2005;137:52–4.
22. Ignacio RC, Klapheke WP, Stephen T, Bond S. Diverticulitis in a child with Williams syndrome: a case report and review of the literature. J Pediatr Surg. 2012;47(9):E33–5. https://doi.org/10.1016/j.jpedsurg.2012.05.036.
23. Allen-Brady K, Cannon-Albright L, Farnham JM, Teerlink C, Vierhout ME, Van Kempen LCL, Kluivers KB, Norton PA. Identification of six loci associated with pelvic organ prolapse using genome-wide association analysis. Obstet Gynecol. 2011;118:1345–53.
24. Sling BA, Jirholt J, Hammond P, Knutsson M, Walentinsson A, Davidson G, Agreus L, Lehmann A, Lagerström-Fermer M. Collagen type III alpha I is a gastro-oesophageal reflux disease susceptibility gene and a male risk factor for hiatus hernia. Gut. 2009;58(8):1063–9. https://doi.org/10.1136/gut.2008.167353.
25. Kluivers KB, Dijkstra JR, Hendriks JCM, Lince SL, Vierhout ME, Van Kempen LCL. COL3A1 2209G>A is a predictor of pelvic organ prolapse. Int Urogynecol J. 2009;20:1113–8.
26. Jorgenson E, Makki N, Shen L, Chen DC, Tian C, Eckalbar WL, Hinds D, Ahituv N, Avins A. A genome-wide association study identifies four novel susceptibility loci underlying inguinal hernia. Nat Commun. 2015;6:10130. https://doi.org/10.1038/ncomms10130.
27. Beasley WD, Beynon J, Jenkins GJS, Parry JM. Reprimo 824 G>C and p53R2 4696 C>G single nucleotide polymorphisms and colorectal cancer: a case-control disease association study. Int J Color Dis. 2008;23:375–81.
28. Connelly TM, Berg AS, Hegarty JP, Deiling S, Brinton D, Poritz LS, Koltun WA. The TNFSF15 gene single nucleotide polymorphism rs7848647 is associated with surgical diverticulitis. Ann Surg. 2014;259:1132–7.
29. Reichert MC, Kupcinskas J, Krawczyk M, et al. A variant of COL3A1 (rs3134646) is associated with risk of developing diverticulosis in white men. Dis Colon Rectum. 2018;61(5):604–11. https://doi.org/10.1097/DCR.0000000000001001.
30. Sigurdsson S, Alexandersson KF, Sulem P, et al. Sequence variants in ARHGAP15, COLQ and FAM155A associate with diverticular disease and diverticulitis. Nat Commun. 2017;8:15789. https://doi.org/10.1038/ncomms15789.
31. Maguire LH, Handelman SK, Du X, Chen Y, Pers TH, Speliotes EK. Genome-wide association analyses identify 39 new susceptibility loci for diverticular disease. Nat Genet. 2018;50:1359–65.
32. Schafmayer C, Harrison JW, Buch S, et al. Genome-wide association analysis of diverticular disease points towards neuromuscular, connective tissue and epithelial pathomechanisms. Gut. 2019;68(5):854–65. https://doi.org/10.1136/gutjnl-2018-317619.

Neuromuscular Function Abnormalities 4

Gabrio Bassotti, Carolina Pellegrini,
and Nunzia Bernardini

4.1 Introduction

Colonic diverticular disease (CDD) is a commonly encountered condition in clinical practice, with clinical manifestations ranging from being completely silent (diverticulosis) to complicated diverticulitis [1–3]. The pathogenesis of CDD and its various clinical manifestations have been related to several pathophysiological mechanisms that, however, have not been fully elucidated to date [4]. An important point to consider is that the etiology of CDD is likely multifactorial, with different biological mechanisms underlying different clinical manifestations [4]. Among these mechanisms, certain importance has been attributed to the presence of neuromuscular dysfunction, and this hypothesis is actually supported by literature evidence [5–7], even though there are still some controversial issues. The various aspects of possible neuromuscular function abnormalities in CDD will be reviewed in this chapter.

G. Bassotti (✉)
Gastroenterology, Hepatology and Digestive Endoscopy Section, Department of Medicine and Surgery, University of Perugia, Perugia, Italy

Gastroenterology and Hepatology Unit, Santa Maria della Misericordia Hospital, Perugia, Italy
e-mail: gabassot@tin.it

C. Pellegrini · N. Bernardini
Department of Pharmacy, University of Pisa, Pisa, Italy

Department of Clinical and Experimental Medicine, University of Pisa, Pisa, Italy
e-mail: c.pellegrini@med.unipi.it; carolina.pellegrini@unipi.it; n.bernardini@med.unipi.it; nunzia.bernardini@unipi.it

© The Author(s), under exclusive license to Springer Nature Switzerland AG 2022

A. Tursi et al. (eds.), *Colonic Diverticular Disease*,
https://doi.org/10.1007/978-3-030-93761-4_4

4.2 Microscopic and Molecular Neuromuscular Abnormalities

The enteric neuromuscular compartment consists of the enteric nervous system (ENS) and muscular layers. The ENS, including the myenteric plexus (or Auerbach's plexus) and the submucosal (Meissner's) plexus, is an intrinsic neuronal semiautonomous network, which regulates digestive functions and cooperates with the central nervous system through sympathetic and parasympathetic pathways [8]. It contains primary afferent neurons, interneurons, motor neurons (protein gene product 9.5 (PGP9.5), and type 1 neuronal nuclear antibodies (HuC/D)-positive), which regulate bowel motility by acting on different effector cells in both the myenteric and muscular compartments, such as the interstitial Cajal cells (ICCs) and the smooth muscle cells (SMCs) [9, 10]. ICCs are the main non-neuronal cells, which coordinate gastrointestinal motility, and can be classified into the following groups: submucosal ICCs (ICCs-SM), located on the submucosal surface of the colonic circular muscle; myenteric ICCs (ICCs-MY), forming a cell network along the myenteric plexus between the longitudinal and circular layers of the *tunica muscularis*; and intramuscular ICCs (ICCs-IM), distributed within the longitudinal and circular muscle layers. ICCs are regarded as pacemaker cells, generating spontaneous and rhythmic electrical activity, and as intermediaries in signal transmission from enteric neurons to smooth muscle cells (SMCs) [8]. SMCs are characterized by three types of filaments: thin actin filaments, thick myosin filaments, and intermediate filaments. The latter link the cytoplasmic dense bodies to dense bands along the inner face of the plasma membrane. In addition, they display gap junctions, including connexins, on the plasma membrane to allow the transmission of signaling molecules from innervated SMCs to noninnervated neighboring SMCs [11]. pS368-Cx43, protein kinase C phosphorylated substrates (PKCps), RhoA, and smooth muscle α-actin (αSMA) regulate gap junction functionality and SMC contractile activity [12, 13]. Another important component of the ENS is represented by the enteric glial cells (EGCs), associated with submucosal and myenteric neurons and also located in proximity to epithelial cells [8, 14, 15]. In addition, EGC terminal endfoot processes run to the epithelial basement membrane and blood capillaries [16]. Notably, EGCs maintain enteric neuron homeostasis, regulate colonic motility, and have been recently considered capable of preserving intestinal epithelial barrier integrity [14, 17, 18]. EGCs (S100β or glial fibrillary acidic protein (GFAP)-positive) release several neurotrophic factors, including glial cell line-derived neurotrophic factor (GDNF) and neuregulin 1 (NR) that, through Ret proto-oncogene (RET) [19] or ErbB2/ErbB3 signaling, respectively, contribute to ENS growth, differentiation and synaptic plasticity, as well as to the regulation of bowel motility [18, 20].

Of interest, CDD patients, including asymptomatic subjects with diverticula and those with symptomatic complicated or uncomplicated diverticulitis, are characterized by substantial molecular and morphological alterations of the enteric neuromuscular compartment that could contribute to bowel dysfunctions, including motor disturbances and visceral hypersensitivity [21–23]. Considering the ENS, both symptomatic and asymptomatic patients display an increased number of nerve fibers in the diverticular area, whereas patients with symptomatic uncomplicated diverticular disease (SUDD) show active nerve fiber outgrowth characterized by extensive axonal sprouting [24]. In addition, complicated DD and SUDD patients are characterized by loss of enteric neurons, hypoganglionosis, and imbalance in myenteric (e.g., acetylcholine, substance P, nitric oxide, vasoactive intestinal polypeptide and serotonin, calcitonin gene-related peptide) and pain-mediating (e.g., galanin, neuropeptide K) neurotransmitters [21, 23, 25–28]. Moreover, significant changes in the density and morphology of ICCs-SM and ICCs-MY in DD patients have been documented [21] (Fig. 4.1). These alterations may account for the dysfunction of the rhythmic activity of intestinal muscle cells observed in CDD patients.

Of note, CDD patients are also characterized by alterations of the number, morphology, and expression of molecular pathways of EGCs that could further contribute to bowel symptoms. In particular, there is evidence of a decrease in the density of S100-positive cells in the myenteric plexus of CDD patients (Fig. 4.2) [21, 26], even though a recent study has documented an increased expression of S100β in both the submucosal and myenteric plexus of CDD patients without changes in EGC numbers, suggesting the occurrence of enteric gliosis in CDD [29]. These discrepancies could be ascribed to different experimental setups, including patient recruitment or the use of different EGC markers. Indeed, EGC subpopulations could be differently affected during the pathophysiological course of CDD [30]. Of note, both symptomatic and asymptomatic CDD patients are characterized by a downregulated mRNA expression and immunoreactivity of GDNF family receptor alpha 1 (GFRα1) and RET in the colonic myenteric plexus, whereas only symptomatic patients display decreased mRNA GDNF levels [31]. These results point out that CDD is associated with alterations at the gene and protein levels of GDNF signaling that could contribute to the alterations of colonic motility. Besides GDNF signaling, a decreased mRNA expression and immunoreactivity of the NRG1-ErbB2/ErbB3 system and nicotinic acetylcholine receptor (nAChR) subunit b4 has been observed

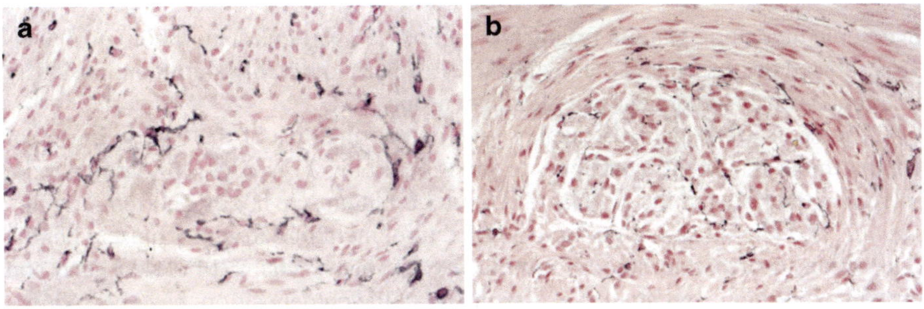

Fig. 4.1 Representative images of ICCs in the myenteric ganglia (ICCs-MY) of colonic specimens from control subjects (**a**) and colonic diverticular disease patients (**b**). CDD specimens contain fewer ICCs, which display abnormal, pruned, and shortened extensions. Immunostaining is done with the anti-c-Kit antibody (CD117), DAB is enhanced with nickel, and nuclear counterstaining is with fast red. Original magnification ×40

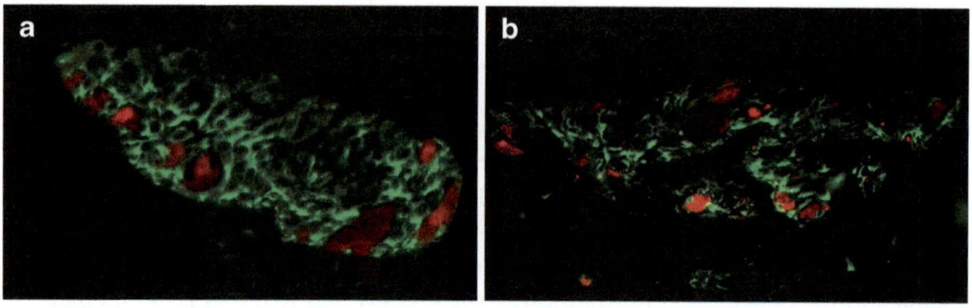

Fig. 4.2 Representative images of double immunofluorescence of HuC/D (red neurons)-GFAP (green glial cells) in the myenteric ganglia of normal (**a**) and colonic diverticular disease (**b**) human colon. A reduced density of S100-positive cells is visible in CDD specimens. Original magnification ×40

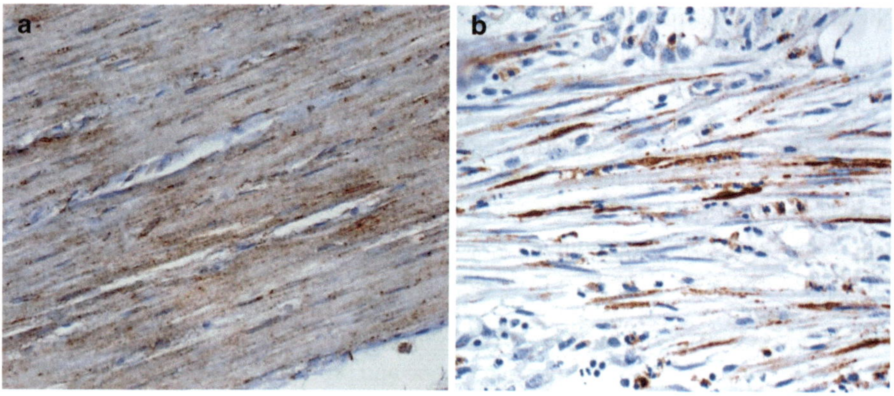

Fig. 4.3 Representative images of Cx43 immunostaining in the *tunica muscularis* of the colon from control subjects (**a**) and colonic diverticular disease patients (**b**). A patchy distribution of Cx43 staining is appreciable in smooth muscle cells of CDD specimens with a lot of Cx43-negative cells and scattered cells with CX43 stockpiles. Original magnification ×40

in colonic myenteric ganglia from CDD patients. In particular, morphological analyses showed decreased and patchy NRG1, ErbB3, and nAChRb4 immunopositivity in both neuronal somata and ganglionic neuropil [32].

Of interest, CDD patients display severe abnormalities of the enteric muscular compartment that could contribute to functional bowel disorders. In particular, an increased thickness of the circular and longitudinal muscle layers, shortening of the *taeniae*, and altered smooth muscle architecture, including irregular muscle bundle orientation, decrease in smooth muscle myosin heavy chain (MYH11) gene and protein expression, and abnormal elastin and collagen deposition, have been documented in patients with both diverticulosis and complicated CDD [33–35]. In addition, a decrease in Cx26, Cx43, PKCps, and RhoA expression has been observed in colonic SMCs from CDD symptomatic patients (Fig. 4.3). These molecular changes in SMCs could facilitate a collapse and/or weakening of tensile strength in the *tunica muscularis* [36]. Others show that CDD patients also display rearrangements in the expression of enteric neurotransmitter receptors in the colonic *tunica muscularis*, in both symptomatic and asymptomatic forms: a decrease in 5HT-4 serotonin receptors was documented in diverticulitis patients [27] along with an upregulation of subtype 3 muscarinic receptors in uncomplicated CDD patients [37].

Of note, alterations of ICCs-IM appearance and distribution in colonic muscle layers from complicated CDD patients have also been detected. In particular, the c-Kit network was rarefied and disarranged as a consequence of morphological alterations of ICCs, which showed curtailed and blunted processes along with a decrease in ICC density in both circular and longitudinal layers [36].

4.3 Abnormal Motility Function

The presence of abnormal colonic motility as a contributing pathogenetic factor in patients with CDD has been suggested long ago. Based on the observation of increased motility in both the basal state and after meal ingestion, the authors hypothesized that increased intraluminal pressures arising in the affected segments might be related to the formation of diverticula [38, 39]. However, the studies subsequently carried out to confirm this hypothesis have yielded (likely due to the heterogeneous methods of recording colonic motility in these patients) conflicting results. In fact, significant increases in motility both basally and after eating in CDD patients, compared to controls, were documented manometrically or electromyographically in some studies [40–43], whereas other investigations did not demonstrate significant differences in colonic motor activity between CDD patients and controls [44–46]. The discrepancies between the above-mentioned studies might, however, be likely due to the heterogeneous methods of recording colonic motility in these patients, short recording periods, different kinds of patients, and the fact that most investigations were actually carried out in the rectum or at the rectosigmoid junction, thereby missing the diverticular area [5].

A few subsequent studies were carried out for investigating more proximal colonic segments for prolonged (24 h) periods of time and for positioning the recording catheters within the diverticular tracts by means of colonoscopy. One study evaluated colonic motility in patients with asymptomatic CDD (diverticulosis); compared to controls, patients with diverticulosis had an overall significant increase in colonic motor activity in the segments harboring diverticula, also showing an exaggerated motor response to meal ingestion, especially in the sigmoid colon [47]. Of interest, in the patients' group, a significant increase in high-amplitude propagated contractions, the manometric equivalent of mass movements, was recorded [48]. Another study, carried out in patients with SUDD revealed that, compared to controls, the diverticular segments of these patients displayed a significant increase in regular contractile pattern duration, mostly represented by activity of 2–3 cycles/min. It is worth noting that in about 30% of patients (but not in controls), this activity was accompanied by pain similar to that experienced at home [49].

However, these studies may be insufficient to draw firm conclusions on the evidence of abnormal colonic motility in CDD patients, as stated in a recent review [50]. Most of the criticisms were related to the technological limitations during recordings obtained with low-resolution manometric techniques. Indeed, recent preliminary evidence provided by high-resolution recordings suggest that, at least for patients with diverticulosis, there could be no significant differences in colonic motility compared to controls [51].

4.4 Abnormal Visceral Perception

Visceral perception has also been quite a neglected topic in CDD, with only a couple of studies addressing the matter. In a first barostat/motility study, diverticular (sigmoid) and non-diverticular (rectal) segments were investigated, comparing patients with diverticulosis and SUDD with healthy controls [52]. Compared to asymptomatic diverticulosis and controls, the perception of rectal distention was increased in SUDD patients; rectal compliance did not show significant differences between the three groups. Moreover, compared to controls, but not asymptomatic diverticulosis, SUDD patients displayed increased sigmoid perception before and after meals, whereas the sigmoid colon compliance was similar between the three groups. These results demonstrated that in patients with SUDD, but not in those with symptomatic diverticulosis, colonic distention evokes increased perception in both the affected diverticular segments and in the unaffected ones (rectum). This increased perception is not related to abnormal colonic wall compliance, suggesting that the colonic abnormalities may be related to motor/perceptive functions and might be responsible for some of the symptoms reported by the patients [52].

This hypothesis was subsequently confirmed in another study in which asymptomatic diverticulosis and SUDD patients were investigated by sigmoidoscopy, followed by biopsy sampling 5–10 days later by rectal barostat testing [53]. Compared to asymptomatic patients, SUDD patients had a lower first-reported threshold to pain, a higher median overall pain score, and a greater relative expression of neurokinin-1 and tumor necrosis factor alpha mRNA. There was a significant correlation between barostat pain scores and neurokinin-1 expression. These results suggested that SUDD patients exhibit visceral hypersensitivity mediated by low-grade inflammation and upregulation of tachykinins [53].

4.5 Conclusions

Overall, both symptomatic and asymptomatic CDDs are associated with ENS neuroplasticity, mainly characterized by rearrangements of enteric neuronal coding, hypoganglionosis, and nerve fiber remodeling along with alterations of the density and morphology of ICCs and EGCs and changes in the expression of neuronal and glial molecular pathways that could lead to abnormal colonic motility and perception and to the development of bowel symptoms. In addition, changes in the enteric muscular compartment, including altered expression of enteric neurotransmitter receptors, decrease in ICCs-IM density, and impaired gap junction pathways in SMCs further contribute to gut dysfunctions associated with CDD.

Acknowledgments This chapter is dedicated to the memory of Professor Corrado Blandizzi, friend and colleague.

Conflict of Interest None declared.

Funding None.

References

1. Cuomo R, Barbara G, Pace F, Annese V, Bassotti G, Binda GA, Casetti T, Colecchia A, Festi D, Fiocca R, Laghi A, Maconi G, Nascimbeni R, Scarpignato C, Villanacci V, Annibale B. Italian consensus conference for colonic diverticulosis and diverticular disease. United European Gastroenterol J. 2014;2:413–42.
2. Annibale B, Lahner E, Maconi G, Usai P, Marchi S, Bassotti G, Barbara G, Cuomo R. Clinical features of symptomatic uncomplicated diverticular disease: a multicenter Italian survey. Int J Color Dis. 2012;27:1151–9.
3. Tursi A, Brandimarte G, Di Mario F, Lanas A, Scarpignato C, Bafutto M, Barbara G, Bassotti G, Binda GA, Biondi A, Biondo S, Cambiè G, Cassieri C, Crucitti A, Dumitrascu DL, Elisei W, Escalante R, Herszènyi L, Kruis W, Kupcinskas J, Lahat A, Lecca PG, Maconi G, Malfertheiner P, Mazzari A, Mearìn F, Milosavljeviċ T, Nardone G, Chavez De Oliveira E, Papa A, Papagrigoriadis S, Pera M, Persiani R, Picchio M, Regula J, Štimac D, Stollman N, Strate LL, Violi A, Walker MM. International consensus on diverticulosis and diverticular disease. Statements from the 3rd international symposium on diverticular disease. J Gastrointestin Liver Dis. 2019;28(suppl 4):57–66.
4. Tursi A, Scarpignato C, Strate LL, Lanas A, Kruis W, Lahat A, Danese S. Colonic diverticular disease. Nat Rev Dis Primers. 2020;6:20. Erratum in: Nat Rev Dis Primers 2020, 6:35. Erratum in: Nat Rev Dis Primers 2020, 6:50
5. Bassotti G, Villanacci V. Colonic diverticular disease: abnormalities of neuromuscular function. Dig Dis. 2012;30:24–8.
6. Bassotti G, Villanacci V, Bernardini N, Dore MP. Diverticular disease of the colon: neuromuscular function abnormalities. J Clin Gastroenterol. 2016;50(Suppl 1):S6–8.
7. Kupcinskas J, Strate LL, Bassotti G, Torti G, Herszènyi L, Malfertheiner P, Cassieri C, Walker MM, Tursi A. Pathogenesis of diverticulosis and diverticular isease. J Gastrointestin Liver Dis. 2019;28(Suppl 4):7–10.
8. Furness JB, Callaghan BP, Rivera LR, Cho HJ. The enteric nervous system and gastrointestinal innervation: integrated local and central control. Adv Exp Med Biol. 2014;817:39–71.
9. Costa M, Brookes SJ, Hennig GW. Anatomy and physiology of the enteric nervous system. Gut. 2000;47(Suppl 4):iv15–9.
10. Bernardini N, Ippolito C, Segnani C, Mattii L, Bassotti G, Villanacci V, Blandizzi C, Dolfi A. Histopathology in gastrointestinal neuromuscular diseases: methodological and ontological issues. Adv Anat Pathol. 2013;20:17–31.
11. Kanczuga-Koda L, Sulkowski S, Koda M, Sobaniec-Lotowska M, Sulkowska M. Expression of connexins 26, 32 and 43 in the human colon—an immunohistochemical study. Folia Histochem Cytobiol. 2004;42:203–7.
12. Rattan S, Phillips BR, Maxwell PJt. RhoA/Rho-kinase: pathophysiologic and therapeutic implications in gastrointestinal smooth muscle tone and relaxation. Gastroenterology. 2010;138:13–8.

13. Ek-Vitorin JF, King TJ, Heyman NS, Lampe PD, Burt JM. Selectivity of connexin 43 channels is regulated through protein kinase C-dependent phosphorylation. Circul Res. 2006;98:1498–505.
14. Bassotti G, Villanacci V, Antonelli E, Morelli A, Salerni B. Enteric glial cells: new players in gastrointestinal motility? Lab Investig. 2007;87:628–32.
15. Bassotti G, Villanacci V, Fisogni S, Rossi E, Baronio P, Clerici C, Maurer CA, Cathomas G, Antonelli E. Enteric glial cells and their role in gastrointestinal motor abnormalities: introducing the neuro-gliopathies. World J Gastroenterol. 2007;13:4035–41.
16. Yu YB, Li YQ. Enteric glial cells and their role in the intestinal epithelial barrier. World J Gastroenterol. 2014;20:11273–80.
17. Aubé AC, Cabarrocas J, Bauer J, Philippe D, Aubert P, Doulay F, Liblau R, Galmiche JP, Neunlist M. Changes in enteric neurone phenotype and intestinal functions in a transgenic mouse model of enteric glia disruption. Gut. 2006;55:630–7.
18. Rao M, Rastelli D, Dong L, Chiu S, Setlik W, Gershon MD, Corfas G. Enteric glia regulate gastrointestinal motility but are not required for maintenance of the epithelium in mice. Gastroenterology. 2017;153:1068–81.
19. Bar KJ, Facer P, Williams NS, Tam PK, Anand P. Glial-derived neurotrophic factor in human adult and fetal intestine and in Hirschsprung's disease. Gastroenterology. 1997;112:1381–5.
20. Barrenschee M, Lange C, Cossais F, Egberts JH, Becker T, Wedel T, Böttner M. Expression and function of neuregulin 1 and its signaling system ERBB2/3 in the enteric nervous system. Front Cell Neurosci. 2015;9:360.
21. Bassotti G, Battaglia E, Bellone G, Dughera L, Fisogni S, Zambelli C, Morelli A, Mioli P, Emanuelli G, Villanacci V. Interstitial cells of Cajal, enteric nerves, and glial cells in colonic diverticular disease. J Clin Pathol. 2005;58:973–7.
22. Gallego D, Espín F, Mikulka J, Šmirg O, Gil V, Faundez-Zanuy M, Jiménez M, Clavé P. In vitro motor patterns and electrophysiological changes in patients with colonic diverticular disease. Int J Color Dis. 2013;28:1413–22.
23. Fornai M, Colucci R, Antonioli L, Ippolito C, Segnani C, Buccianti P, Marioni A, Chiarugi M, Villanacci V, Bassotti G, Blandizzi C, Bernardini N. Role of cyclooxygenase isoforms in the altered excitatory motor pathways of human colon with diverticular disease. Br J Pharmacol. 2014;171:3728–40.
24. De Simone V, van Baarle L, Matteoli G. Neurite outgrowth in symptomatic uncomplicated diverticular disease. Neurogastroenterol Motil. 2019;31:e13680.
25. Iwase H, Sadahiro S, Mukoyama S, Makuuchi H, Yasuda M. Morphology of myenteric plexuses in the human large intestine: comparison between large intestines with and without colonic diverticula. J Clin Gastroenterol. 2005;39:674–8.
26. Wedel T, Büsing V, Heinrichs G, Nohroudi K, Bruch HP, Roblick UJ, Böttner M. Diverticular disease is associated with an enteric neuropathy as revealed by morphometric analysis. Neurogastroenterol Motil. 2010;22:407–14, e93-4
27. Böttner M, Barrenschee M, Hellwig I, Harde J, Egberts JH, Becker T, Zorenkov D, Wedel T. The enteric serotonergic system is altered in patients with diverticular disease. Gut. 2013;62:1753–62.
28. Pauza AG, Rysevaite-Kyguoliene K, Malinauskas M, Lukosiene JI, Alaburda P, Stankevicius E, Kupcinskas J, Saladzinskas Z, Tamelis A, Pauziene N. Alterations in enteric calcitonin gene-related peptide in patients with colonic diverticular disease: CGRP in diverticular disease. Auton Neurosci. 2019;216:63–71.
29. Cossais F, Leuschner S, Barrenschee M, Lange C, Ebsen M, Vogel I, Böttner M, Wedel T. Persistent increased enteric glial expression of S100β is associated with low-grade inflammation in patients with diverticular disease. J Clin Gastroenterol. 2019;53:449–56.
30. Boesmans W, Lasrado R, Vanden Berghe P, Pachnis V. Heterogeneity and phenotypic plasticity of glial cells in the mammalian enteric nervous system. Glia. 2015;63:229–41.
31. Tursi A. Current and evolving concepts on the pathogenesis of diverticular disease. J Gastrointest Liver Dis. 2019;28:225–35.

32. Barrenschee M, Cossais F, Bottner M, Egberts JH, Becker T, Wedel T. Impaired expression of neuregulin 1 and nicotinic acetylcholine receptor beta4 subunit in diverticular disease. Front Cell Neurosci. 2019;13:563.
33. Wess L, Eastwood MA, Wess TJ, Busuttil A, Miller A. Cross linking of collagen is increased in colonic diverticulosis. Gut. 1995;37:91–4.
34. Matrana MR, Margolin DA. Epidemiology and pathophysiology of diverticular disease. Clin Colon Rect Surg. 2009;22:141–6.
35. Hellwig I, Böttner M, Barrenschee M, Harde J, Egberts JH, Becker T, Wedel T. Alterations of the enteric smooth musculature in diverticular disease. J Gastroenterol. 2014;49:1241–52.
36. Mattii L, Ippolito C, Segnani C, Battolla B, Colucci R, Dolfi A, Bassotti G, Blandizzi C, Bernardini N. Altered expression pattern of molecular factors involved in colonic smooth muscle functions: an immunohistochemical study in patients with diverticular disease. PLoS One. 2013;8:e57023.
37. Golder M, Burleigh DE, Belai A, Ghali L, Ashby D, Lunniss PJ, Navsaria HA, Williams NS. Smooth muscle cholinergic denervation hypersensitivity in diverticular disease. Lancet. 2003;361:1945–51.
38. Parks TG, Connell AM. Motility studies in diverticular disease of the colon. Gut. 1969;10:534–42.
39. Ritchie JA. Movement of segmental constrictions in the human colon. Gut. 1971;12:350–5.
40. Suchowiecky M, Clarke DD, Bhasker M, Perry RJ, Snape WJ Jr. Effect of secoverine on colonic myoelectric activity in diverticular disease of the colon. Dig Dis Sci. 1987;32:833–40.
41. Trotman IF, Misiewicz JJ. Sigmoid motility in diverticular disease and the irritable bowel syndrome. Gut. 1988;29:218–22.
42. Cortesini C, Pantalone D. Usefulness of colonic motility study in identifying patients at risk for complicated diverticular disease. Dis Colon Rectum. 1991;34:339–42.
43. Shafik A, Ahmed I, Shafik AA, El Sibai O. Diverticular disease: electrophysiologic study and a new concept of pathogenesis. World J Surg. 2004;28:411–5.
44. Kratzsch KH. Results of electromyography studies of the rectosigmoid. Dtsch Z Verdau Stoffwechselkr. 1985;45:45–51.
45. Katschinski M, Lederer P, Ellermann A, Ganzleben R, Lux G, Arnold R. Myoelectric and manometric patterns of human rectosigmoid colon in irritable bowel syndrome and diverticulosis. Scand J Gastroenterol. 1990;25:761–8.
46. Viebig RG, Pontes JF, Michelsohn NH. Electromanometry of the rectosigmoid in colonic diverticulosis. Arq Gastroenterol. 1994;31:135–44.
47. Bassotti G, Battaglia E, Spinozzi F, Pelli MA, Tonini M. Twenty-four hour recordings of colonic motility in patients with diverticular disease: evidence for abnormal motility and propulsive activity. Dis Colon Rectum. 2001;44:1814–20.
48. Bassotti G. 1907-2020: more than one century of colonic mass movements in humans. Am J Physiol Gastrointest Liver Physiol. 2021;320:G117–24.
49. Bassotti G, Battaglia E, De Roberto G, Morelli A, Tonini M, Villanacci V. Alterations in colonic motility and relationship to pain in colonic diverticulosis. Clin Gastroenterol Hepatol. 2005;3:248–53.
50. Jaung R, Robertson J, O'Grady G, Milne T, Rowbotham D, Bissett IP. Limited evidence of abnormal intra-colonic pressure profiles in diverticular disease—a systematic review. Color Dis. 2017;19:O168–76.
51. Jaung R, Varghese C, Lin AY, Paskaranandavadivel N, Du P, Rowbotham D, Dinning P, O'Grady G, Bissett I. High-resolution colonic manometry pressure profiles are similar in asymptomatic diverticulosis and controls. Dig Dis Sci. 2021;66:832–42.
52. Clemens CH, Samsom M, Roelofs J, van Berge Henegouwen GP, Smout AJ. Colorectal visceral perception in diverticular disease. Gut. 2004;53:717–22.
53. Humes DJ, Simpson J, Smith J, Sutton P, Zaitoun A, Bush D, Bennett A, Scholefield JH, Spiller RC. Visceral hypersensitivity in symptomatic diverticular disease and the role of neuropeptides and low grade inflammation. Neurogastroenterol Motil. 2012;24:318-e163.

5 Changes in Colonic Structure and Mucosal Inflammation

Pellegrino Crafa and Salvador J. Diaz-Cano

5.1 Introduction

Diverticula are sac-like protrusions of the mucosal and submucosal layers through weak colonic wall areas ("locus minoris resistentiae"). These areas mainly include the points where intramural blood vessels, the perforating arteries ("vasa recta"), are brought into the mucosa to distribute blood by punching through the circular muscular layer. So defined, the existence of diverticula is a congenital or an acquired anomaly whose etiology has just begun to be understood but, because of its multifactorial condition, still has some unclear points. The study of changes in the structure of the colon and inflammation of the mucosa is the starting point for understanding the sequence of events that leads to the formation of diverticula and, consequently, to the setting of proper treatment of the pathology. In Western industrialized countries, the site most affected by diverticular disease is the left colon, but, in the Asian population, right-sided diverticulosis is more common. The incidence reported is in 17.5% of the general population, and it represents up to 42% of all endoscopic diagnosis, increasing steadily with age, reaching around 30% at 65 years, 50% in those over 75 years, and 71% in those aged ≥80 years [1]. No difference has been found in the sex distribution of diverticulosis [2]. Left-sided diverticulosis almost invariably involves the sigmoid colon and may extend proximally,

P. Crafa (✉)
Department of Pathology, "Ospedale Maggiore" University Hospital, University of Parma, Parma, Italy
e-mail: pellegrino.crafa@unipr.it

S. J. Diaz-Cano
Queen Elizabeth Hospital, Birmingham, UK

Department of Pathology and Molecular Pathology, King's Health Partners, University of London, London, UK
e-mail: sjdiazcano@doctors.org.uk

© The Author(s), under exclusive license to Springer Nature Switzerland AG 2022
A. Tursi et al. (eds.), *Colonic Diverticular Disease*,
https://doi.org/10.1007/978-3-030-93761-4_5

but the involvement of the ascending colon and cecum occurs in fewer than 10% of cases. The extraperitoneal rectum is not affected [3]. Left-sided diverticulosis is also known as pulsion diverticulosis. The demographic profile of the typical patient with diverticulosis perfectly matches the natural history of diverticular disease. According to Laplace's law in organs with a distensible wall, it is commonly believed that high colonic pressure will develop tension in response to the elongation, thus leading to the development of diverticula at the weakest point of the colonic tissue. However, there is no validated theory to support these claims; even severe mechanical stress is a significant factor driving tissue remodeling [4, 5]. Patel et al. developed an experimental model on swine's descending colon based on simultaneous inflation and extension tests evaluating the result obtained using the Finite Element (FE) software. This approach simulates a physical phenomenon occurring during diverticula formations and reports the results with a computational model using a numerical mathematical technique to prove that the mechanical stress could be critical in diverticulum genesis and in the increase of the diverticulum's volume [6]. The model was designed keeping in mind the typical anisotropic nature of the colonic tissue, which in turn depends on its microscopic characteristics. Thus, the model has shown that the highest stress values are concentrated around the luminal side of the pouch's neck. The increase in stress increases with increasing pressure until it reaches two to three times the maximum values observed in a normal colon. A significant elevation of stress could occur in a colon with diverticulosis than in a normal colon, which implicates elevated stresses in this condition that are responsible for diverticular wall remodeling. In this manner, computational structural mechanics can investigate potential changes in stress distribution that could be introduced in the colonic tissue due to the presence of a pouch-like structure. More interesting, the analysis shows a correlation between stress elevation and size of the pouch. It is known that pouch size increases over time in diverticulosis and that mechanical stress is a significant factor driving biological tissue remodeling. These two elements would explain the overall pouch size increase in response to elevated stress values around the pouch, leading to a vicious cycle where the pouch size is further increased. The distance from the center of the pouch (zone of influence) increases with pressure, reaching a plateau value after a specific pressure elevation that correlates with the area of the pouch neck, suggesting that the size of the pouch neck is more important than the surface area of the pouch itself in pouches under high stress and with a greater zone of influence. Besides, a significant luminal pressure drop would be necessary to restore stress to an average level, explaining the low effectiveness of a high-fiber diet as a stand-alone treatment solution once pouches are developed. A diverticulum is expected to be more compliant than a normal tissue constituted by only the mucosal and submucosal layers. The mucosa has been reported to be extremely expansible, and the submucosa could withstand deformations four to five times greater than the muscular layer [7]. Notably, even if the colon is a collapsible tube with curves, the stress values would undoubtedly change, but the high-stress value observed at the neck of the pouch with a relative increase in pressure and pouch size will not change. Luminal pressure (pressure on the inner wall of the tissue with an external force equal to zero) values above 1.5 kPa lead to permanent tissue damage. The computational simulations pushing this value to visualize the evolution of stress values and luminal pressure might explain the variation in diverticular shape and volume. Moreover, it might also try to explain tissue remodeling until a complication appears.

5.2 Muscle Thickening and Mucosal Inflammation

Morson [8] demonstrated a marked abnormal muscle thickening in colonic diverticulosis without inflammation, and Golder reported occasional neutrophils and plasma cells and a diffuse lymphocytic infiltrate mainly localized to the luminal side of the lamina propria, findings consistent with a chronic inactive inflammatory infiltrate, a natural defense mechanism of a normal large bowel mucosa [9]. It was suggested that thickening of the muscularis propria is caused by two factors: (1) aging or more extended periods of low dietary fiber intake and (2) high intraluminal pressure. The muscle thickening might be associated with rigidity or decreased strength of the colonic wall in diverticulosis.

5.3 Mesenchymal Alteration

The etiology and pathogenesis of diverticular disease are multifactorial. Various aspects can also be understood at the time of macroscopic evaluation (Figs. 5.1 and 5.2) of colectomy samples removed for diverticular disease: a considerable thickening of the muscular layer, peri-diverticular fibrosis, which means an increase in elastin content together with elastosis [10], and increased intraluminal pressure within the sigmoid colon of persons with diverticulosis during periods of

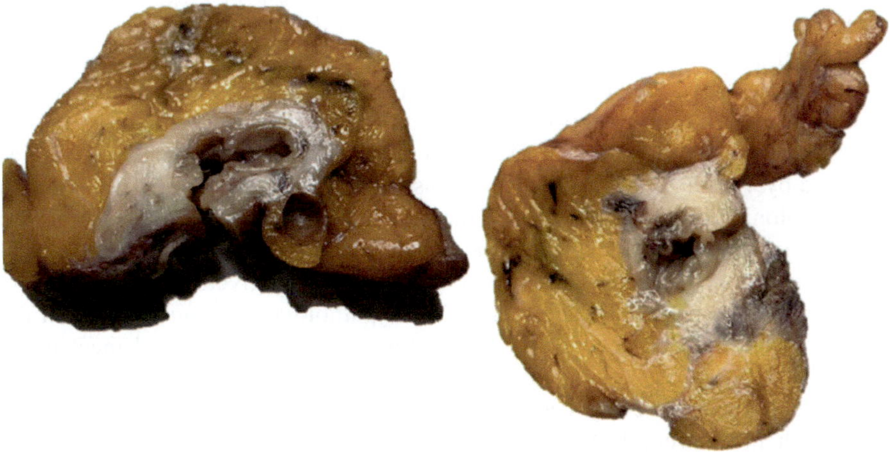

Fig. 5.1 Cut section: thickening of the colonic wall near a diverticulum

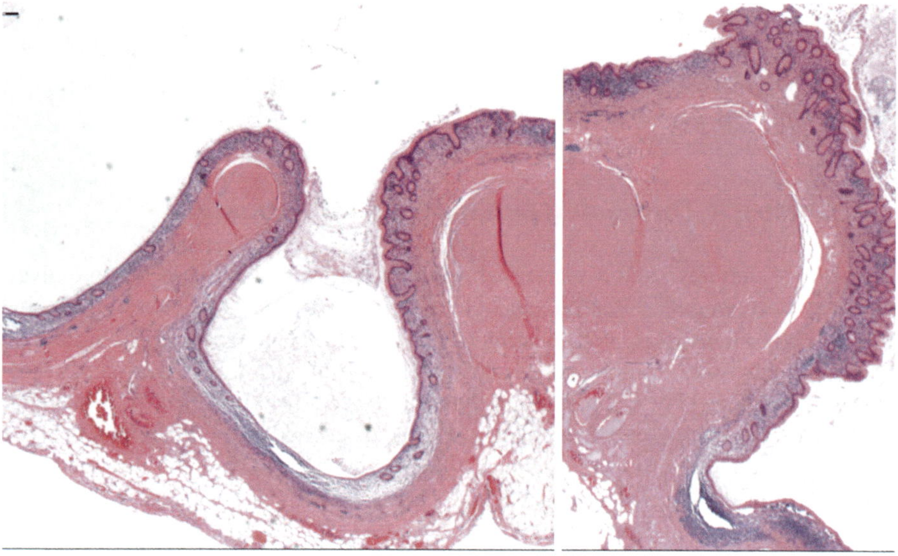

Fig. 5.2 Diverticula (hematoxilin & eosin-stained section)

peak contraction, resulted in pressures of up to 90 mmHg, a value nine times higher than those in normal colons [11], demonstrated by the increase in thickness of the circular and longitudinal muscular layers together with a progressive increase in the thickness of collagen and elastin tissues of the colon wall [12]. The latter feature is related to the deficiency in dietary fiber consumption and genetic factors [13]. Collagen is the most abundant protein in mammals, and one of its primary functions is to maintain the structural integrity of connective tissues [14]. The mechanical properties of the colon wall depend not only on the individual components of its various layers but also on the relationships they contract with each other. Whiteway and Morson [10] observed that the elastin content of the taenia coli in patients with diverticular disease is twofold higher than that in controls. The elastin was documentable between the muscle cells, warping the typical fascicular pattern of the taenia coli. This variation of the viscoelastic properties of the colon is related to the decrease in the integrity of the connective tissue, as reported by Watters et al., which is responsible for a reduction in tensile strength in the colonic wall with age, particularly in the distal colon. An extracellular matrix provides the maintenance of the integrity and flexibility of the colonic wall with its components such as collagen, elastin, and proteoglycans [15], which are, however, subject to rehash due to age. Thus, pathological aging changes in the colonic wall could be secondary to a decline in the structural and mechanical integrity of the various layers of the large bowel wall [15]. Given that the development of colonic diverticulosis, as known, is a function of age and declining colonic wall mechanical strength, the latter should be addressed partly due to changes in the collagen structure [16].

5.3.1 Decrease of Collagen I and Increase of Collagen III

Notably, collagen is the most abundant extracellular matrix protein, which is implied in the mechanical stability of the connective tissue and is responsible for the tensile strength of tissues. Fibrillar collagens are synthesized as precursors (procollagens) containing different extra domains known as pro-peptides. After extracellular cleavage of both ends, collagen molecules are assembled into collagen fibers, where covalent cross-links form between the adjacent collagen molecules. The most important types are collagen I, found in mature tissues, and collagen III; collagen I is the critical structural component of several tissues. It is expressed in almost all connective tissues, and it is the predominant component of the interstitial membrane. It is also responsible for forming mature tissues, whereas collagen III, a homotrimer consisting of only one collagen alpha chain, shows less mechanical strength [17]. Mature collagen type I was significantly lower in the diverticulitis group, whereas immature collagen type III was higher than in controls. Therefore, the collagen ratio (I/III) was significantly lower in the diverticulitis group. The amount of collagen and its structure is regulated mainly by matrix metalloproteinases (MMPs). These are a family of enzymes, zinc-containing neural endopeptidases, which are structurally related neutral proteinases that use either disulfides or calcium ions to stabilize the enzyme's structure. MMPs are secreted as inactive zymogens with structural pro-forms; the activation of these zymogens requires double proteolytic cleavage of the pro-domain at the N-terminal of the MMP. They have crucial roles in many physiological situations [18]. MMP activity is regulated by interactions with members of the tissue inhibitor of matrix metalloproteinase (TIMP) family, generating an inactive MMP/TIMP complex. Remarkably, TIMPs may also play a role in the activation process of MMPs by binding to the hemopexin-like domains of adjacent MMPs, thus favoring a reciprocal activation. Moreover, TIMPs are secreted in proenzyme forms requiring extracellular activation from various cell types, including macrophages, T cells, and myofibroblasts, stimulated by cytokines and other factors [19]. MMPs can virtually degrade all extracellular matrix components. Thus, MMPs directly determine the synthesis, deposition, and remodeling of collagen types I and III in all tissues [20]. Among the MMPs, MMP-1 and MMP-3 are the principal enzymes that can cleave fibrillar type I, II, and III collagens. MMP-1 cleaves both ECM and non-ECM substrates such as collagen, gelatin, laminin, complement C1q, IL-1β, and TNF-α, suggesting a crucial role in inflammatory and fibrotic responses. The MMP-3 enzyme degrades collagen types II, III, IV, IX, and X, proteoglycans, fibronectin, laminin, and elastin. MMP-3 can also activate other MMPs such as MMP-1, MMP-7, and MMP-9, rendering MMP-3 crucial to connective tissue remodeling [21]. Stumpf et al. found a statistically significant reduction in the expression of MMP-1 in the diverticulitis group. Downregulation of MMP-1 may be necessary for the development of diverticulitis because proteases act not only in proteolysis, inflammation, and invasion but also in angiogenesis and even growth [22]. MMP-1 and MMP-3 are abundant in granulation tissues of gastrointestinal ulcers [23]. A considerable number of polymorphonuclear leukocytes, immune-positive for MMP-9, were observed throughout the intestinal wall of Crohn's disease, implying its role in connective tissue remodeling. MMP-3 is markedly overexpressed at inflamed sites in patients with ulcerative colitis or Crohn's disease, whereas TIMP-1 remains unaltered, suggesting that excess MMP-3 might be responsible for loss of mucosal integrity in these conditions [24]. Mimura et al. demonstrated an increasing trend in the amount of collagen in both uncomplicated and complicated diverticulosis than in controls. Both TIMP-1 and TIMP-2 were significantly higher in the muscular layer of complicated diverticulosis than in controls [25]. The finding that the mRNA of TIMP-1 was higher, with a decreasing trend in such order, in complicated diverticulosis, uncomplicated diverticulosis, and controls, might suggest that the expression of their mRNA is related to the clinical course of diverticula. Macrophage-like and fibroblast-like cells (TIMP-1- and TIMP-2-positive cells) were frequently encountered around the blood vessel areas in the muscular layer and serosa. This suggests that these cells could be sources of TIMPs in this disease. They could infiltrate the inflamed areas where extracellular matrix deposition was required for tissue remodeling, thus affecting the turnover of the extracellular matrix and creating a predisposition that has formation of colonic diverticula as an outcome. It is a prolonged process, usually taking 40 years, undergoing periods of exacerbation and remission of inflammation. Thus, it could involve extensive MMP-driven remodeling of the connective tissue and possibly chronic inflammation, causing an increase in TIMPs and facilitating the excess deposit of the extracellular matrix in the pathogenesis of diverticular disease.

5.3.2 Cross-Linking Between Collagen Fibers

Collagen is known to have intermolecular and intramolecular cross-links, which stabilize and strengthen the tissue in which it is located. Two cross-linking pathways have been identified in collagen, one based on lysine aldehydes and the other on hydroxylysine aldehydes, producing allysine and hydroxylysine, respectively. The reaction of either type of aldehyde with the e-amino group of lysine or hydroxylysine results in the production of reducible intermolecular cross-links. Initially, all reactions produce a Schiff base-type cross-link, also known as an aldimine-type linkage. These intermediate forms are susceptible to cleavage by diluting acid. Hydroxyallysine-derived intermediate cross-links can also undergo a further spontaneous reaction to form a ketamine-type structure in vivo (known as the Amadori rearrangement). The ability of the intermediate cross-link to create the acid-stable ketamine depends on whether it is derived from allysine and hydroxylysine or from hydroxylysine and lysine. The first of these is unable to form the ketamine, whereas the second can do this. The ketamine-type cross-link is stable for weak acids. The number of acid-labile cross-links decreases with maturation of the tissue [26]. A healthy colon has both propulsive and storage functions and needs to withstand the extremes of pressure in the large bowel – equivalent to 100–150 mmHg [27]. The intrinsic strength of the bowel wall is believed to be independent of the submucosal layer. Wess et al. [16] found significantly different levels of mature cross-linked collagen in healthy colons from individuals over 60 years and in colons from subjects of the same age showing diverticulosis. As the number of collagen cross-linkage increases, the corresponding tissue becomes stiffer [28]. These observations may explain the onset of high intraluminal pressures because of changes in the colonic wall in patients with diverticular disease. Early-onset diverticula have been reported in patients with connective tissue diseases such as Ehlers–Danlos syndrome and Marfan syndrome [29]. Despite this increased thickness of muscle coats, however, the colonic wall is reported to have a lowered resistance to distension in diverticulosis. Watters et al. [15] showed that both the tensile and the burst strength of the human colonic wall depend on the integrity of the submucosa. Thomson et al. [14, 30] showed that colonic submucosal structures undergo aging changes in both standard and diverticular colons. These changes include differences between the right and left sides of the colon as an increase in the number of fibrils and a decrease in the fibril diameter in the left colon compared with those in the right colon. Acid insolubility increases after 40 years—an exciting finding as colonic diverticulosis is rare before that age. This relationship was more strongly significant in the sigmoid colon, which is the predominant location for the development of colonic diverticula. These results also indicate that colonic collagen from subjects affected by colonic diverticulosis is less acid-soluble than that from healthy colons of those over 60 years ($p < 0\ 05$), suggesting that the collagen from colonic diverticulosis colons has a higher number of cross-links than that from the unaffected colonic tissue. The solubility of collagen in weak acids is known to decrease with advancing age in specific tissues, such as the skin, vascular adventitia, and chordae tendineae of the heart valves [28]. Thomson et al. have shown an increase in the collagen fibril numbers and decreased collagen fibril diameter in the left colon of patients with diverticular disease [14]. Colonic collagen is in a dynamic state, given that it is continuously produced and degraded. Aging is associated with increased cross-linking between collagen molecules, which results in decreased solubility in weak acids, increasing stiffness and resistance to enzymic digestion in vitro [26].

5.4 Nervous Alteration

Since the gut is regarded as the second brain, the search for nervous alteration or running change has a logical background. Short-lived recurrent abdominal pain is a common and debilitating symptom reported by a third of patients with symptomatic diverticular disease, suggesting that visceral hypersensitivity might play a role [31]. Patients with symptomatic diverticular disease demonstrate visceral hypersensitivity to rectal balloon distension because of peripheral sensitization, with both inflammatory and neurochemical factors playing a role [31]. This finding is associated with an increase in the expression of the inflammatory cytokines IL-6 and TNF-α and an upregulation of the neuropeptide receptor NK1. Prior inflammation, in the form of episodes of acute diverticulitis, is associated with a fourfold increase in the risk of reporting recurrent abdominal pain in patients with diverticulosis, with such patients also having inflammatory changes present in resection specimens [32]. An increase in substance P and galanin-secreting neurons in mucosal biopsies of patients with prior episodes of acute diverticulitis has also been demonstrated [33]. This finding suggests that both inflammation and variation in neuropeptide secretions may be necessary for generating symptoms in patients with diverticulitis. Both these mechanisms may be responsible for peripheral sensitization leading to visceral hypersensitivity, as previous studies have separately demonstrated changes in inflammation, enteric nerves, and sensitization [31, 32], suggesting that patients with the symptomatic disease have distinct abnormalities in motor function and inflammatory and neural changes that differ from asymptomatic patients. Simpson et al. [33] focused on the structural and luminal changes in the condition, particularly the role of high-pressure colonic contractions. Similar amplitude contractions are also present in healthy volunteers but are not reported to be painful [34], suggesting that visceral hypersensitivity is an essential determinant of symptoms. Humes [35] demonstrated an increased expression of genes producing inflammatory proteins such as IL-6 and TNF-α in symptomatic than in asymptomatic patients. The increase in inflammatory gene expression and cell-to-cell interaction suggests that these patients have a low-grade inflammation associated with visceral hypersensitivity. In a normal gastrointestinal tract, vagal activity regulates exocrine function, promotes bowel motility, and initiates feedback signals to the central nervous system. The vagal signal is carried through the cholinergic and muscarinic pathways, whereas the sympathetic signal is carried through the adrenergic pathways [36]. The idea that chafing of vagal innervation leads to vagal hypersensitivity in the recipient organ may explain why baseline motility is normal in diverticular disease, but amplified colonic motility mimicking irritable bowel syndrome is seen postprandially. In this setting, dysfunctional bowel contractions are believed to contribute to gaps in tissue planes between muscle fibers, through which mucosal herniations are believed to occur. Notably, the heightened smooth muscle contractions in diverticular disease have been attributed to cholinergic receptor overexpression, and not excess vagal innervation [37]. Yun et al. [36] hypothesized that the vagal withdrawal of diverticulosis may represent a specific local manifestation of the aging-related global retreat of vagal innervation from recipient organs. This global phenomenon is likely to be an evolutionary maladaptation that has been unmasked by the rapid expansion of human lifespan during the last few centuries [38]. A loss of enteric neurons is a common histopathological feature within the spectrum of gastrointestinal neuromuscular pathology and diverticular disease (DD) [39]. In addition, Barrenschee et al. [40] reported a significant reduction in the myenteric neuronal number per 100 mm intestinal length and an average in neuronal number per ganglion in patients with DD. In contrast, Iwase et al. [41] observed a reduction in the number and size of myenteric ganglion cells per cm in both patients with asymptomatic diverticula and DD. In this case, the observed reduction might involve glial rather than neuronal cells. Immunohistochemistry shows a reduction in both the neuropil and the somata of myenteric neurons for GDNF family receptor alpha 1 (GFRα1) and REarranged during Transfection (RET), which provide evidence for the involvement of glial cells and neurons in the case of GFRα1. For RET, immunohistochemistry indicates only a reduction in myenteric neurons with its processes, given that RET is not expressed in glial cells. However, a quantitation analysis exhibited a similar reduction in receptor expression in both diverticulosis and DD. This indicates that the reduced receptor expression is an early event within the pathogenic process, most likely provoked by an impaired glial cell line-derived neurotrophic factor (GDNF) system. GDNF is a potent neurotrophic factor for various neuronal cell populations in the central and peripheral nervous systems and in the enteric nervous system (ENS), which continues during the progression of the disease. Novel concepts consider that patients with DD exhibit disturbed intestinal motility patterns [34, 42], morphological alteration in the ENS (oligoneuronal hypoganglionosis) [41, 43], remodeling in the nerve tissue, and impaired neuromuscular communication and disturbed enteric neurotransmission [9, 44]. These alterations in patients with DD might lead to uncoordinated contractions and high pressure, thus producing and triggering the formation of diverticula. It is suggested that enteric neuromuscular changes may result from remodeling processes after acute inflammation since several neuropeptides, found to be increased after acute inflammation, were also increased in symptomatic but not in inflamed DD [33]. Thus, in the case of DD, a reduced GDNF expression could also be explained because of previous inflammation that damaged the ENS or the intestinal musculature. However, Barrenschee [40] demonstrated that downregulation of the components of the GDNF system already occurs in earlier stages of this illness, namely, in asymptomatic diverticulosis, where no inflammatory events could be observed before having strengthened the hypothesis that the disturbed GDNF system could be the primary trigger for the reduced neuronal number rather than for inflammatory processes.

5.5 Mucosal Alteration and Markers of Histological Inflammation

Diverticula comprise mucosa pouches, surrounded by loose fibro fatty tissues in the subserosal layer or the adventitia of the colon. There is a residual strand instead of a fully formed muscularis mucosae, usually accompanied by an increase in the number and size of lymphoid follicles within the mucous lining [45], as a local response to fecal stasis, like that seen in the vermiform appendix or diversion proctocolitis [46]. The histology of diverticula is directly related to the degree of inflammation and injury to the mucosa [47]. Commonly, it has the histological feature of a normal colonic mucosa. However, most times, there is an increase in the lymphoplasmacytic mononuclear chronic cellular infiltrate in the lamina propria coupled with mucin depletion, cryptitis, architectural distortion, Paneth cell metaplasia, and formation of lymphoglandular complexes (Fig. 5.3). Erosions and ulcers (Fig. 5.4) can complete the histological picture, and fecal material escaping into the mucosa or subserosa may elicit a foreign body granuloma. The mucosal changes are usually confined to the diverticula but may extend to the ostia, whereas the surrounding mucosa, in most cases, is histologically normal. In severely shortened thick-walled segments of the bowel with diverticulosis, the redundant mucosa is bent into characteristic polypoid folds (Fig. 5.5). Microscopically, the folds show vascular

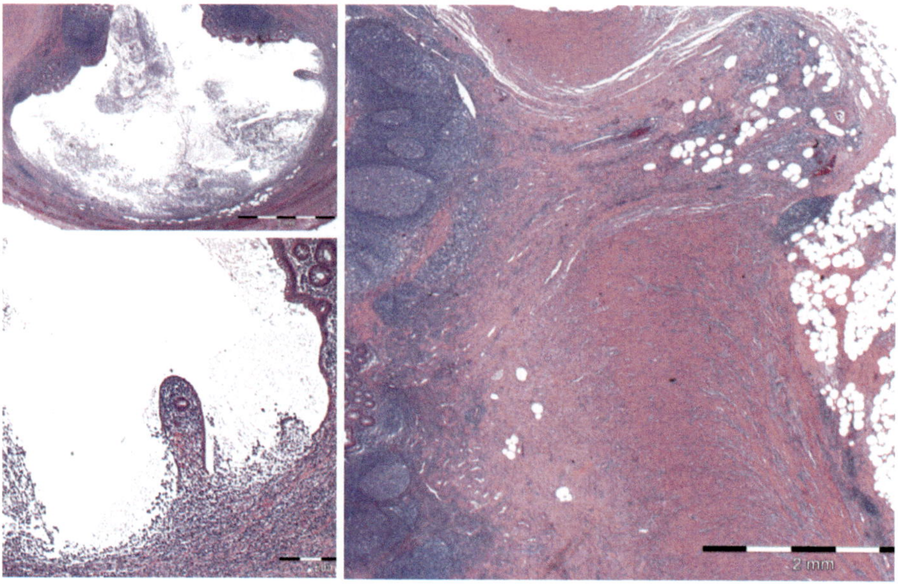

Fig. 5.3 Progressive damage of the epithelial lining and inflammatory reaction extending to the adjacent soft tissues

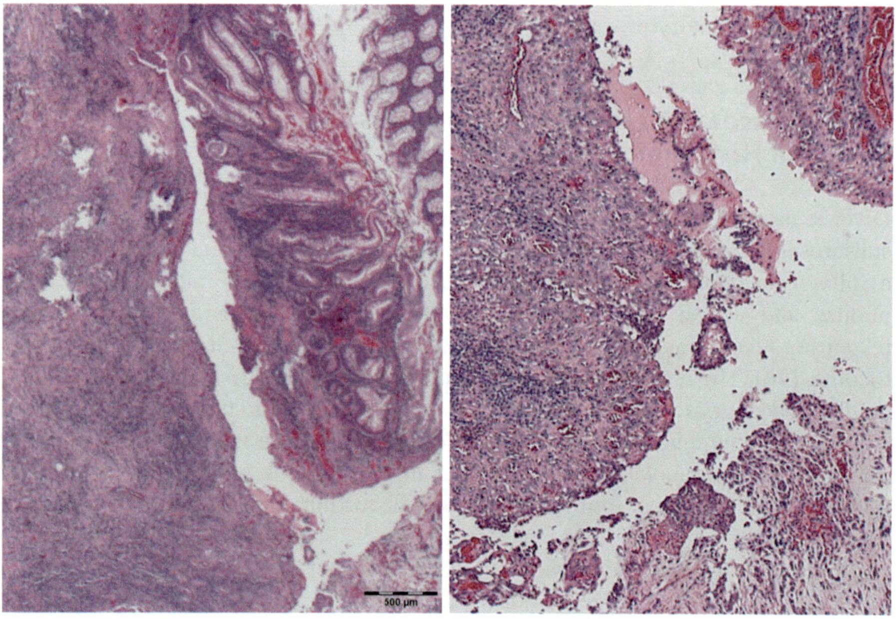

Fig. 5.4 Abscess in diverticular disease

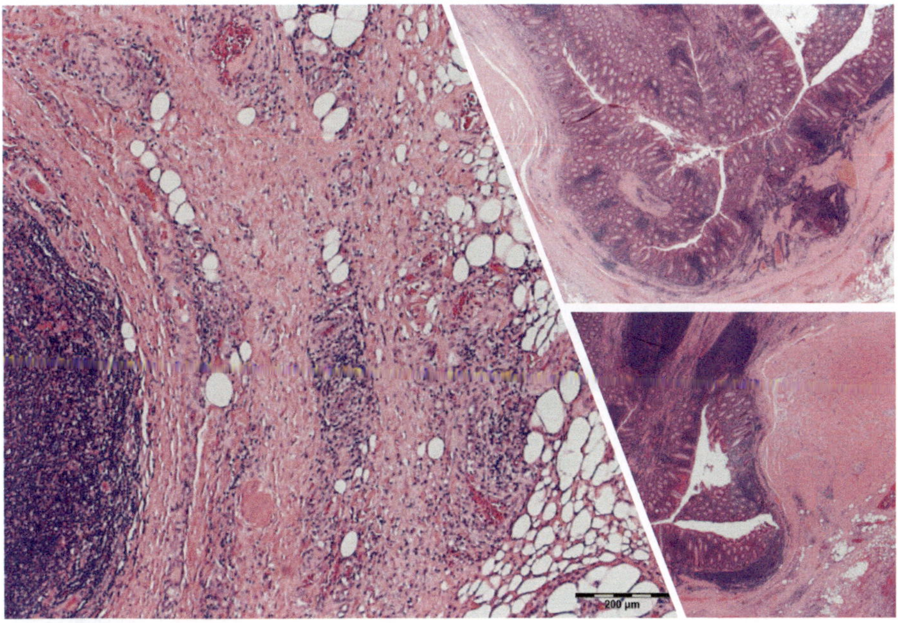

Fig. 5.5 Chronic diverticulitis, fibrosis, and mucosal polypoid fold

congestion, mucosal edema, and hemosiderin deposition, which follows acute bleeding [47]. The characteristic features of mucosal prolapse, including crypt hyperplasia, muscularization of the lamina propria, and superficial erosions, are commonly present [48]. In a small proportion of patients with sigmoid diverticulosis or diverticulitis (estimated to be from 0.3 to 1.3%), the mucosa between the diverticula of surgically removed diverticulitis specimens is grossly erythematous, granular, and friable. It thus resembles the colonic mucosa in a chronic inflammatory bowel disease [49]. Most patients (75–80%) with diverticulosis will remain asymptomatic throughout their lifetime. Diverticulitis is the most common cause of symptoms, affecting 10–25% of patients with diverticulosis [50]. Obstruction of the neck of a diverticulum with fecal matter is believed to cause distension of the diverticulum responsible for the compression of the vasa recta deployed on the convexity of the pouch, resulting in focal ischemia of the mucosa, thus leading to local inflammation, mucus stack, and bacterial overgrowth. Hemorrhage is a common complication of diverticular disease accounting for more than 40% of lower gastrointestinal bleeding episodes in some series [51]. Mucosal ulceration could lead to gradual and mild bleeding, whereas erosion of the vasa recta, which traverses the circular muscle, may cause a rapid hemorrhage. Inflammation of the diverticulum may lead to a peri-diverticular abscess within the colonic subserosa, and this can cause serositis, adhesions, and formation of an inflammatory mass that may ultimately heal by fibrosis, causing a stricture and an obstruction or adhesion to the nearby organ(s)

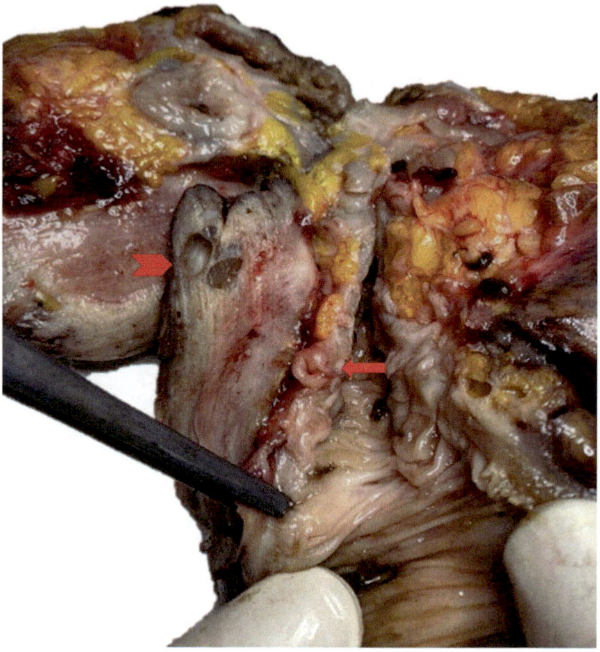

Fig. 5.6 Adhesion between the colon and uterus. Arrow: diverticulum; arrowhead: uterus with Naboth's cysts

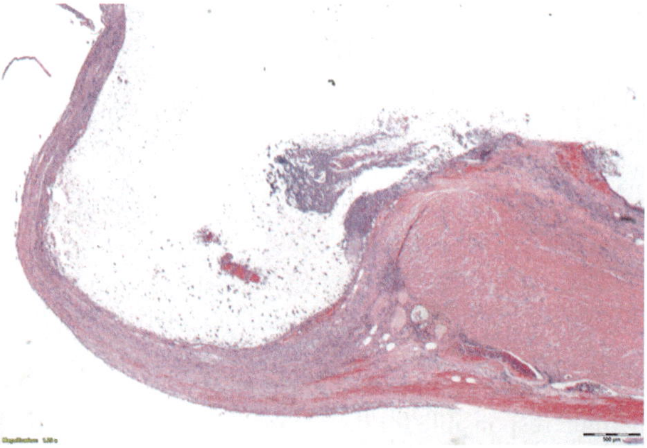

Fig. 5.7 Thinning of the diverticulum wall preceding perforation

(Fig. 5.6) till fistula formation. Inflamed diverticula can perforate, causing purulent peritonitis (Figs. 5.7 and 5.8), or can undergo rupture in the free peritoneal cavity, causing fecal peritonitis. The infection can also spread systemically, causing bacteremia or sepsis. Chronic low-grade inflammation has also been reported within and around diverticula in participants who underwent sigmoid resection for symptomatic uncomplicated diverticular disease (SUDD) but not diverticulitis [52]. These findings correlate with the overexpression of TNF-α in participants with a history of diverticulitis and diverticular disease [53]. When diverticulosis becomes

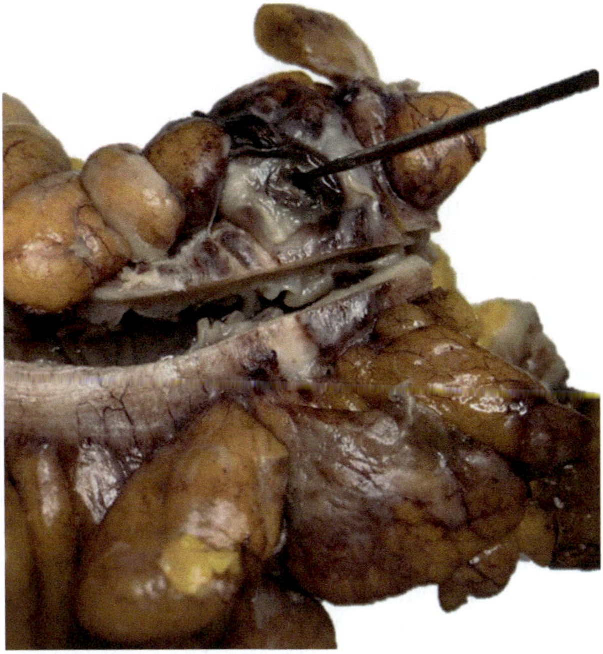

Fig. 5.8 Perforation of a diverticulum with an induced fibrin-purulent reaction covering the colonic serosa

symptomatic, it is called DD. The most common conventional complication of DD is diverticulitis, which is essentially a pericolic inflammatory process that originates within the diverticula and extends into the surrounding tissues but spares the non-diverticular colonic mucosa. DD may show a low-grade microscopic inflammation related to the severity of the disease [54]. Tumor necrosis factor-alpha (TNF-α) is overexpressed concerning the severity of the histological inflammation [55]. It is also overexpressed in segmental colitis-associated diverticulosis (SCAD), which is considered a 'bridge' between a classical IBD and a complication of a long-lasting DD [56]. The presence of an inflammatory infiltrate was assessed by a semiquantitative lymphocytic and neutrophil count on ten colonic fields with a high-power field (HPF) technique at 40× magnification, assessed at the bottom and on the whole crypts [57]. Hematoxylin–eosin staining was performed to assess the histology of the sigmoid tract. Count lymphocyte assay (CLA) for T cells was performed using anti-CD3 (pan-T) monoclonal antibodies. Lymphocyte infiltration was graded as: Score 0 (normal) = 3–5 cells; Score 1 (mild) = 6–8 cells; Score 2 (moderate) = 9–10 cells; and Score 3 (severe) = >10 cells. The neutrophilic infiltrate was also evaluated to assess active or nonactive inflammation using a semiquantitative grading: Score 0 (absence of neutrophilic infiltrate) = nonactive; Score 1 (focal presence of neutrophil) = mild; Score 2 (presence of neutrophil intermediate between 1 and 3) = moderate; and Score 3 (diffuse neutrophilic infiltrate) = severe. Neutrophils were localized using anti-CD15 monoclonal antibodies. As the severity of histological inflammation is based on the severity of the neutrophil infiltrate, the choice to assess only the acute infiltrate may be considered adequate in such a context [55]. According to Pucilowska et al. [58], acute injury on the colonic mucosa causes normal mesenchymal cells to be activated to a fibrogenic phenotype with consequent normal healing of fibrosis. During normal healing, excess extracellular matrix deposition is prevented by post-transcriptional or post-translation regulation of collagen, reversal of the fibrogenic phenotype, or selective death of fibrogenic cells. If these events do not occur or are not sufficiently active or if the fibrogenic cell population expands, fibrosis may occur. However, in a recent study, Järbrink-Sehgal et al. [59] have assessed all colonic segment biopsies, from left to right, using standard endoscopic forceps. The corresponding hematoxylin and eosin-stained slides were investigated for either the presence or the absence of markers of histological inflammation, such as surface epithelium, mucin depletion, Paneth cells, cryptitis or crypt abscesses, apoptosis of the epithelium, normal architecture/crypt branching, chronic inflammatory gradient from the base to the surface, basal plasmacytosis, and granulomas. The number of lymphoid aggregates, follicles, and neutrophils was counted in the lamina propria, and intraepithelial lymphocytes were counted/100 colonocytes [60]. The surface epithelium and chronic inflammatory gradient were intact in all participants, and basal plasmacytosis and granulomas were absent in all samples. There was a trend of increased numbers of cecal lymphoid aggregates in cases vs. controls ($P = 0.07$), but no other associations between diverticulosis and inflammatory markers were found. Kealy et al. [61] reported that the density of microscopic lymph follicles and aggregates increased in the necropsied colons of patients with diverticular disease than in those without, suggesting that lymphoid follicles may be weak points in the mucosa and that diverticula could develop at these points. The Järbrink-Sehgal population-based study, assessing the whole colon for inflammation, regardless of diverticula localization, complements the findings by Peery et al. [59, 62], demonstrating the absence of colonic mucosal inflammation in diverticulosis or symptomatic diverticulosis, therefore questioning the role of chronic low-grade inflammation in diverticula's genesis. Similarly, in the symptomatic diverticulosis subanalysis, Järbrink-Sehgal et al. [59] found no association between symptomatic diverticulosis with abdominal pain or diarrhea and serological or mucosal inflammation throughout the colon. These findings uphold other findings of an absence of colonic mucosal inflammation in the sigmoid, using serological immune markers and histological cytokine levels in patients with symptomatic diverticulosis and SUDD compared with controls without diverticulosis [63]. The same conclusion was drawn by Peery et al. [62] in a large colonoscopy-based study of individuals without a history of diverticulitis or overt peri-diverticular inflammation. It was found that colonic diverticulosis was not associated with mucosal inflammation and no association was found between colonic diverticulosis and chronic gastrointestinal symptoms. There was no evidence for mucosal inflammation in individuals with diverticulosis and chronic gastrointestinal symptoms, the so-called symptomatic uncomplicated diverticular disease.

5.6 Segmental Colitis-Associated Diverticulosis (SCAD)

As the name suggests, SCAD is a colonic inflammatory disorder that occurs in patients with superimposable characteristics mimicking the clinical and endoscopic features of inflammatory bowel diseases, such as Crohn's disease and ulcerative colitis. By definition, SCAD is a pathological entity characterized by a chronic inflammatory response involving the interdiverticular mucosa of the colonic segment involved. The rectum, by definition, is free of inflammation [64]. A nonspecific, nongranulomatous, and localized inflammatory process involving the sigmoid colon (i.e., 'sigmoiditis') and sparing the rectum and a more proximal colon defines this pathology. The true prevalence of the disease is probably underestimated, with an incidence varying between 0.3 and 1% [61, 65, 66]; however, a Dutch retrospective study reported an incidence as high as 8% [67]. SCAD is now viewed as a specific inflammatory pathology paired with diverticulosis whose etiology is still not entirely known [66, 68]. Most cases occur in males, with rectal bleeding being the most frequent initial presentation (hematochezia: more than 70%). Usually, the entity is almost exclusively a disorder of the elderly, often after the age of 50 years [69]. SCAD represents a distinct clinical and pathological entity sharing some features with other forms of inflammatory bowel diseases (IBDs). The pathogenesis of SCAD is multifactorial and includes genetic susceptibility, alteration in the colonic microbiome, local ischemia, and mucosal prolapse [61, 70, 71]. SCAD is pathologically defined by a nonspecific segmental or localized nongranulomatous inflammatory process, usually confined to the sigmoid colon. The right colon and rectal inflammatory sparing are confirmed by histologically normal mucosa in the endoscopically documented left diverticular ostia. When it is present, the perianal disease, a marker more suggestive of Crohn's disease, is also missing. In more than 60% of patients with recurrent SCAD, the second episode of the disease had clinical evidence more than a decade after the initial clinical episode, indicating that the disease often seems to be a self-limited inflammatory process that resolves with no future disease episodes or requirement for ongoing treatment. Increased TNF-α concentrations have been reported in Crohn's disease and ulcerative colitis, and SCAD [69]. The hematoxylin and eosin-stained specimens of the inflamed colonic tract were used to evaluate either the whole mucosal damage or the activity of the inflammation. Mucosal damage was reflected by a score representing the mean value of the single scores of the following histological characteristics: polymorphonuclear infiltration of the epithelium and lamina propria, crypt abscesses, loss of glandular parallelism, crypt shortening and ramification, mucus epithelial depletion, and involvement of the muscularis mucosae and submucosa. Each histology score ranged from 0 (normal) to 3 (severe). The inflammation activity was expressed by the total number of neutrophils in the lamina propria, counted with software in five high-power fields, selected based on high cellular density. The inflammation activity was considered mild ($\geq$5 and <10 cells/mm^2), moderate ($\geq$10 and <15 cells/mm^2), or severe ($\geq$15 cells/mm^2) [69]. In SCAD, biopsies were collected from the interdiverticular mucosa, which, by definition, is affected by the disease [65, 70].

The endoscopic classification of SCAD was based on a score formulated by Tursi et al. The disease was classified into four different endoscopic patterns (types A, B, C, and D), mirroring the symptoms reported by patients. Patients with milder lesions (types A and C) report mild abdominal pain or diarrhea. In contrast, more severe lesions (types B and D) are always accompanied by abdominal pain, rectal bleeding, or sometimes subocclusive attacks (type D) [70]. Moreover, Tursi et al. [72] showed a lower rate of recurrence in patients with mild endoscopic and clinical patterns (types A and C) compared with patients with severe endoscopic and clinical patterns at entry (types B and D). Four different endoscopic patterns (Table 5.1) are recognized, associated with peculiar histological characteristics [61, 70, 73–75]. Type A is characterized endoscopically by red patches involving colonic folds and diverticular sparing. Types B and D are characterized endoscopically by ulcerative colitis (UC)-like changes with erosions and hyperemic areas involving the colonic folds and severe inflammation involving the overall diverticula containing the mucosa, respectively. Type C is characterized by Crohn's disease-like changes, with isolated aphthous ulcers and transmural inflammatory changes [74].

On light microscopy, histological features include cryptitis, crypt abscesses, and expansion of the lamina propria by mononuclear cells, sometimes arranged in prominent basal lymphoid aggregates. Features of chronicity, including basal lymphoplasmacytosis, crypt distortion, and Paneth cell metaplasia, are usually seen. A granulomatous cryptolytic reaction (Figs. 5.9 and 5.10) confined to the damaged crypts might also be seen. In general, the inflammatory infiltrate is limited to the mucosa. Histological features in SCAD appear in variable combinations [65]. A correlation with the clinical and endoscopic characteristics, not histology alone, is essential for establishing the correct diagnosis in cases of suspected SCAD [46, 72]. Occasionally, histological features of ischemic colitis could lead to the speculation that a small percentage of SCAD might represent a type of ischemic colitis because diverticula in such areas could favor, by compression of the vasa recta, ischemic lesions. Biopsies of the rectum should be histologically normal and, in this regard, are mandatory. In patients who must undergo segmental resection for control of symptoms, the resected sigmoid colons show the features described above, along with the bowel's luminal surface and contiguous diverticular pouches. However, the

Table 5.1 Relationship between macroscopic (endoscopic) and microscopic (histological) morphological features

	Endoscopic pattern (%)	Pairing histological features
A	Crescentic fold disease (52%)	Mild lymphoid and neutrophil infiltrate; sparing of the glandular structure
B	Mild-to-moderate UC-like (30–40%)	Active inflammatory infiltrate, glandular distortion, reduction of goblet cells, intraepithelial abscesses, rectal sparing
C	Crohn's–colitis-like (11%)	Active and chronic inflammation with prominent lymphoid follicles, sometimes micro-fistulas in the mucosa and/or cryptolytic granulomas but no epithelioid granulomas.
D	Severe ulcerative colitis-like (7%).	Heavy acute and chronic inflammatory infiltrate, glandular distortion with massive depletion of goblet cells, cryptitis with cryptic abscesses, rectal sparing

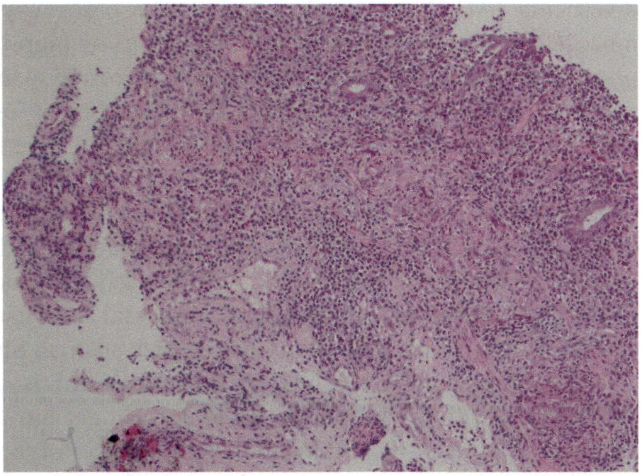

Fig. 5.9 Segmental colitis-associated diverticolosis type C: active and chronic inflammation with cryptolytic granulomas but no epithelioid granulomas

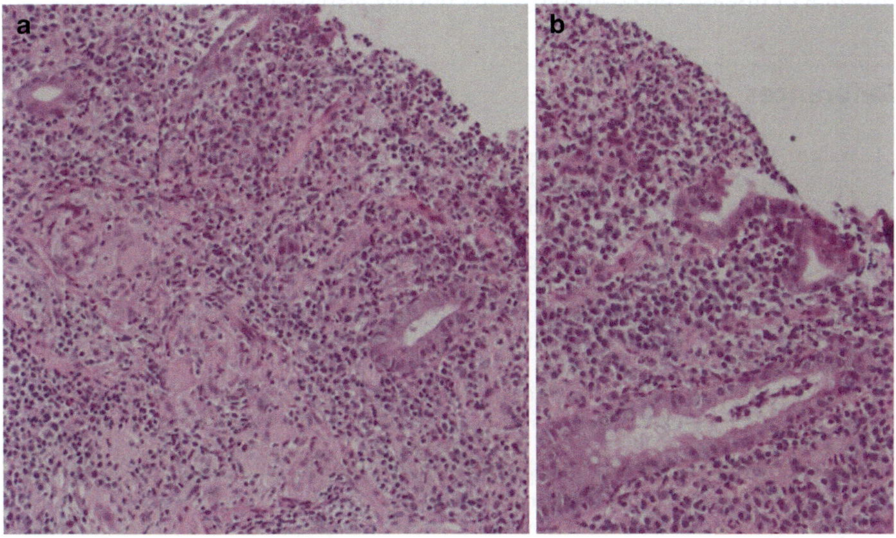

Fig. 5.10 (**a**) Details of a cryptolitic granulomatous reaction. Foreign-body giant cells are scattered around the colonic glands. (**b**) Cryptic abscess and erosion of the mucosal surface

extension of acute inflammation into the bowel wall near the diverticula, with abscess formation, fibrosis, and often perforation, is absent. Some patients with true diverticulitis develop an inflammatory reaction that mimics Crohn's disease [49] in patients without previous or present evidence of Crohn's disease elsewhere in the gastrointestinal tract. The resection specimens demonstrate a Crohn's-like reaction to the inflamed diverticula. It can be challenging to differentiate diverticular disease-associated segmental colitis from ulcerative colitis or occasionally from Crohn's colitis. Clinically, the rectum is infrequently spared in ulcerative colitis, and the inflammatory process extends beyond the segment of the bowel involved by the diverticula [64]. Even in ulcerative colitis cases with rectal sparing, the rectal mucosa shows some quiescent colitis features on biopsy with fibrosis of the lamina propria, basal plasmacytosis, and distortion of the glandular architecture. Crohn's patients usually have involvement of different bowel segments as well. In addition, since cryptolytic granulomas represent sigmoid diverticulitis, caution should be exercised to avoid an inappropriate diagnosis of Crohn's disease [49]. Histological observation of a significant increase in immunohistochemical TNF-α expression in patients with SCAD [72] allows for correct differential diagnosis of SCAD concerning other forms of chronic colitis, particularly UC and CD. Other entities in the differential diagnosis, emphasizing segmental left-sided colitis that might mimic ulcerative colitis, include infectious entities such as Shigella and Salmonella species, NSAID-associated colitis, and diversion colitis. Endoscopists must provide pathologists with the information that the patient has a diverticular disease, communicate sparing of the rectum and the remainder of the bowel, and obtain biopsies from both the involved segment of the bowel and the spared rectum so that the distribution of disease can be histologically documented [64].

References

1. Walker MM, Harris AK. Pathogenesis of diverticulosis and diverticular disease. Min Gastroenterol Dietol. 2017;63(2):99–109.
2. Jun S, Stollman N. Epidemiology of diverticular disease. Best Pract Res Clin Gastroenterol. 2002;16:529–42.
3. West BA. The pathology of diverticulosis: classical concepts and mucosal changes in diverticula. J Clin Gastroenterol. 2006;40:S126–31.
4. Patel B, Guo X, Noblet J, Chambers S, Gregersen H, Kassab GS. Computational analysis of mechanical stress in colonic diverticulosis. Sci Rep. 2020;10:6014. https://doi.org/10.1038/s41598-020-63049-w.
5. Swartz MA, Tschumperlin DJ, Kamm RD, Drazen JM. Mechanical stress is communicated between different cell types to elicit matrix remodeling. Proc Natl Acad Sci U S A. 2001;98:6180–5.
6. Patel B, et al. Constitutive modeling of the passive inflation-extension behavior of the swine colon. J Mech Behav Biomed Mater. 2018;77:176–86.
7. Egorov V, Schastlivtsev I, Prut E, Baranov A. Mechanical properties of the human gastrointestinal tract. J Biomech. 2002;35:1417–25.
8. Morson BC. The muscle abnormality in diverticular disease of the colon. Proc R Soc Med. 1963;56:798–803.
9. Golder M, Burleigh DE, Belai A, Ghali L, Ashby D, Lunniss PJ, Navsaria HA, Williams NS. Smooth muscle cholinergic denervation hypersensitivity in diverticular disease. Lancet. 2003;361:1945–51.
10. Whiteway J, Morson BC. Elastosis in diverticular disease of the sigmoid colon. Gut. 1985;26:258–66.
11. Painter NS, Truelove SC, Ardran GM, Tuckey M. Segmentation and the localization of intraluminal pressures in the human colon, with special reference to the pathogenesis of colonic diverticula. Gastroenterology. 1965;49:169–77.
12. Wess L, Eastwood MA, Edwards CA, Busuttil A, Miller A. Collagen alteration in an animal model of colonic diverticulosis. Gut. 1996;38(5):701–6.
13. Frieden JH, Morgenstern L. Sigmoid diverticulitis in identical twins. Dig Dis Sci. 1985;30:182–3.

14. Thomson HJ, Busuttil A, Eastwood MA, Smith AN, Elton RA. Submucosal collagen changes in the normal colon and in diverticular disease. Int J Colorect Dis. 1987;2:208–13.
15. Watters DA, Smith AN, Eastwood MA, Anderson KC, Elton RA, Mugerwa JW. Mechanical properties of the colon: comparison of the features of the African and European colon in vitro. Gut. 1985;26:384–92.
16. Wess L, Eastwood MA, Wess TJ, Busuttil A, Miller A. Cross linking of collagen is increased in colonic diverticulosis. Gut. 1995;37(1):91–4.
17. Fleischmajer R, Perlish JS, Burgeson RE, Shaikh-Bahai F, Timpl R. Type I and type III interactions during fibrillogenesis. Ann N Y Acad Sci. 1990;580:161.
18. Birkedal-Hansen H, Moore WG, Bodden MK, et al. Matrix metalloproteinases: a review. Crit Rev Oral Biol Med. 1993;4:197–250.
19. MacDonald TT, Pender SL. Proteolytic enzymes in inflammatory bowel disease. Inflamm Bowel Dis. 1998;4:157–64.
20. Saarialho-Kere UK, Kovacs SO, Pentland AP, Olerud JE, Welgus HG, Parks WC. Cell-matrix interactions modulate interstitial collagenase expressions by human keratinocytes actively involved in wounding healing. J Clin Invest. 1993;902:2858.
21. Docherty AJ, Murphy G. The tissue metalloproteinase family and the inhibitor TIMP: a study using cDNAs and recombinant proteins. Ann Rheum Dis. 1990;49(Suppl 1):469–79.
22. Stumpf M, Cao W, Klinge U, Klosterhalfen B, Kasperk R, Schumpelick V. Increased distribution of collagen type III and reduced expression of matrix metalloproteinase 1 in patients with diverticular disease. Int J Color Dis. 2001;16(5):271–5.
23. Saarialho-Kere UK, Vaalamo M, Puolakkainen P, Airola K, Parks WC, Karjalainen-Lindsberg ML. Enhanced expression of matrilysin, collagenase, and stromelysin-1 in gastrointestinal ulcers. Am J Pathol. 1996;148:519–26.
24. Heuschkel RB, MacDonald TT, Monteleone G, Bajaj-Elliott M, Smith JA, Pender SL. Imbalance of stromelysin-1 and TIMP-1 in the mucosal lesions of children with inflammatory bowel disease. Gut. 2000;47:57–62.
25. Mimura T, Bateman AC, Lee RL, Johnson PA, McDonald PJ, Talbot IC, et al. Up-regulation of collagen and tissue inhibitors of matrix metalloproteinase in colonic diverticular disease. Dis Colon Rectum. 2004;47(3):371–9.
26. Robins SP, Shimokomaki M, Bailey AJ. The chemistry of the collagen cross-links. Age related changes in the reducible components of intact bovine collagen fibres. Biochem J. 1973;131:771–80.
27. Fry RD, Shemesh EL. Perforation of the rectum and sigmoid colon during barium-enema examination. Management and prevention. Dis Colon Rectum. 1989;32:759–64.
28. Schnider SL, Kohn RR. Effects of age and diabetes mellitus on the solubility of collagen from human skin, tracheal cartilage and dura mater. Exp Gerontol. 1982;17:185–94.
29. Beighton PH, Murdoch JL, Votteler T. Gastrointestinal complications of the Ehlers-Danlos syndrome. Gut. 1969;10:1004.
30. Thomson JH, Busuttil A, Eastwood MA, Smith AN, Elton RA. The submucosa of the human colon. J Ultrastr Res. 1987;96:22–30.
31. Clemens CHM, Samsom M, Roelofs J, van Berge Henegouwen GP, Smout AJPM. Colorectal visceral perception in diverticular disease. Gut. 2004;53:717–22.
32. Horgan AF, McConnell EJ, Wolff BG, The S, Paterson C. Atypical diverticular disease: surgical results. Dis Colon Rectum. 2001;44:1315–8.
33. Simpson J, Sundler F, Humes DJ, Jenkins D, Scholefield JH, Spiller RC. Post inflammatory damage to the enteric nervous system in diverticular disease and its relationship to symptoms. Neurogastroenterol Motil. 2009;21:847–58.
34. Bassotti G, Battaglia E, De Roberto G, Morelli A, Tonini M, Villanacci V. Alterations in colonic motility and relationship to pain in colonic diverticulosis. Clin Gastroenterol Hepatol. 2005;3:248–53.
35. Humes DJ, Simpson J, Smith J, Sutton P, Zaitoun A, Bush D, et al. Visceral hypersensitivity in symptomatic diverticular disease and the role of neuropeptides and low grade inflammation: symptomatic diverticular disease. Neurogastroenterol Motil. 2012;24(4):318–e163.

36. Yun AJ, Bazar KA, Lee PY. A new mechanism for diverticular diseases: aging-related vagal withdrawal. Med Hypotheses. 2005;64(2):252–5.
37. Tomita R, Tanjoh K, Fujisaki S, Fukuzawa M. Physiological studies on nitric oxide in the right side of the colon of patients with diverticular disease. Hepato-Gastroenterology. 1999;46:2839–44.
38. Lee PY, Yun AJ, Bazar KA. Conditions of aging as manifestations of sympathetic bias unmasked by loss of parasympathetic function. Med Hypotheses. 2004;62(6):868–70.
39. Knowles CH, De Giorgio R, Kapur RP, Bruder E, Farrugia G, Geboes K, et al. The London classification of gastrointestinal neuromuscular pathology: report on behalf of the Gastro 2009 International Working Group. Gut. 2010;59(7):882–7.
40. Barrenschee M, Wedel T, Lange C, Hohmeier I, Cossais F, Ebsen M, Vogel I, Bottner M. No neuronal loss, but alterations of the GDNF system in asymptomatic diverticulosis. PLoS One. 2017;12(2):e0171416. https://doi.org/10.1371/journal.pone.0171416.
41. Iwase H, Sadahiro S, Mukoyama S, Makuuchi H, Yasuda M. Morphology of myenteric plexuses in the human large intestine: comparison between large intestines with and without colonic diverticula. J Clin Gastroenterol. 2005;39(8):674–8.
42. Gallego D, Espin F, Mikulka J, Smirg O, Gil V, Faundez-Zanuy M, et al. In vitro motor patterns and electrophysiological changes in patients with colonic diverticular disease. Int J Color Dis. 2013;28(10):1413–22.
43. Deduchovas O, Saladzinskas Z, Tamelis A, Pavalkis D, Pauziene N, Pauza DH. Morphologic pattern of myenteric neural plexus in colonic diverticular disease. A whole-mount study employing histochemical staining for acetylcholinesterase. Ann Anat. 2008;190(6):525–30.
44. Barrenschee M, Bottner M, Harde J, Lange C, Cossais F, Ebsen M, et al. SNAP-25 is abundantly expressed in enteric neuronal networks and upregulated by the neurotrophic factor GDNF. Histochem Cell Biol. 2015;143(6):611–23.
45. Sadiq M, Mahmood S. Sadiq morphological study of reactive follicular hyperplasia lymph node. PJMHS. 2014;8(2):398–402.
46. Haque S, Eisen RN, West AB. The morphologic features of diversion colitis: studies of a pediatric population with no other disease of the intestinal mucosa. Hum Pathol. 1993;24:211–9.
47. Ludeman L, Warren BF, Shepherd NA. The pathology of diverticular disease. Best Pract Res Clin Gastroenterol. 2002;16:543–62.
48. Kelly JK. Polypoid prolapsing mucosal folds in diverticular disease. Am J Surg Pathol. 1991;15:871–8.
49. Goldstein NS, Leon-Armin C, Mani A. Crohn's colitis-like changes in sigmoid diverticulitis specimens is usually an idiosyncratic inflammatory response to the diverticulosis rather than Crohn's colitis. Am J Surg Pathol. 2000;24:668–75.
50. Fearnhead NS, Mortensen NJ. Clinical features and differential diagnosis of diverticular disease. Best Pract Res Clin Gastroenterol. 2002;16:577–93.
51. Longstreth GF. Epidemiology and outcome of patients hospitalized with acute lower gastrointestinal hemorrhage: a population-based study. Am J Gastroenterol. 1997;92:419–24.
52. Goldstein NS, Ahmad E. Histology of the mucosa in sigmoid colon specimens with diverticular disease: observations for the interpretation of sigmoid colonoscopic biopsy specimens. Am J Clin Pathol. 1997;107:438–44.
53. Tursi A, Elisei W, Brandimarte G, et al. Musosal tumour necrosis factor A in diverticular disease of the colon is overexpressed with disease severity. Color Dis. 2012;14:e258–63.
54. Tursi A, Brandimarte G, Elisei W, et al. Assessment and grading of mucosal inflammation in colonic diverticular disease. J Clin Gastroenterol. 2008;42:699–703.
55. Strober W, Fuss IJ. Proinflammatory cytokines in the pathogenesis of inflammatory bowel diseases. Gastroenterology. 2011;140:1756–67.
56. Tursi A. Segmental colitis associated with diverticulosis: complication of diverticular disease or autonomous entity? Dig Dis Sci. 2011;56:27–34.
57. Tursi A, Brandimarte G, Elisei W, Giorgetti GM, Inchingolo CD, Aiello F. Faecal calprotectin in colonic diverticular disease: a case–control study. Int J Color Dis. 2009;24:49–55.

58. Pucilowska JB, Williams KL, Lund PK. Fibrogenesis. IV. Fibrosis and inflammatory bowel disease: cellular mediators and animal models. Am J Physiol Gastrointest Liver Physiol. 2000;279:G653–9.
59. Järbrink-Sehgal ME, Rassam L, Jasim A, Walker MM, Talley NJ, Agréus L, et al. Diverticulosis, symptoms and colonic inflammation: a population-based colonoscopy study. Am J Gastroenterol. 2019;114(3):500–10.
60. Feakins RM, British Society of Gastroenterology. Inflammatory bowel disease biopsies: updated British Society of Gastroenterology reporting guidelines. J Clin Pathol. 2013;66:1005–26.
61. Kealy WF. Lymphoid tissue and lymphoid-glandular complexes of the colon: relation to diverticulosis. J Clin Pathol. 1976;29:245–9.
62. Peery AF, Keku TO, Addamo C, et al. Colonic diverticula are not associated with mucosal inflammation or chronic gastrointestinal symptoms. Clin Gastroenterol Hepatol. 2018;16:884–91.e1.
63. Elli L, Roncoroni L, Bardella MT, et al. Absence of mucosal inflammation in uncomplicated diverticular disease. Dig Dis Sci. 2011;56:2098–103.
64. Villanacci V, Regiani-Bonetti L, Leoncini G, Parente P, Cadei M, Albarello L, Mandelli G, Caputo A. Histopathology of Non-IBD colitis. A practical approach from the Italian Group for the study of the gastrointestinal tract (GIPAD). Pathologica. 2021;113(1):54–65.
65. Freeman HJ. Natural history and long-term clinical behavior of segmental colitis associated with diverticulosis (Scad Syndrome). Dig Dis Sci. 2008;53:2452–7.
66. Koutroubakis IE, Antoniou P, Tzardi M, Kouroumalis EA. The spectrum of segmental colitis associated with diverticulosis. Int J Color Dis. 2005;20:28–32.
67. Hadithi M, Cazemier M, Meijer GA, Bloemena E, Felt-Bersma RJ, Mulder CJ, Meuwissen SG, Pena AS, van Bodegraven AA. Retrospective analysis of old-age colitis in the Dutch inflammatory bowel disease population. World J Gastroenterol. 2008;14:3183–7.
68. Freeman HJ. Segmental colitis associated diverticulosis syndrome. World J Gastroenterol. 2016;22(36):8067–9.
69. Hassan C, Zullo A, Ierardi E, Burattini O, De Francesco V, Morini S. Tumour necrosis factor a downregulation and therapeutic response to infliximab in a case of segmental colitis associated with diverticula. Gut. 2006;55(4):589–90.
70. Tursi A, Elisei W, Brandimarte G, Giorgetti GM, Lecca PG, Di Cesare L, Inchingolo CD, Aiello F. The endoscopic spectrum of segmental colitis associated with diverticulosis. Color Dis. 2010;12:464–70.
71. Stollman N, Picchio M, Biondo S, Lahat A, Dumitrascu DL, Regula J, Walker M. Critical issues on diverticular disease. J Gastrointestin Liver Dis. 2019;28(Suppl 4):35–7.
72. Tursi A, Elisei W, Giorgetti GM, Inchingolo C, Nenna R, Picchio M, Brandimarte G. Segmental colitis associated with diverticulosis: a 5-year follow-up. Int J Color Dis. 2012;27:179–85.
73. Tursi A, Elisei W, Brandimarte G, Giorgetti GM, Inchingolo CD, Nenna R, Ieraldi E. Tumour necrosis factor-alpha expression in segmental colitis associated with diverticulosis is related to the severity of the endoscopic damage. Dig Liver Dis. 2011;43:374–9.
74. Schembri J, Bonello J, Christodoulou DK, Katsanos KH, Ellul P. Segmental colitis associated with diverticulosis: is it the coexistence of colonic diverticulosis and inflammatory bowel disease? Ann Gastroenterol. 2017;30:257–61.
75. Tursi A, Inchingolo CD, Picchio M, et al. Histopathology of segmental colitis associated with diverticulosis resembles inflammatory bowel diseases. J Clin Gastroenterol. 2015;49:350–1.

Microbiota Changes

6

Loris R. Lopetuso and Paola Mastromarino

6.1 Introduction

The gastrointestinal (GI) tract represents a dynamic network where several players form a cross-talking functional unit [1–4]. In this scenario, GI functions are carried out in an active environment inhabited by 1 kg of commensal microbes that include more than three million genes [2, 3]. They belong to the three domains of life, *Bacteria*, *Archaea*, and *Eukarya* [4–6], as well as to viral particles [7, 8]. Culture-independent molecular techniques, by analysis using phylogenetic arrays, next-generation 16S rRNA sequencing, and metagenomic sequencing derived from human mucosal biopsies, luminal contents, and feces, have shown that four major microbial phyla (*Firmicutes*, *Bacteroides*, *Proteobacteria*, and *Actinobacteria*) represent 98% of the intestinal microbiota and fall into three main groups of strict extremophile anaerobes: *Bacteroides*, *Clostridium* cluster *XIVa* (also known as the Clostridium coccoides group), and *Clostridium* cluster *IV* (also known as the Clostridium leptum group) [5, 6, 9–16].

L. R. Lopetuso (✉)
CEMAD Digestive Disease Center, Dipartimento di Scienze Mediche e Chirurgiche, Fondazione Policlinico Universitario "A. Gemelli" IRCCS, Università Cattolica del Sacro Cuore, Rome, Italy

Department of Medicine and Ageing Sciences, "G. d'Annunzio" University of Chieti-Pescara, Chieti, Italy

Center for Advanced Studies and Technology (CAST), "G. d'Annunzio" University of Chieti-Pescara, Chieti, Italy
e-mail: lorislopetuso@libero.it

P. Mastromarino
Department of Public Health and Infectious Diseases, "Sapienza" University, Rome, Italy
e-mail: paola.mastromarino@uniroma1.it

© The Author(s), under exclusive license to Springer Nature Switzerland AG 2022

A. Tursi et al. (eds.), *Colonic Diverticular Disease*,
https://doi.org/10.1007/978-3-030-93761-4_6

An intricate and mutualistic symbiosis modulates the relationship between the host and the gut microbiota [10, 17, 18]. This relationship is constantly challenged by several factors such as rapid turnover of the intestinal epithelium and the overlaying mucus, exposure to peristaltic activity, food molecules, gastric, pancreatic, and biliary secretions, defense molecules, drugs, pH and redox potential variations, and exposure to transient bacteria from the oral cavity and esophagus, and can lead to the collapse of the microbial community structure [16]. On the other hand, resident microbes perform several useful functions, including maintaining barrier function, synthesis and metabolism of nutrients, drug and toxin metabolism, and behavioral conditioning [1]. The gut microbiota are also involved in the digestion of energy substrates, production of vitamins and hormones [19], protection from pathogenic bacteria by consuming nutrients and producing molecules that inhibit their growth [20–22], production of nutrients for mucosal cells [23–25], augmenting total and pathogen-specific mucosal IgA levels upon infection [26, 27], and modulating immune system development and immunological tolerance [28].

Unfavorable alterations in microbiota composition, known as dysbiosis, have been implicated in the chronic gut and also in systemic immune disorders [29, 30] and even in cancers [13, 31–33].

Despite these findings, the current literature regarding the exact impact of a gut microbiota dysbiosis in GI and extraintestinal diseases is at present ambiguous. Thus, translational microbiota applications in terms of diagnosis and treatment are still limited. This may be not only due to the use of different analysis techniques and sample collection but also due to the study design that usually focuses only on a specific disease, without considering other pathological conditions that often affect the same part of the GI tract.

In this scenario, diverticular disease (DD) may also be a condition in which luminal microbial factors could play a role in the development of symptoms and complications. Here, we critically explore the association between the gut microbiota and diverticular diseases, touching upon the potential areas of future development for research and clinical practice in this field.

6.2 Gut Barrier and the Gut Microbiota

The intestinal barrier is a functional unit, organized as a multilayer system, in which it is possible to recognize two main parts: a superficial physical barrier, which prevents bacterial adhesion and regulates paracellular diffusion to the underlying host tissues, and a deeper functional barrier, which is able to discriminate commensal bacteria from pathogens and is responsible for immunological tolerance to commensal and immune response to pathogen microorganisms [1]. Every day, thousands of compounds derived from food and microorganisms come in contact with the intestinal mucosa. This interaction requires a complex defense system that separates intestinal contents from the host tissues, regulates nutrient absorption, and allows tolerance between the resident bacterial flora and the mucosal immune system, while inhibiting translocation of infectious agents to the inner tissues. The commensal gut microbiota constitute the anatomical barrier, along with the mucosal layer and the intestinal epithelial monolayer. The deeper, inner layer is represented by GALT. GALT represents both isolated and aggregated lymphoid follicles and is one of the largest lymphoid organs, containing up to 70% of the body's total number of immunocytes, and is involved in responding to pathogenic microorganisms and in providing immune tolerance to commensal bacteria. The ability of GALT to interact with luminal antigens rests on specific mucosal immune cells (i.e., dendritic cells and M cells), primarily localized to Peyer's patches within the ileum, which are intimately positioned at the mucosal–environmental interface and internalize both microorganisms and macromolecules. These specialized immune cells have the ability to present antigens to naïve T lymphocytes, which subsequently produce cytokines and activate mucosal immune responses, when needed. Thus, the mucosal immune system participates in the maintenance of gut microbial communities by directly monitoring the luminal environment by constant sampling through M cells that overlie lymphoid follicles and through dendritic cells that reside within the lamina propria. The interaction of these cellular components sustains the delicate equilibrium needed to maintain intestinal homeostasis, thus establishing a state of immunological tolerance toward antigens from food and commensal bacteria. Many factors can alter this balance, including alterations in the gut microflora, modifications of the mucosal layer, and epithelial damage, leading to increased intestinal permeability and translocation of luminal contents to the underlying mucosa.

6.3 Role of the Gut Microbiota in Diverticular Disease

It has been proposed that stagnation of microbe-rich content in diverticular pockets could promote dysbiosis. This can happen together with a mucosal barrier leakage and microbial translocation through the thin mucosal diverticular layer, which can lead to a frank perforation, local or systemic flogosis, and septic complications. The observations that small bowel diverticula are connected to bacterial overgrowth and that the majority of colonic diverticular complications are due to bacteria, benefiting from antibiotic therapy or fecal stream diversion, broadly sustain the importance of gut microbiota involvement in DD pathogenesis [34, 35]. Despite this rationale, there are no solid available data. Indeed, studies are importantly flawed by a reduced sample size, different methodological techniques and enrolment plans, and insufficient clinical definitions. Future research should focus on the crosstalk between the gut microbiota and local tissue disease, with/without the inclusion of symptoms evaluation. This could help in extrapolating disease-related biomarkers and specific medical therapy. Undoubtedly, an integrated approach including sequencing and metabolomic analysis would definitely open new horizons in this field.

Taking into account these points and the conflicting nature of the studies, the few available findings indicate some interesting concepts. Asymptomatic diverticulosis, and thus the early phase of the pathogenesis, does not seem to be linked to a consistent microbial impairment. Conversely, important variations that evolve into SCAD or acute diverticulitis can occur in the disease spectrum. In these situations, a depletion of anti-inflammatory taxa has been underlined, such as *Clostridium cluster IV*, Lactobacilli, and Bacteroides. Vice versa, an increased abundance of Bifidobacteria, Enterobacteriaceae, and *Akkermansia* seems to occur in DD, with no clear clinical significance. These taxa could directly exert both anti-inflammatory (Bifidobacteria, *Akkermansia*) and proinflammatory (Enterobacteriaceae) actions or may play a role in homeostatic activity in response to variations of the mucosal habitat. These evidences suggest the notion that the gut microbiota could be implicated in the progression of diverticulosis to DD and diverticulitis but not in the pathogenesis of diverticula. Following this assumption, the gut microbiota can possess a particular pathophysiological weight in SUDD and diverticulitis, thus representing a potential therapeutic target in these phases [36, 37]. In fact, SUDD has been linked to a different fecal [36] and urinary [38] metabolomics asset compared with DD [37]. Moreover, acute alterations in the gut microbiota can exert a role in the complications of DD [39]. Notably, fecal microbiota transplantation for the *Clostridium difficile* infection has been associated with the induction of diverticulitis, thus proposing a crucial role of intestinal microbes in the pathogenesis of this acute disease [40].

Overall, few evidences sustain a potential role of the gut microbiota in the pathophysiology of DD, with a structured network between the intestinal barrier and the entire organism.

6.4 Gut Microbiota Profile in Diverticular Disease: Studies on the Fecal Microbiota

So far, few studies have evaluated the fecal microbiota in patients with diverticulosis or DD. A study cohort of 28 patients with SUDD evidenced that the relative abundance of *Ruminococcus* and *Roseburia* was positively and negatively associated, respectively, with an increased bloating severity score, whereas that of *Cyanobacterium* was consistently correlated with pain intensity [41]. At the same time, a higher abundance of *Pseudobutyrivibrio*, *Bifidobacterium*, and *Christensenellaceae* families together with gut microbiota biodiversity was positively correlated with fecal calprotectin. Another small case series of patients with DD showed a higher presence of *Roseburia*, *Veillonella*, *Haemophilus*, and *Streptococcus* [42], whereas a study cohort including patients with asymptomatic diverticulosis, SUDD, and healthy controls found a substantial similarity among groups of the overall fecal gut microbiota community. However, asymptomatic diverticulosis was mainly associated with a lower presence of *Clostridium cluster* IV, whereas SUDD showed a decreased abundance of *Fusobacterium* and *Lactobacillaceae* [35]. Controversial and conflicting results were constantly evidenced by further studies in this field. Indeed, Tursi et al. showed no differences in gut microbiota composition among SUDD, asymptomatic diverticulosis, and controls. Only *Akkermansia muciniphila* evidenced a higher, but not significant, abundance trend in SUDD. This was linked to a different metabolic asset, such as a lower N-acetyl compound and isovalerate levels in SUDD [43]. Notably, this setting differs from that detected in IBDs, where *Akkermansia* is generally reduced and not increased [44]. *A. muciniphila* is a symbiotic member of the gut microbiota, belonging to the Verrucomicrobia phylum, and has been correlated with several pathological conditions [45]. This bacterium has an essential role in maintaining intestinal homeostasis, owing to a strong interplay between both the host cells and the gut microbial community. It is crucial for guaranteeing proper mucus production and thickness [46, 47]. This property to degrade the mucus also has other beneficial effects, since it leads to the production of oligosaccharides, amino acids, propionate, acetate, and important vitamins and cofactors, which become useful for other microbial commensals [48, 49]. Emerging studies on animal models have indicated its ability to modulate genes implicated in immune response regulatory processes [50]. *A. muciniphila* can also release vesicles with an anti-inflammatory activity on intestinal cells and dampen the severity of colitis in mice [51]. A variation in the abundance of this bacterium has been shown in fecal and intestinal samples of patients affected by various pathologies [46, 52]. The alteration of the *A. muciniphila* level has been proposed as a crucial common microbial dysbiotic marker of the disease [44]. In this field, in a pilot study, *A. muciniphila* levels correlated with the presence and severity of symptoms in patients with SUDD, which were linked also to the levels of specific microbial metabolites [53].

Finally, a small study cohort suggested that the reduction of *Collinsella aerofaciens, Collinsella stercoris, and Bacteroides fragilis* was associated with DD, even if without statistical significance [54]. Interestingly, *Bacteroides fragilis* has been consistently included in the pathophysiological mechanisms of gut inflammation [55].

Overall, these data suggest a potential correlation between gut microbiota features (i.e., *A. muciniphila* and *Bacteroides fragilis* imbalance) and a potential role in modulating mucosal inflammation in DD. However, the reduced sample size and the highly heterogeneous study design do not allow to draw definitive and clear conclusions on the active involvement of the gut microbiota in the pathophysiological process.

6.5 Gut Microbiota Profile in Diverticular Disease: Studies on the Intestinal Mucosal Microbiota

On the basis of these assumptions, the evaluation of the mucosa-associated microbiota may represent a more reliable representation of the microbial community in DD. Indeed, fecal microbiota composition can have a high variability linked to stool consistency and number of bowel movements, as well as to stool moisture. Moreover, DD is generally localized to limited segments of the colon, which can harbor specific microbial communities, different from the adjacent normal areas. Finally, the diverticular pockets may be characterized by unique habitats that can represent a crucial player in the progression of diverticulosis toward a symptomatic disease [37].

In this scenario, Enterobacteriaceae is highly represented in colonic mucosal biopsies obtained from DD patients [56]. These findings were confirmed in a cohort

Table 6.1 Main gut microbiota changes involved in diverticular disease

Gut microbiota	Gut mycobiome	Gut virome
Increased:	*Increased:*	*Increased:*
Akkermansia muciniphila	Exophiala and Agaricales	Human cytomegalovirus in diverticulitis
Bacteroides/ Prevotella		Expression of antiviral response genes in earlier-onset diverticulitis
Bifidobacterium longum		
Bifidobacterium animalis		
Proteobacteria		
Enterobacteriaceae		
Microbacteriaceae		
Roseburia hominis		
Decreased:		
Clostridium cluster IV		
Clostridium cluster IX		
Fusobacterium		
Lactobacillaceae		

of nine patients with SCAD, confirming the notion that indicates the overgrowth of Enterobacteriaceae as one of the most important characteristics of severe dysbiosis consequent to mucosal flogosis [57, 58]. A further evaluation on few patients evidenced an association between acute diverticulitis and a higher abundance of *Bifidobacterium longum* [59], which has been associated with a potential anti-inflammatory activity in experimental models and thus with a possible homeostatic mechanism [37]. Another study did not find significant differences between controls and asymptomatic diverticulosis. Interestingly, SUDD had a significantly lower proportion of *Akkermansia* [35]. Finally, a larger cohort evidenced no differences between healthy controls and diverticulosis with a substantial overlap, except for a mild higher biodiversity and an increase of Proteobacteria and Comamonadaceae [60].

Again, as mentioned above, the results are highly conflicting, but they suggest a potential role of the gut microbiota in the disease spectrum that goes from asymptomatic diverticulosis to DD, with a fascinating interplay between mucosa-associated commensals and the mucosal immune system (Table 6.1).

6.6 Gut Microbiota Profile in Diverticular Disease: Mycobiome and Virome

While on one side studies on bacterial communities are fragmented, on the other side, the involvement of human fungal communities in DD is completely understudied. However, even in this field, the regional colonization of microbial communities seems to have a crucial importance. Preliminary studies in diverticulitis patients showed an increased abundance of Exophiala in diseased tissues, whereas Agaricales was evidenced in the adjacent normal mucosa [61].

The human gut virome could play an important role in modulating the immune response and could be deeply implicated in chronic immune disorders, such in IBDs [62]. In this context, human cytomegalovirus was detected in intestinal cells obtained from patients with diverticulitis [63]. Furthermore, earlier-onset diverticulitis subjects (<42 years old) showed a higher expression of antiviral response genes than did later-onset patients (>65 years old), indicating a possible involvement of host response to viral infection in defining a subgroup of earlier-onset diverticulitis patients.

6.7 Conclusions

DD is a common condition that can evolve to symptomatic and then to severe complications. Several hypotheses on its pathogenesis have been formulated. In this scenario, novel immunological pathways particularly connected to gut microbiota alterations are becoming available, and their involvement in the clinical course of the disease is highly plausible. Despite these findings, data remain controversial and conflicting and are too preliminary for drawing any useful conclusions for clinical practice. Future clinically oriented research will definitely represent a fascinating occasion to identify potential microbial targets for achieving personalized disease management and for translating the microbiological concepts into clinical practice.

References

1. Scaldaferri F, Pizzoferrato M, Gerardi V, Lopetuso L, Gasbarrini A. The gut barrier: new acquisitions and therapeutic approaches. J Clin Gastroenterol. 2012;46 Suppl:S12–7.
2. Leser TD, Molbak L. Better living through microbial action: the benefits of the mammalian gastrointestinal microbiota on the host. Environ Microbiol. 2009;11(9):2194–206.
3. Neish AS. Microbes in gastrointestinal health and disease. Gastroenterology. 2009;136(1):65–80.
4. Scanlan PD, Marchesi JR. Micro-eukaryotic diversity of the human distal gut microbiota: qualitative assessment using culture-dependent and -independent analysis of faeces. ISME J. 2008;2(12):1183–93.
5. Eckburg PB, Bik EM, Bernstein CN, Purdom E, Dethlefsen L, Sargent M, et al. Diversity of the human intestinal microbial flora. Science. 2005;308(5728):1635–8.
6. Gill SR, Pop M, Deboy RT, Eckburg PB, Turnbaugh PJ, Samuel BS, et al. Metagenomic analysis of the human distal gut microbiome. Science. 2006;312(5778):1355–9.
7. Zhang T, Breitbart M, Lee WH, Run JQ, Wei CL, Soh SW, et al. RNA viral community in human feces: prevalence of plant pathogenic viruses. PLoS Biol. 2006;4(1):e3.
8. Breitbart M, Haynes M, Kelley S, Angly F, Edwards RA, Felts B, et al. Viral diversity and dynamics in an infant gut. Res Microbiol. 2008;159(5):367–73.
9. Hold GL, Pryde SE, Russell VJ, Furrie E, Flint HJ. Assessment of microbial diversity in human colonic samples by 16S rDNA sequence analysis. FEMS Microbiol Ecol. 2002;39(1):33–9.

10. Backhed F, Ley RE, Sonnenburg JL, Peterson DA, Gordon JI. Host-bacterial mutualism in the human intestine. Science. 2005;307(5717):1915–20.
11. Ley RE, Backhed F, Turnbaugh P, Lozupone CA, Knight RD, Gordon JI. Obesity alters gut microbial ecology. Proc Natl Acad Sci U S A. 2005;102(31):11070–5.
12. Ley RE, Peterson DA, Gordon JI. Ecological and evolutionary forces shaping microbial diversity in the human intestine. Cell. 2006;124(4):837–48.
13. Frank DN, St Amand AL, Feldman RA, Boedeker EC, Harpaz N, Pace NR. Molecular-phylogenetic characterization of microbial community imbalances in human inflammatory bowel diseases. Proc Natl Acad Sci U S A. 2007;104(34):13780–5.
14. Rajilic-Stojanovic M, Smidt H, de Vos WM. Diversity of the human gastrointestinal tract microbiota revisited. Environ Microbiol. 2007;9(9):2125–36.
15. Tap J, Mondot S, Levenez F, Pelletier E, Caron C, Furet JP, et al. Towards the human intestinal microbiota phylogenetic core. Environ Microbiol. 2009;11(10):2574–84.
16. Manson JM, Rauch M, Gilmore MS. The commensal microbiology of the gastrointestinal tract. Adv Exp Med Biol. 2008;635:15–28.
17. McCracken VJ, Lorenz RG. The gastrointestinal ecosystem: a precarious alliance among epithelium, immunity and microbiota. Cell Microbiol. 2001;3(1):1–11.
18. Lievin-Le Moal V, Servin AL. The front line of enteric host defense against unwelcome intrusion of harmful microorganisms: mucins, antimicrobial peptides, and microbiota. Clin Microbiol Rev. 2006;19(2):315–37.
19. Sekirov I, Russell SL, Antunes LC, Finlay BB. Gut mircobiota in health and disease. Physiol Rev. 2010;90:859–904.
20. Silva AM, Barbosa FHF, Duarte R, et al. Effect of Bifidobacterium longum ingestion on experimental salmonellosis in mice. J Appl Microbiol. 2004;97:29–37.
21. Truusalu K, Mikelsaar R-H. Eradication of Salmonella Typhimurium infection in a murine model of typhoid fever with the cimbination of probiotic Lactobacillus fermentum ME-3 and ofloxacin. BMC Microbiol. 2008;8:132.
22. Searle LE, Best A, Nunez A, Salguero FJ, Johnson L, Weyer U, et al. A mixture containing galactooligosaccharide, produced by the enzymic activity of Bifidobacterium bifidum, reduces Salmonella enterica serovar Typhimurium infection in mice. J Med Microbiol. 2009;58(Pt 1):37–48.
23. Martens EC, Roth R, et al. Coordinate regulation of glycan degradation and polysaccharide capsule biosynthesis by a prominent gut symbiont. J Biol Chem. 2009;284:18445–57.
24. Burger van Paassen N, VAea. The regulation of intestinal mucin MUC2 expression by short chain fatty acid: implications for epithelial pretection. Biochem J. 2009;420:211–9.
25. Dharmani P, Srivastava V, Kissoon-Singh V, Chadee K. Role of intestinal mucins in annate host defense mechanisms against pathogens. J Innamte Immun. 2009;1:123–35.
26. Galdeano CM, Perdigon G. The probiotic bacterium Lactobacillus casei induces activation of the gut mucosal immune system through innate immunity. Clin Vaccine Immunol. 2006;13(2):219–26.
27. Leblanc J, Fliss I, Matar C. Induction of a humoral immune response following an Escherichia coli O157:H7 infection with an immunomodulatory peptidic fraction derived from Lactobacillus helveticus-fermented milk. Clin Diagn Lab Immunol. 2004;11(6):1171–81.
28. Allen CA, Torres AG. Host-microbe communication within the GI tract. Adv Exp Med Biol. 2008;635:93–101.
29. Parashar UD, Gibson CJ, Bresee JS, Glass RI. Rotavirus and severe childhood diarrhea. Emerg Infect Dis. 2006;12(2):304–6.
30. Scaldaferri F, Nardone O, Lopetuso LR, Petito V, Bibbo S, Laterza L, et al. Intestinal gas production and gastrointestinal symptoms: from pathogenesis to clinical implication. Eur Rev Med Pharmacol Sci. 2013;17(Suppl 2):2–10.
31. Swidsinski A, Ladhoff A, Pernthaler A, Swidsinski S, Loening-Baucke V, Ortner M, et al. Mucosal flora in inflammatory bowel disease. Gastroenterology. 2002;122(1):44–54.
32. Hill DA, Artis D. Intestinal bacteria and the regulation of immune cell homeostasis. Annu Rev Immunol. 2010;28:623–67.

33. Sartor RB. Microbial influences in inflammatory bowel diseases. Gastroenterology. 2008;134(2):577–94.
34. Jacobs DO. Clinical practice. Diverticulitis. N Engl J Med. 2007;357(20):2057–66.
35. Barbara G, Scaioli E, Barbaro MR, Biagi E, Laghi L, Cremon C, et al. Gut microbiota, metabolome and immune signatures in patients with uncomplicated diverticular disease. Gut. 2017;66(7):1252–61.
36. Scaioli E, Colecchia A, Marasco G, Schiumerini R, Festi D. Pathophysiology and therapeutic strategies for symptomatic uncomplicated diverticular disease of the colon. Dig Dis Sci. 2016;61(3):673–83.
37. Ticinesi A, Nouvenne A, Corrente V, Tana C, Di Mario F, Meschi T. Diverticular disease: a gut microbiota perspective. J Gastrointestin Liver Dis. 2019;28(3):327–37.
38. Tursi A, Mastromarino P, Capobianco D, Elisei W, Miccheli A, Pratico G, et al. Urinary metabolic profiling and symptomatic uncomplicated diverticular disease of the colon. Clin Res Hepatol Gastroenterol. 2017;41(3):344–6.
39. Skoldberg F, Olen O, Ekbom A, Schmidt PT. Appendectomy and risk of subsequent diverticular disease requiring hospitalization: a population-based case-control study. Dis Colon Rectum. 2018;61(7):830–9.
40. Mandalia A, Kraft CS, Dhere T. Diverticulitis after fecal microbiota transplant for C. difficile infection. Am J Gastroenterol. 2014;109(12):1956–7.
41. Kvasnovsky CL, Leong LEX, Choo JM, Abell GCJ, Papagrigoriadis S, Bruce KD, et al. Clinical and symptom scores are significantly correlated with fecal microbiota features in patients with symptomatic uncomplicated diverticular disease: a pilot study. Eur J Gastroenterol Hepatol. 2018;30(1):107–12.
42. Ponziani FR, Scaldaferri F, Petito V, Paroni Sterbini F, Pecere S, Lopetuso LR, et al. The role of antibiotics in gut microbiota modulation: the eubiotic effects of rifaximin. Dig Dis. 2016;34(3):269–78.
43. Tursi A, Mastromarino P, Capobianco D, Elisei W, Miccheli A, Capuani G, et al. Assessment of fecal microbiota and fecal metabolome in symptomatic uncomplicated diverticular disease of the colon. J Clin Gastroenterol. 2016;50(Suppl 1):S9–S12.
44. Lopetuso LR, Quagliariello A, Schiavoni M, Petito V, Russo A, Reddel S, et al. Towards a disease-associated common trait of gut microbiota dysbiosis: the pivotal role of Akkermansia muciniphila. Dig Liver Dis. 2020;52(9):1002–10.
45. Lopez-Siles M, Enrich-Capo N, Aldeguer X, Sabat-Mir M, Duncan SH, Garcia-Gil LJ, et al. Alterations in the abundance and co-occurrence of Akkermansia muciniphila and Faecalibacterium prausnitzii in the colonic mucosa of inflammatory bowel disease subjects. Front Cell Infect Microbiol. 2018;8:281.
46. Belzer C, de Vos WM. Microbes inside—from diversity to function: the case of Akkermansia. ISME J. 2012;6(8):1449–58.
47. Alam A, Leoni G, Quiros M, Wu H, Desai C, Nishio H, et al. The microenvironment of injured murine gut elicits a local pro-restitutive microbiota. Nat Microbiol. 2016;1:15021.
48. Derrien M, Vaughan EE, Plugge CM, de Vos WM. Akkermansia muciniphila gen. nov., sp. nov., a human intestinal mucin-degrading bacterium. Int J Syst Evol Microbiol. 2004;54(Pt 5):1469–76.
49. van Passel MW, Kant R, Zoetendal EG, Plugge CM, Derrien M, Malfatti SA, et al. The genome of Akkermansia muciniphila, a dedicated intestinal mucin degrader, and its use in exploring intestinal metagenomes. PLoS One. 2011;6(3):e16876.
50. Derrien M, Van Baarlen P, Hooiveld G, Norin E, Muller M, de Vos WM. Modulation of mucosal immune response, tolerance, and proliferation in mice colonized by the Mucin-Degrader Akkermansia muciniphila. Front Microbiol. 2011;2:166.
51. Kang CS, Ban M, Choi EJ, Moon HG, Jeon JS, Kim DK, et al. Extracellular vesicles derived from gut microbiota, especially Akkermansia muciniphila, protect the progression of dextran sulfate sodium-induced colitis. PLoS One. 2013;8(10):e76520.

52. Everard A, Belzer C, Geurts L, Ouwerkerk JP, Druart C, Bindels LB, et al. Cross-talk between Akkermansia muciniphila and intestinal epithelium controls diet-induced obesity. Proc Natl Acad Sci U S A. 2013;110(22):9066–71.
53. Laghi L, Mastromarino P, Elisei W, Capobianco D, Zhu CL, Picchio M, et al. Impact of treatments on fecal microbiota and fecal metabolome in symptomatic uncomplicated diverticular disease of the colon: a pilot study. J Biol Regul Homeost Agents. 2018;32(5):1421–32.
54. Lopetuso LR, Petito V, Graziani C, Schiavoni E, Paroni Sterbini F, Poscia A, et al. Gut microbiota in health, diverticular disease, irritable bowel syndrome, and inflammatory bowel diseases: time for microbial marker of gastrointestinal disorders. Dig Dis. 2018;36(1):56–65.
55. Jiang F, Meng D, Weng M, Zhu W, Wu W, Kasper D, et al. The symbiotic bacterial surface factor polysaccharide A on Bacteroides fragilis inhibits IL-1beta-induced inflammation in human fetal enterocytes via toll receptors 2 and 4. PLoS One. 2017;12(3):e0172738.
56. Linninge C, Roth B, Erlanson-Albertsson C, Molin G, Toth E, Ohlsson B. Abundance of Enterobacteriaceae in the colon mucosa in diverticular disease. World J Gastrointest Pathophysiol. 2018;9(1):18–27.
57. Sassone-Corsi M, Nuccio SP, Liu H, Hernandez D, Vu CT, Takahashi AA, et al. Microcins mediate competition among Enterobacteriaceae in the inflamed gut. Nature. 2016;540(7632):280–3.
58. Lupp C, Robertson ML, Wickham ME, Sekirov I, Champion OL, Gaynor EC, et al. Host-mediated inflammation disrupts the intestinal microbiota and promotes the overgrowth of Enterobacteriaceae. Cell Host Microbe. 2007;2(3):204.
59. Gueimonde M, Ouwehand A, Huhtinen H, Salminen E, Salminen S. Qualitative and quantitative analyses of the bifidobacterial microbiota in the colonic mucosa of patients with colorectal cancer, diverticulitis and inflammatory bowel disease. World J Gastroenterol. 2007;13(29):3985–9.
60. Jones RB, Fodor AA, Peery AF, Tsilimigras MCB, Winglee K, McCoy A, et al. An aberrant microbiota is not strongly associated with incidental colonic diverticulosis. Sci Rep. 2018;8(1):4951.
61. Schieffer KM, Sabey K, Wright JR, Toole DR, Drucker R, Tokarev V, et al. The microbial ecosystem distinguishes chronically diseased tissue from adjacent tissue in the sigmoid colon of chronic, recurrent diverticulitis patients. Sci Rep. 2017;7(1):8467.
62. Lopetuso LR, Ianiro G, Scaldaferri F, Cammarota G, Gasbarrini A. Gut virome and inflammatory bowel disease. Inflamm Bowel Dis. 2016;22(7):1708–12.
63. Hollink N, Dzabic M, Wolmer N, Bostrom L, Rahbar A. High prevalence of an active human cytomegalovirus infection in patients with colonic diverticulitis. J Clin Virol. 2007;40(2):116–9.

Environmental Factors and Lifestyles

7

Maria Ellionore Jarbrink-Sehgal and David Humes

7.1 Introduction

According to the significant prevalence of diverticulosis and diverticular disease, the environmental and lifestyle factors in the natural history of diverticular disease have been extensively investigated. Environmental factors (such as geography, urbanization, and migration) and lifestyle factors (such as diets, physical activity, voluptuary habits, and drug use) may play a role in the spectrum of diverticular disease, even if the evidence supporting their role is not always clear.

7.2 Lifestyle Factors

7.2.1 Diet

Diverticular disease was first described as a "deficiency disease of Western Civilization" after researchers observed a greater prevalence of diverticulosis in Western industrial countries compared to developing countries in Africa. An association was also described between the introduction of roller milling in Britain (which removed two-thirds of the remaining fibers in flour) and an increase in the prevalence of the disease [1].

M. E. Jarbrink-Sehgal
Department of Gastroenterology, Veterans Affairs Medical Center, Baylor College of Medicine, Houston, TX, USA
e-mail: maria.jarbrink-sehgal@bcm.edu

D. Humes (✉)
Nottingham Digestive Diseases Centre and National Institute for Health Research (NIHR), Nottingham Biomedical Research Centre, Nottingham University Hospitals NHS Trust, University of Nottingham, Nottingham, UK
e-mail: david.humes@nottingham.ac.uk

© The Author(s), under exclusive license to Springer Nature Switzerland AG 2022

A. Tursi et al. (eds.), *Colonic Diverticular Disease*,
https://doi.org/10.1007/978-3-030-93761-4_7

Migration studies report an increased risk of diverticular disease in immigrants who have left low-prevalence areas and adopted Western dietary patterns and lifestyles over time after settlement [2]. Explanatory mechanisms for diets affecting diverticular disease are unclear, but alterations in stool bulk, stool transit time, intracolonic pressures, and alterations in the gut microbiome have all been suggested [3–6].

7.2.2 Fibers

Several well-characterized large prospective cohort studies have confirmed the benefits of a high-fiber diet in reducing the risk of diverticular disease [7–10]. However, the impact of the amount and source of fiber intake, such as fruit and vegetable fibers vs. cereal fibers, on the risk of diverticular disease has varied in these studies. A recent systematic review and meta-analysis (including 5 prospective cohort studies with 19,282 cases of diverticular disease and 865,829 participants) has found a pooled risk reduction of 26% (RR 0.74, 95% CI 0.71–0.78), 44% (RR 0.56, 95% CI 0.37–0.84), and 26% (RR 0.74, 95% CI 0.67–0.81) per 10 g/day of total fiber intake, fruit fiber intake, and cereal fiber intake, respectively [11]. Furthermore, a high dietary fiber intake of 40 g/day reduced the risk of diverticular disease by 58%, thus confirming an inverse linear association between the amount of fiber intake and diverticular disease. Fruit fiber, followed by vegetable fiber (excluding potato fiber), and cereal fiber seemed to be the most beneficial. In the same meta-analysis, a low cereal fiber consumption was linked to a slightly increased risk of diverticular disease but protective when consumed at a level of 15–30 g daily [11]. The authors concluded that further studies were required on the types of fibers and the risk of diverticular disease and diverticulitis.

However, the role of fibers in symptomatic uncomplicated diverticular disease (SUDD) remains unclear. A recent systematic review has evaluated the role of diet in the treatment of SUDD, but significant heterogeneity among included studies and differences in quality, methodology, and therapeutic regimens or outcome measurements precluded a conclusion on whether fibers are indeed beneficial in the symptom improvement treatment of SUDD [12].

Similarly, the relationship between fibers and diverticulosis is unclear. In contrast to the historical link between a low-fiber diet and diverticulosis [4], a large cross-sectional study found no correlation between the low-fiber diet and asymptomatic diverticulosis [13]. In fact, a high fiber intake was associated with an increased prevalence of diverticulosis compared to participants with a low fiber intake. Similarly, no association between consumption and amount of vegetables, fermented vegetables (kimchi), fruits, and fruit juice intake and diverticulosis was shown in a Korean cross-sectional study [14].

7.2.3 Nuts, Seeds, Corn, and Popcorn

In contradiction to the previous common advice to avoid nuts, seeds, and popcorn to lower the risk of diverticular disease, a large prospective Health Professional Follow-Up cohort study including 47,228 men found that nuts, seeds, and popcorn seemed safe to consume. In fact, during the 18 years of follow-up, a high nut and popcorn consumption (at least twice a week) was associated with a lower risk of diverticulitis (HR 0.80, 95% CI 0.63–1.01 for nuts and HR 0.72, 95% CI 0.56–0.92 for popcorn) when compared to men with the lowest intake (less than once per month). No significant association was noted between eating corn and diverticulitis or between nut, corn, or popcorn ingestion and diverticular hemorrhage [15].

7.2.4 Vegetarian Diet and Diverticular Disease

A large prospective UK study found that vegetarians had a 31% lower risk (RR 0.69, 95% CI 0.55–0.86) of diverticular disease (hospital admission and death) than did meat eaters [7].

7.2.5 Meat

The Health Professionals Follow-Up study, a large prospective study including 46, 461 men, has recently reported that men with the highest total red meat consumption had a 58% increased risk of incident diverticulitis (RR 1.58, 95% CI 1.19–2.11) than did men with the lowest red meat intake [16]. The risk seemed independent of the amount with a plateaued effect after six servings per week. The authors further reported that unprocessed red meat, including beef, pork, and lamb, was associated with a higher risk of diverticulitis than processed red meat such as bacon, hot dogs, salami, bologna, sausages, poultry, and fish. Finally, and very interestingly, substituting one serving of unprocessed meat per day with either poultry or fish independently reduced the risk of diverticulitis by 20% (RR 0.80, 95% CI 0.63–0.99) [16].

In summary, dietary recommendations should include avoidance of red meat, especially unprocessed meat, substitution of red meat with poultry or fish, and consumption of a diet rich in fruit and vegetable fibers. A high fiber intake is recommended (i.e., >26 g daily), but preferably >30 g daily for the highest risk reduction for diverticulitis. Nuts, seeds, and popcorn are safe to consume in patients with diverticular disease.

7.3 Obesity

Large observational studies have found that a body mass index (BMI) of 25 or above (overweight and obese) increases the risk of diverticular disease including mild-to-severe diverticulitis [7, 17–23], complicated diverticular disease with abscess/perforation [20, 24], emergency surgery, and diverticular hemorrhage [19], in both genders. The large prospective Health Professionals Follow-Up Study found that men in the obese category (BMI 30 kg/m^2 or above) were two and threefold more likely to develop diverticulitis and diverticular hemorrhage, respectively, compared to men with a BMI of <21 kg/m^2 (RR 1.78, 95% CI 1.08–2.94 and RR 3.19, 95% CI 1.45–7.00) [19]. In addition, the type of body fat seems to play a role in diverticular disease. For example, a higher waist circumference and waist–hip ratio, both indirect markers of central obesity and visceral fat, have been associated with significantly increased risks of diverticulitis and diverticular hemorrhage when compared with men in the lowest quintile for both categories even after adjustment for the BMI [19]. Visceral fat has further been linked to a more severe diverticular disease and higher likelihood to require emergency surgery, with postoperative complications and longer hospitalizations [25]. The reported mechanisms of this may be related to a proinflammatory state induced by the visceral fat [26].

The strong association between obesity and diverticular disease has been further demonstrated in a recent meta-analysis, including 6 prospective cohort studies, 28,915 cases of diverticular disease, and 1,636,777 controls, finding a 28% (RR 1.28, 95% CI 1.18–1.40), 31% (RR 1.31, 95% CI 1.09–1.56), and 20% (RR 1.20, 95% CI 1.04–1.40) increase in the relative risk of diverticular disease, diverticulitis, and diverticular disease complications, respectively, per each 5 unit increase in the BMI [27]. There was a linear association between the BMI and diverticular disease but not with complicated diverticular disease. Underweight participants (BMI <18) had an increased risk of complicated diverticular disease compared to those with normal BMI, who had the lowest risk.

Early exposure to obesity and weight gain during adulthood also seems to play a role in developing diverticular disease. In a large population-based cohort of conscripts, exposure to a BMI of 25 or higher in late adolescence was associated with a twofold increased risk of diverticular disease requiring hospitalization compared to conscripts with normal BMI [23]. Similarly, in the prospective Nurses' Health Study, a weight gain of 20 kg or more during adulthood was associated with a 73% increased risk of diverticulitis when compared to women maintaining their weight from the age of 18 [28].

Finally, in contrast to the well-established role of obesity in diverticular disease, studies examining the role of obesity in diverticulosis are discordant. Two prospective studies, including a Korean colonoscopy study [14] and a large US cohort study [19], were unable to find a significant association between obesity and diverticulosis. Conversely, obesity (BMI 30 kg/m^2 or more) was found to be independently associated with diverticulosis in both a retrospective Israeli case–control study [29] and a recent US colonoscopy study [30].

In summary, although conflicting evidence exists on the association between obesity and diverticulosis, there is robust evidence that obesity, specifically central obesity, is an independent risk factor for all types of diverticular disease, ranging from mild-to-severe diverticulitis, complicated diverticular disease, need for emergency surgery, and diverticular hemorrhage. Visceral body fat is more hazardous than subcutaneous body fat. Recommendations for early adoption of healthy lifestyles and avoidance of adulthood weight gain are supported by epidemiological studies to minimize the risk of future diverticular disease.

7.4 Physical Activity

Various studies support an inverse correlation between high physical activity and incidence of diverticular disease ranging from mild-to-severe diverticular disease [20, 23, 27, 31, 32]. Strenuous physical activity (28 or more metabolic equivalents of task (METs) per week) has been associated with a 34% risk reduction for diverticular disease and up to 39% risk reduction for diverticular hemorrhage when compared to those in the least active quintile of activity [20, 23, 32]. Conversely, physical inactivity (30 min or less per day) was associated with a 42% increased risk of diverticular disease requiring hospitalizations (RR 1.42, 95% CI 1.18–1.69) but not with complicated diverticular disease [20].

A recent meta-analysis with 5 prospective cohort studies, 2080 cases with diverticular disease, and 147, 869 participants, has further supported the benefits of physical activity in diverticular disease [27]. The findings included a 24% (RR 0.76, 95% CI 063–0.93) risk reduction for diverticular disease in participants with high vs low physical activity in adulthood and a 26% (RR 0.74, 95% CI 0.57–0.97) risk reduction when comparing the highest vs the lowest level of vigorous physical activity [27].

In summary, early adoption of a healthy lifestyle with high or vigorous exercise more than three times weekly is associated with a reduced risk of significant diverticular disease.

7.5 Smoking

Several studies have found a positive association between smoking and both symptomatic [7, 18, 33–35] and complicated diverticular disease (perforation and/or abscess) [33, 35]. Most recently, a meta-analysis, including 5 studies with 6076 cases among 385,291 participants, has found a 36% (RR 1.36, 95% CI 1.15–1.61), 17% (RR 1.17, 95% CI 1.05–1.31), and 29% (RR 1.29, 95% CI 1.05–1.31) increased risk of incident diverticular disease among current, former, and ever smokers, respectively, and has further supported a dose-dependent association with 11% increased risk per 10 cigarettes per day (RR 1.11, 95% CI 0.99–1.25) [35]. Additionally, although the number of included studies was small (3 with a total of 1118 cases of complications among 292, 965 participants), current smokers had a three to fourfold higher likelihood of having complicated diverticular disease compared to nonsmokers [35]. This further strengthened the previous report where a two to threefold increased risk of complicated diverticular disease was noted among current male smokers, especially among heavy smokers and those smoking more than 15 cigarettes per day [34].

However, the relationship between smoking and diverticulosis per se is less clear. Although few studies have found an association between smoking and diverticulosis, cross-sectional design and confounding variables limited their validity [14, 36].

In summary, strong data support that smoking cessation should be recommended or at least smoking should be reduced, as it has been associated with diverticular disease, in particular complicated disease, and there is evidence of a dose-dependent relationship.

7.6 Alcohol

To date, conflicting data exist on the relationship between alcohol and diverticular disease.

Two large population-based studies from Denmark [37] and Sweden [23] reported a threefold and 43% increased risk of symptomatic diverticular disease requiring hospitalization among patients with previous admission for alcoholism when compared to the general population and among late adolescents with risky alcohol use compared to those without alcohol use, respectively. Conversely, two prospective population-based studies from the UK and US found no independent associations between alcohol consumption and self-reported diverticular disease or hospital admissions for diverticular disease [7, 17]. A recent systematic review has found alcohol to be associated with diverticular hemorrhage (OR 3.3, 95% CI 1.3–8.5) for moderate and heavy drinkers but not with recurrent diverticular disease or complications [38].

The relationship between alcohol use and diverticulosis is similarly unclear. Although three colonoscopy-based cross-sectional studies from Korea [14], Lebanon [39], and Taiwan [40] found a positive association with the presence of diverticulosis, a recent meta-analysis including 6 studies and 53,644 participants has not [41].

7.7 Medications

Several medications have been implicated in diverticular disease, in particular with complicated perforated diverticular disease and diverticular hemorrhage.

7.7.1 NSAIDs

Multiple studies confirm a significantly increased risk of diverticulitis and diverticular hemorrhage with NSAID use. For example, regular aspirin use has been associated with a 25 and 70% increased risk of diverticulitis and diverticular hemorrhage, respectively, compared to nonusers (HR 1.25, 95% CI 1.05–1.47 and HR 1.70, 95% CI 1.21–2.39, respectively) [42]. Similar positive associations were noted between nonaspirin NSAID use and diverticulitis and diverticular hemorrhage when compared to nonusers. The highest risk group, however, comprised individuals with high aspirin use (2–5.9 of 325 mg tablets per week, 4–6 days per week), with a two and threefold increased likelihood to develop incident diverticulitis and diverticular hemorrhage, respectively (HR 2.32, 95% CI 1.34–4.02 and HR 3.13, 95% CI 1.34–4.02, respectively) [42]. This strong association between NSAIDs and diverticular hemorrhage has since been confirmed in two meta-analyses [43, 44].

The use of NSAIDs has also been well linked to complicated diverticular disease with perforation and abscess formation. In a UK database study, Humes et al. found increased odds among current and previous NSAID users (OR 1.51, 95% CI 0.98–2.31 and OR 1.62, 95% CI 1.39–1.90, respectively [24]. A prospective cohort study further found 87% increased risk of diverticular perforation among NSAID users [42]. Additionally, a meta-analysis including 8 studies found a pooled OR of 2.49 (95% CI 1.98–3.14) for diverticular perforation among NSAID users [43].

7.7.2 Opioids and Corticosteroids

Perforated diverticular disease has strongly been associated with current opioids (OR 2.16, 95% CI 1.55–3.01) and oral corticosteroids (OR 2.74, 95% CI 1.63–4.61) [24]. However, oral corticosteroid use has not been associated with diverticular hemorrhage in a recent meta-analysis with three studies included (pooled OR 1.95, 95% CI 0.64–5.93) [43].

7.7.3 Statins

Statin use may be protective against complicated diverticular disease and diverticular disease requiring surgical treatment, at least in subjects aged 65 years or older. In a UK database study, statin use was associated with a 56% risk reduction for perforated diverticular disease in current users, but no association was found in ever users (OR 0.44, 95% CI 0.20–0.95) [24]. However, statin use had no effect on uncomplicated diverticular disease in a large prospective Swedish population-based case–control study [45]. Additionally, a recent retrospective study from New Zealand has found no effect of statin use on diverticulitis requiring hospitalization nor on complicated or recurrent diverticulitis [46]. However, an age-stratified subanalysis found a significant risk reduction in diverticulitis, complicated diverticular disease, and recurrent disease among subjects aged 65 years or older (RR 0.47, 95% CI 0.34–0.67; RR 0.35, 95% CI 0.19–0.64; RR 0.36, 95% CI 0.14–0.95) [46].

7.7.4 Other Medications

Selective serotonin reuptake inhibitor (SSRI) use has been associated with a decreased risk of diverticulitis, complicated diverticular disease, and recurrent disease [46]. Calcium channel blocker use has been associated with increased odds for diverticular hemorrhage in a recent meta-analysis including three case–control studies (pooled OR 2.50, 95% CI 1.44–4.35) [43] but not with perforating diverticular disease [24].

In summary, the above-mentioned lifestyle factors are modifiable with evidence that adherence to a healthy lifestyle reduces the risk of future diverticulitis by 50% with adoption of a low-risk lifestyle [47].

7.8 Environmental Risk Factors

To date, studies evaluating the role of environmental factors, such as geographical and seasonal variability, urbanization, and crowded living, in diverticulosis and diverticular disease are few and discordant [2, 7, 48–53].

7.8.1 Socioeconomic Status, Urbanization, and Education

High socioeconomic status (SES) and urbanization were found to be associated with diverticulosis in an early Greek study [48]. However, recent data have been conflicting. A US study showed low SES to be linked to emergent presentation of diverticular disease and worse disease on admission [54]. In addition, two Swedish adult population-based studies found discordant results. The first study found low SES to be associated with a lower risk of hospitalization for both uncomplicated and complicated diverticular disease admissions compared to those with the highest income [53], whereas another found an increased risk [2]. In contrast, a Swedish population-based study of conscripts in late adolescence found no association between SES during childhood and future diverticular disease requiring hospitalization [55].

Similar discordant study results exist on the association between urban vs rural areas of living and diverticular disease. Two adult population-based studies found positive associations between rural residency and risk of uncomplicated diverticular disease and diverticular disease requiring hospitalization, when compared to urban living [2, 53], whereas the Swedish population-based conscript study did not [55].

The influence of education on diverticular disease has been similarly contradicting.

One large prospective UK cohort study found higher education level (higher secondary level and university degree vs. some secondary school) to be protective against future hospitalizations from diverticular disease [7]. In a similar vein, Nikberg et al. found low education level to be associated with increased risk of uncomplicated and complicated diverticular disease needing hospital admission [53]. However, two Swedish population-based studies in adult and late adolescent populations found no association [2, 55].

7.8.2 Geographical and Seasonal Factors

Geographical and seasonal variances have been reported to play a role in diverticulitis-associated admissions. A US study found lower age-adjusted rates of diverticulitis-associated admissions in the West (50.4/100,000) compared to those in the Northeast (77.7/100,000), South (73.9/100,000), and Midwest (71.0/100,000). The Northeast was noted to have the highest increase in admission for diverticular disease (39%), followed by the Midwest [49]. In addition, low UV areas in the US have been reported to have a higher rate of diverticulitis admissions, diverticular abscess (12.0 vs. 9.7%; $P < 0.001$), and colectomies for diverticular disease compared to high UV areas. Paradoxically, summer was the season with the highest rate of diverticulitis admissions compared to winter months (748 vs. 645 per 100,000; $P < 0.001$). The admission rate difference was more pronounced in areas with the greatest UV fluctuations throughout the year and among patients older than 60 years of age, Caucasians, and rural patients compared to their respective reference groups [49].

Seasonal variance seems to exist in other parts of the world as well. A recent multinational database study, including three geographically distinct populations from the United Kingdom, Australia, and the US, has found a 22–24% maximal increase in admissions during peak summer months in all three countries [52]. However, diverticular hemorrhage was not associated with any geographical or seasonal variance [49].

References

1. Painter NS. Diverticular disease of the colon--a disease of the century. Lancet. 1969;2(7620):586–8.
2. Hjern F, Johansson C, Mellgren A, Baxter NN, Hjern A. Diverticular disease and migration--the influence of acculturation to a Western lifestyle on diverticular disease. Aliment Pharmacol Ther. 2006;23(6):797–805.
3. Wrick KL, Robertson JB, Van Soest PJ, Lewis BA, Rivers JM, Roe DA, et al. The influence of dietary fiber source on human intestinal transit and stool output. J Nutr. 1983;113(8):1464–79.
4. Painter NS, Burkitt DP. Diverticular disease of the colon: a deficiency disease of Western civilization. Br Med J. 1971;2(5759):450–4.
5. Barbara G, Scaioli E, Barbaro MR, Biagi E, Laghi L, Cremon C, et al. Gut microbiota, metabolome and immune signatures in patients with uncomplicated diverticular disease. Gut. 2017;66(7):1252–61.
6. Tursi A, Scarpignato C, Strate LL, Lanas A, Kruis W, Lahat A, et al. Colonic diverticular disease. Nat Rev Dis Primers. 2020;6(1):20.
7. Crowe FL, Appleby PN, Allen NE, Key TJ. Diet and risk of diverticular disease in Oxford cohort of European prospective investigation into cancer and nutrition (EPIC): prospective study of British vegetarians and non-vegetarians. BMJ. 2011;343:d4131.
8. Crowe FL, Balkwill A, Cairns BJ, Appleby PN, Green J, Reeves GK, et al. Source of dietary fibre and diverticular disease incidence: a prospective study of UK women. Gut. 2014;63(9):1450–6.

9. Mahmood MW, Abraham-Nordling M, Håkansson N, Wolk A, Hjern F. High intake of dietary fibre from fruit and vegetables reduces the risk of hospitalisation for diverticular disease. Eur J Nutr. 2019;58(6):2393–400.
10. Strate LL, Keeley BR, Cao Y, Wu K, Giovannucci EL, Chan AT. Western dietary pattern increases, and prudent dietary pattern decreases, risk of incident diverticulitis in a prospective cohort study. Gastroenterology. 2017;152(5):1023–30.e2.
11. Aune D, Sen A, Norat T, Riboli E. Dietary fibre intake and the risk of diverticular disease: a systematic review and meta-analysis of prospective studies. Eur J Nutr. 2020;59(2):421–32.
12. Carabotti M, Annibale B, Severi C, Lahner E. Role of fiber in symptomatic uncomplicated diverticular disease: a systematic review. Nutrients. 2017;9(2):161.
13. Peery AF, Barrett PR, Park D, Rogers AJ, Galanko JA, Martin CF, et al. A high-fiber diet does not protect against asymptomatic diverticulosis. Gastroenterology. 2012;142(2):266–72 e1.
14. Song JH, Kim YS, Lee JH, Ok KS, Ryu SH, Moon JS. Clinical characteristics of colonic diverticulosis in Korea: a prospective study. Korean J Intern Med. 2010;25(2):140–6.
15. Strate LL, Liu YL, Syngal S, Aldoori WH, Giovannucci EL. Nut, corn, and popcorn consumption and the incidence of diverticular disease. JAMA. 2008;300(8):907–14.
16. Cao Y, Strate LL, Keeley BR, Tam I, Wu K, Giovannucci EL, et al. Meat intake and risk of diverticulitis among men. Gut. 2018;67(3):466–72.
17. Aldoori WH, Giovannucci EL, Rimm EB, Wing AL, Trichopoulos DV, Willett WC. A prospective study of alcohol, smoking, caffeine, and the risk of symptomatic diverticular disease in men. Ann Epidemiol. 1995;5(3):221–8.
18. Rosemar A, Angerås U, Rosengren A. Body mass index and diverticular disease: a 28-year follow-up study in men. Dis Colon Rectum. 2008;51(4):450–5.
19. Strate LL, Liu YL, Aldoori WH, Syngal S, Giovannucci EL. Obesity increases the risks of diverticulitis and diverticular bleeding. Gastroenterology. 2009;136(1):115–22.e1.
20. Hjern F, Wolk A, Håkansson N. Obesity, physical inactivity, and colonic diverticular disease requiring hospitalization in women: a prospective cohort study. Am J Gastroenterol. 2012;107(2):296–302.
21. Korda RJ, Liu B, Clements MS, Bauman AE, Jorm LR, Bambrick HJ, et al. Prospective cohort study of body mass index and the risk of hospitalisation: findings from 246361 participants in the 45 and up study. Int J Obes. 2013;37(6):790–9.
22. Jamal Talabani A, Lydersen S, Ness-Jensen E, Endreseth BH, Edna TH. Risk factors of admission for acute colonic diverticulitis in a population-based cohort study: the north Trondelag health study. Norway World J Gastroenterol. 2016;22(48):10663–72.
23. Järbrink-Sehgal ME, Schmidt PT, Sköldberg F, Hemmingsson T, Hagström H, Andreasson A. Lifestyle factors in late adolescence associate with later development of diverticular disease requiring hospitalization. Clin Gastroenterol Hepatol. 2018;16(9):1474–1480.e1.
24. Humes DJ, Fleming KM, Spiller RC, West J. Concurrent drug use and the risk of perforated colonic diverticular disease: a population-based case-control study. Gut. 2011;60(2):219–24.
25. Docimo S, Lee Y, Chatani P, Rogers AM, Lacqua F. Visceral to subcutaneous fat ratio predicts acuity of diverticulitis. Surg Endosc. 2017;31(7):2808–12.
26. Murray KA-O, Hoad CL, Garratt J, Kaviani M, Marciani L, Smith JK, et al. A pilot study of visceral fat and its association with adipokines, stool calprotectin and symptoms in patients with diverticulosis. (1932--6203 (Electronic)). PLoS One. 2019;14(5):e0216528.
27. Aune D, Sen A, Leitzmann MF, Norat T, Tonstad S, Vatten LJ. Body mass index and physical activity and the risk of diverticular disease: a systematic review and meta-analysis of prospective studies. Eur J Nutr. 2017;56(8):2423–38.
28. Ma W, Jovani M, Liu PH, Nguyen LH, Cao Y, Tam I, et al. Association between obesity and weight change and risk of diverticulitis in women. Gastroenterology. 2018;155(1):58–66.e4.
29. Kopylov U, Ben-Horin S, Lahat A, Segev S, Avidan B, Carter D. Obesity, metabolic syndrome and the risk of development of colonic diverticulosis. Digestion. 2012;86(3):201–5.
30. Peery AF, Keil A, Jicha K, Galanko JA, Sandler RS. Association of Obesity with Colonic Diverticulosis in women. Clin Gastroenterol Hepatol. 2020;18(1):107–14.e1.

31. Aldoori WH, Giovannucci EL, Rimm EB, Ascherio A, Stampfer MJ, Colditz GA, et al. Prospective study of physical activity and the risk of symptomatic diverticular disease in men. Gut. 1995;36(2):276–82.
32. Strate LL, Liu YL, Aldoori WH, Giovannucci EL. Physical activity decreases diverticular complications. Am J Gastroenterol. 2009;104(5):1221–30.
33. Hjern F, Wolk A, Håkansson N. Smoking and the risk of diverticular disease in women. Br J Surg. 2011;98(7):997–1002.
34. Humes DJ, Ludvigsson JF, Jarvholm B. Smoking and the risk of hospitalization for symptomatic diverticular disease: a population-based cohort study from Sweden. Dis Colon Rectum. 2016;59(2):110–4.
35. Aune D, Sen A, Leitzmann MF, Tonstad S, Norat T, Vatten LJ. Tobacco smoking and the risk of diverticular disease—a systematic review and meta-analysis of prospective studies. Color Dis. 2017;19(7):621–33.
36. Yamamichi N, Shimamoto T, Takahashi Y, Sakaguchi Y, Kakimoto H, Matsuda R, et al. Trend and risk factors of diverticulosis in Japan: age, gender, and lifestyle/metabolic-related factors may cooperatively affect on the colorectal diverticula formation. PLoS One. 2015;10(4):e0123688.
37. Tønnesen H, Engholm G, Moller H. Association between alcoholism and diverticulitis. Br J Surg. 1999;86(8):1067–8.
38. Carabotti M, Falangone F, Cuomo R, Annibale B. Role of dietary habits in the prevention of diverticular disease complications: a systematic review. Nutrients. 2021;13(4):1288.
39. Sharara AI, El-Halabi MM, Mansour NM, Malli A, Ghaith OA, Hashash JG, et al. Alcohol consumption is a risk factor for colonic diverticulosis. J Clin Gastroenterol. 2013;47(5):420–5.
40. Wang FW, Chuang HY, Tu MS, King TM, Wang JH, Hsu CW, et al. Prevalence and risk factors of asymptomatic colorectal diverticulosis in Taiwan. BMC Gastroenterol. 2015;15:40.
41. Jaruvongvanich V, Sanguankeo A, Upala S. Association between alcohol consumption and diverticulosis and diverticular bleeding: a systematic review and meta-analysis. Hawaii J Med Public Health. 2017;76(8):211–9.
42. Strate LL, Liu YL, Huang ES, Giovannucci EL, Chan AT. Use of aspirin or nonsteroidal anti-inflammatory drugs increases risk for diverticulitis and diverticular bleeding. Gastroenterology. 2011;140(5):1427–33.
43. Kvasnovsky CL, Papagrigoriadis S, Bjarnason I. Increased diverticular complications with nonsteriodal anti-inflammatory drugs and other medications: a systematic review and meta-analysis. Color Dis. 2014;16(6):O189–96.
44. Yuhara H, Corley DA, Nakahara F, Nakajima T, Koike J, Igarashi M, et al. Aspirin and non-aspirin NSAIDs increase risk of colonic diverticular bleeding: a systematic review and meta-analysis. J Gastroenterol. 2014;49(6):992–1000.
45. Sköldberg F, Svensson T, Olén O, Hjern F, Schmidt PT, Ljung R. A population-based case-control study on statin exposure and risk of acute diverticular disease. Scand J Gastroenterol. 2016;51(2):203–10.
46. O'Grady M, Clarke L, Turner G, Doogue M, Purcell R, Pearson J, et al. Statin use and risk of acute diverticulitis: a population-based case-control study. Medicine (Baltimore). 2020;99(20):e20264.
47. Liu PH, Cao Y, Keeley BR, Tam I, Wu K, Strate LL, et al. Adherence to a healthy lifestyle is associated with a lower risk of diverticulitis among men. Am J Gastroenterol. 2017;112(12):1868–76.
48. Manousos O, Day NE, Tzonou A, Papadimitriou C, Kapetanakis A, Polychronopoulou-Trichopoulou A, et al. Diet and other factors in the aetiology of diverticulosis: an epidemiological study in Greece. Gut. 1985;26(6):544–9.
49. Nguyen GC, Sam J, Anand N. Epidemiological trends and geographic variation in hospital admissions for diverticulitis in the United States. World J Gastroenterol. 2011;17(12):1600–5.
50. Fares A. Global patterns of seasonal variation in gastrointestinal diseases. J Postgrad Med. 2013;59(3):203–7.

51. Maguire LH, Song M, Strate LL, Giovannucci EL, Chan AT. Association of geographic and seasonal variation with diverticulitis admissions. JAMA Surg. 2015;150(1):74–7.
52. Adler JT, Chang DC, Chan AT, Faiz O, Maguire LH. Seasonal variation in diverticulitis: evidence from both hemispheres. Dis Colon Rectum. 2016;59(9):870–7.
53. Nikberg M, Ji J, Leppert J, Sundquist K, Chabok A. Socioeconomic characteristics and comorbidities of diverticular disease in Sweden 1997-2012. Int J Color Dis. 2017;32(11):1591–6.
54. Csikesz NG, Singla A, Simons JP, Tseng JF, Shah SA. The impact of socioeconomic status on presentation and treatment of diverticular disease. J Gastrointest Surg. 2009;13(11):1993–2001; discussion -2
55. Järbrink-Sehgal ME. Epidemiological and pathophysiological studies on diverticular disease in the colon. Thesis for doctoral degree (Ph.D.). Karolinska Institutet, Stockholm, Sweden, 2018. Available at https://openarchive.ki.se/xmlui/bitstream/handle/10616/46474/Thesis_Ellionore_Jarbrink_Sehgal.pdf?sequence=3&isAllowed=y.

Part III

Clinical Features

Symptomatic Uncomplicated Diverticular Disease

8

Cristina Maria Sabo, Dan L. Dumitrascu, and Ingvar Bjarnason

Abbreviations

AD	Asymptomatic diverticulosis
AUD	Acute diverticulitis
CD	Colonic diverticulosis
DD	Diverticular disease
SCAD	Segmental colitis associated with diverticulosis
SUDD	Symptomatic uncomplicated diverticular disease
IBS	Irritable bowel syndrome

8.1 Introduction

Diverticulosis is characterized by the presence of pockets called "diverticula", which form when the colonic mucosa and submucosa herniate through defects in the muscular layer at the weakest point on the colonic wall – the sites of penetration by blood vessels of the colon wall [1]. A diverticulum was first described anatomically by Littre in 1770, according to a book by Morgagni. In 1896, Mayo operated on a patient with a colovesical fistula, secondary to diverticulitis [2]. Diverticular disease (DD) is defined as the presence of diverticulosis. DD is the most common

C. M. Sabo · D. L. Dumitrascu (✉)
2nd Medical Department, Iuliu Hațieganu University of Medicine and Pharmacy Cluj Napoca, Napoca, Romania
e-mail: cristina.marica90@yahoo.com; ddumitrascu@umfcluj.ro

I. Bjarnason
Department of Gastroenterology, King's College Hospital, London, UK
e-mail: Ingvarbjarnason@mac.com

© The Author(s), under exclusive license to Springer Nature Switzerland AG 2022
A. Tursi et al. (eds.), *Colonic Diverticular Disease*,
https://doi.org/10.1007/978-3-030-93761-4_8

condition affecting the large bowel in the Western world. DD (and diverticulitis in a special way) is one of the most common reasons for ambulatory visits (2,500,000 clinic visits) and hospital admissions (≈200,000 hospital admissions) in the USA and is associated with significant impairment of quality of life. Consequently, DD is associated with significant economic burden in direct health-care expenditures and in indirect costs to society (estimated at $4 billion dollars per year) [3]. Recent studies have reported an increase in the incidence of diverticulitis among age groups 18–44 and 45–64 years (incidence per 1000 population: 0.151–0.251 and 0.659–0.777, respectively), and, additionally, these patients had a more aggressive form of disease, with a fivefold increase in the risk of complications, such as fistula, compared with the age group 45–64 years [4, 5].

Many perceive diverticulosis to be an asymptomatic disease although this is controversial. About 15–20% develop diverticulitis with complications (hemorrhage, inflammation, pericolonic abscesses with or without perforation, strictures, fistulas, and perforation), but most episodes of diverticulitis are uncomplicated and some of these patients may develop what is termed "symptomatic uncomplicated diverticular disease" (SUDD). However, some also use this concept to describe patients without a clear-cut episode of diverticulitis who have recurrent left iliac fossa (LIF) pain amongst other symptoms and who are shown to have diverticulosis without macroscopic inflammation [6].

8.2 Terminology

The literature is replete with terms of unclear meaning, such as DD, symptomatic diverticulosis, and symptomatic uncomplicated diverticular disease (SUDD). According to the current accepted definitions, the following terminology is used to describe diverticulosis and its complications (Table 8.1) [4, 7–9]. However, there is scope for clarification of these terms, to simplify them, and this may have implications in guiding treatment.

Table 8.1 Terminology used for describing different scenarios in which diverticula may be detected [4, 7–9]

Diverticulosis: Presence of colonic diverticula
Diverticular disease: Clinically significant and symptomatic diverticulosis (a) Symptomatic uncomplicated diverticular disease (SUDD): Symptoms (episodes of abdominal pain) attributed to diverticulosis in the absence of any visible inflammation or diverticulitis (b) Diverticulitis: Macroscopic inflammation of diverticula, often associated with pericolonic inflammation • Uncomplicated • Complicated: Abscess, peritonitis, obstructions, fistulas, or hemorrhage
Segmental colitis associated with diverticulosis (SCAD): a form of chronic diverticulitis that occurs in the colon surrounded by multiple diverticula

8.3 Clinical Presentation and Differential Diagnosis

Diverticulosis refers to the presence of asymptomatic colonic diverticula [8]. Among patients who develop colonic diverticulosis, more than 80–85% remain asymptomatic during their lifetime. Only 20% of those affected develop symptoms, the so-called "diverticular disease" [7–10]. The overarching term "diverticular disease" implies that the pathological lesion (diverticulosis) rises to the level of an illness [8]. The majority of patients have an uncomplicated form of diverticular disease and are only discovered because they show up during investigation of other conditions, such as during colonoscopy, which is performed for colorectal screening purposes, etc. The vast majority of these patients have no specific symptoms attributable to diverticulosis; some may clinically present IBS symptoms, but both conditions are extremely common. In all, 15–20% develop a clinical course of diverticulitis, including that which may be associated with complications (requiring surgery for perforations, abscesses, and fistulas) [11] or not; the latter has a complex natural history, that is, many remain asymptomatic, others get recurrent diverticulitis, and others get the so-called SUDD.

8.4 History

Asymptomatic uncomplicated DD refers to the presence of diverticulosis without any symptoms or complications of the disease. Most often this is an incidental finding in asymptomatic patients undergoing gastrointestinal evaluation for other indications [12]. A careful history does not associate the vast majority with specific symptoms, but, in some cases, the patients may have preexisting IBS-like symptoms.

Symptomatic uncomplicated diverticular disease (SUDD) is classically perceived as a subtype of DD characterized by recurrent abdominal symptoms such as lower abdominal pain, bloating, tenesmus, and changes in bowel habits attributed to diverticula, in the absence of other macroscopical alterations (colitis or diverticulitis) [9, 12, 13]. Abdominal symptoms may be similar to those of irritable bowel syndrome (IBS) due to similar pathophysiological mechanisms underlying both disease processes, including visceral hypersensitivity [14, 15]. This of course raises the question whether the symptoms are due to IBS, with the diverticula being an incidental finding, or whether the symptoms are genuinely related to the diverticula. Clemens et al. [16] showed that SUDD patients had hyperalgesia in the sigmoid colon with diverticula, but so do many patients with IBS. However, it is suggested that some abdominal pain features could be used to differentiate these two disorders. A key distinction between pain related to SUDD and IBS is localization of the pain – SUDD patients have episodes of pain typically located in left iliac fossa, lasting 24 h, whereas IBS patients generally complain of diffuse/generalized pain. IBS patients experience diarrhea and/or constipation, whereas in SUDD, constipation is the rule and patients may experience tenderness in the left iliac fossa. Another diagnostic feature in IBS is the relief of pain by defecation or flatulence, which is not seen in SUDD patients [17]. However, sometimes it is impossible to differentiate SUDD from IBS based on the symptoms [18]. Physical examination on SUDD may be completely normal, may show a distended and pressure-sensitive abdomen, or a "palpable and pressure-sensitive roll" may often be found in the left lower quadrant [8].

The problem of distinguishing between these two conditions (in the absence of an episode of diverticulitis) is substantial. The above-mentioned SUDD symptoms have some of the hallmarks of recurrent mild (or ongoing) episodes of diverticulitis. Rectal hypersensitivity estimations do not distinguish this from IBS, and investigations (usually carried out during a time when the patient is relatively asymptomatic) do not demonstrate intestinal inflammation (i.e., negative imaging studies for inflammation, but fecal calprotectin may be marginally raised). This is clearly a situation that requires more research.

The differential diagnosis of lower abdominal pain includes many conditions with overlapping signs and symptoms and can be challenging for the practitioner. Table 8.2 reviews the common differential diagnoses for lower abdominal pain, and Table 8.3 [19] reviews the differential diagnosis between IBS and SUDD.

Table 8.2 Differential diagnoses for lower abdominal pain

Irritable bowel syndrome
Acute infectious bowel diseases
Inflammatory bowel diseases – Crohn's disease, ulcerative colitis
Ischemic colitis or drug-induced colitis (e.g., antibiotics, NSAIDs, etc.)
Acute appendicitis
Hernias (abdominal wall hernia, inguinal hernia)
Gynecological disease – Adnexitis, ovarian cyst, tubal pregnancy, etc
Urological diseases – Ureteral colic, cystitis, pyelonephritis, etc
Malignant diseases – Colon carcinoma, ovarian tumor
Diseases of the retroperitoneum – Abscess, hematoma, aneurysm, etc

Table 8.3 Factors differentiating SUDD from IBS [19]

Factors orienting to:	IBS	SUDD
Age: Older	–	+
Age: Younger	+	–
Sex: Male	–	+
Sex: Female	+	–
Positive Rome IV criteria	+	–
Pain: Periumbilical	+	–
Pain: Left lower quadrant	–	+
Pain: Frequent episodes	+	–
Pain: Long periods of remission	–	+
Pain: Nocturnal	–	+
Fecal inflammatory markers, usually positive	–	+

8.5 What Causes the Transition from Asymptomatic Diverticulosis to Symptomatic Diverticular Disease?

The causes of symptom development, in some patients, are still unclear and largely speculative.

One hypothesis is that motility alteration may be the cornerstone of symptom occurrence. Colonic motility is impaired in those patients and is mainly linked to serotonin imbalance in the muscular layer [20]. In fact, it is known that gene expression profiles of the serotonergic system and distribution of the serotonin type 4 receptor (5HT4R) are decreased in the circular muscular layer and myenteric ganglia of patients with SUDD [21], but a cause-and-effect relationship has not yet been established.

Another postulated mechanism for the development of symptoms is the presence, at least in a subgroup of patients with diverticulosis, of intestinal bacterial overgrowth, a putative mechanism responsible for low-grade inflammation. This bacterial overgrowth, aided by the fecal stasis inside the diverticula, could contribute to intermittent or chronic low-grade inflammation that, together with increasing nerve fiber sprouting [22] and smooth muscle hypertrophy [23], can lead to symptom occurrence. In addition, dysbiosis seems to play a role in SUDD occurrence. In a descriptive, cross-sectional pilot study, Barbara and colleagues [24] showed a depletion of microbiota members with anti-inflammatory activity (including *Clostridium cluster* IV, *Clostridium cluster* IX, *Fusobacterium*, and *Lactobacillaceae*) associated with mucosal macrophage infiltration (>70% increase in colonic macrophages) in patients with diverticular disease. However, the depletion of these bacteria from the intestinal microbiota is nonspecific. Another pilot study [25] analyzed data from stool samples obtained from 44 women (15 patients with SUDD without a history of diverticulitis, 13 with asymptomatic diverticulosis (AD), and 16 healthy controls (HCs)). By assessing the fecal microbiota and metabolome, the authors found that the three groups do not show colonic bacterial overgrowth ($p = 0.449$) with no difference in the *Bacteroides/Prevotella*, *Clostridium coccoides*, *Bifidobacterium*, *Lactobacillus*, and *Escherichia coli* subgroups. Interestingly, the amount of *A. muciniphila*, a species having a mucolytic effect on colonic mucus, was significantly higher in the SUDD group (-3.56 ± 1.27, $P = 0.044$) and in the AD group (-3.41 ± 1.13, $p = 0.019$) than in the HC group (-4.57 ± 1.05). Moreover, the SUDD group was characterized by low levels of valerate ($P = 0.009$), butyrate ($P = 0.047$), and choline ($P = 0.009$) and by high levels of *N*-acetyl-glucosamine ($P < 0.001$) and an unidentified compound (U1) ($P = 0.003$). In both SUDD and AD groups, a correlation between *Akkermansia* levels and several SCFAs was found (isovalerate, valerate, and formate). Moreover, a pilot study [26] found that there is a significant relationship between higher expression of *Akkermansia muciniphila* and symptom occurrence in SUDD.

Several studies confirm the hypothesis that low-grade inflammation may also play a key role in determining the clinical behavior of DD: fecal calprotectin is statistically increased in SUDD patients versus asymptomatic diverticulosis (AD) patients, healthy controls, or IBS patients [27, 28], but most studies show that fecal calprotectin is increased in about 15% of patients with IBS, so it is by itself not a good discriminatory marker. Nevertheless, proinflammatory cytokines such as TNF-α and microscopic inflammatory infiltrates (lymphocytic and neutrophilic inflammatory infiltrates) are increased in DD and seem to be correlated with the severity of the disease [29–31]. Despite these findings, SUDD is still questioned. However, to our minds, it is a key part of the DD spectrum. Finally, not only do low-grade intestinal inflammation, dysbiosis, and serotonergic system have a role in the occurrence of SUDD but also lifestyle factors may explain the development of symptoms – diet (meat, nuts, corn, and seed intake), smoking, alcohol consumption, obesity, physical activity, and drug intake. There is evidence suggesting that certain types of meat, higher alcohol consumption, and smoking increase the risk of diverticulosis and diverticular disease [32–34]. In addition, obesity seems to be linked to diverticular disease complications but not to diverticulosis occurrence [35–37].

8.6 SUDD or IBS "FOLLOWING ACUTE DIVERTICULITIS?"?

Of course, there is a dilemma: is it SUDD or IBS in DD, particularly after a diverticulitis episode? It is not always easy to decide, however, and there are several aspects orienting the diagnosis toward one of the two (Table 8.3) [19].

Following a documented uncomplicated diverticulitis episode, many patients experience ongoing symptoms. These have not been systematically investigated, but there are a number of different possibilities. First, there is a syndrome characterized by recurrent, usually mild, LIF pain, constipation, and tenderness. These episodes are characteristically treated with courses of antibiotics and some of them are associated with increased fecal calprotectin. To our minds, these are best classified as recurrent mild diverticulitis. The second is an ongoing problem with what is mostly a pre-diverticulitis IBS and which has been exacerbated by the diverticulitis episode. Last but not least, there is a possibility that post diverticulitis, symptoms present clinically as de novo IBS (that have all the features of IBS but not the LIF-dominant pain and tenderness). This may present a form of postinflammatory IBS. This is a relatively new concept, based on an old one. Originally, Truelove described a number of patients with severe gastroenteritis that developed a symptom complex that was indistinguishable from IBS. Since then, there is an opinion that one of the possible consequences of enteropathogenic infections by invasive bacteria, protozoa, and viruses is a symptom complex that meets the clinical criteria for IBS. The cause of this is incompletely understood and the natural history is somewhat different from classic IBS with a much higher recovery rate, and it is usually much milder. The overall incidence of this so-called postinfectious IBS varies from 2–5% to 5–40% after certain infections [38].

The criteria for postinfectious IBS [38] are clear:

1. Recurrent abdominal pain, on average, at least 1 day per week in the last 3 months, with symptom onset at least 6 months before diagnosis, associated with two of the following: (a) defecation, (b) a change in the frequency of stool, and (c) a change in the form (appearance) of stool;

2. Symptom development immediately after resolution of acute infectious gastroenteritis;
3. Infectious gastroenteritis defined by a positive stool culture in a symptomatic individual or by the presence of two of the following acute symptoms (when stool culture is not available): (a) fever, (b) vomiting, and (c) diarrhea;
4. Should not meet the criteria for IBS before the onset of acute illness.

A noticeable feature is that more than 50% undergo spontaneous remission within 4–6 years, whereas the rest seem to have ongoing symptoms with a low rate of remission.

After an episode of acute diverticulitis, we know that symptoms may persist, and this syndrome has been initially defined as "post-diverticulitis IBS". Cohen et al. [39] found that, in a population with a mean age > 60 years, the prevalence of IBS following an episode of acute diverticulitis was 4.7-fold higher than that in controls (95% CI 1.6–14.0; $p = 0.006$), and that the mood disorder was 2.2-fold more higher than that in controls (95% CI 1.4–3.5; $p < 0.001$); Yamada et al. [15] found that IBS was observed in 7.5% of people with a prior episode of acute diverticulitis. Moreover, left-sided (odds ratio 3.1) and bilateral diverticulosis (odds ratio 2.6), but not right-sided disease, were associated with a higher risk of IBS. These studies hypothesized that the de novo occurrence of IBS could have a pathogenetic mechanism similar to that causing the so-called "post-infectious" IBS. However, those patients do not have characteristics that fulfill the IBS criteria. Kvasnovsky et al. [40] followed up 245 patients after an episode of acute diverticulitis for 45 months and found that abdominal symptoms persisted for more than 3 months in 53% of this population. Younger age and C-reactive protein (CRP) <50 mg/L were found to be the predictors of symptom persistence, and 6% of those people underwent surgery. Neither surgery may be considered an option for resolving symptoms. Two studies found that about 25% of patients who had elective surgery due to symptoms following acute diverticulitis suffered from persistent symptoms (painful constipation, painful abdominal distension, abdominal cramps, frequent painful diarrhea, fecal incontinence, and fecal urgency) [41, 42]. To our minds, these symptoms are best classified as "post-diverticulitis SUDD". Several factors support this hypothesis – generally, those patients who do not meet the IBS criteria [43] have an increased expression of IL-10 [44]; TNF-α and several other proinflammatory cytokines that are overexpressed [45] have a persistent submucosal inflammation [46]. According to all these findings, the recent third International Symposium on Diverticular Disease has defined SUDD post-acute diverticulitis as "*a chronic inflammatory disease with prolonged chronic symptoms, high levels of systemic serum inflammatory markers, high levels of tissue inflammatory cytokine and chronic inflammatory infiltrates in the affected colonic tissue*. [Evidence level: 2C; Recommendation Grade: B]" [6]. Recently, a clinical score, named the diverticular clinical score (DICS), has been developed and validated to assess post-diverticulitis SUDD-related symptom severity [47]; further studies have to confirm its impact on monitoring post-diverticulitis SUDD in clinical practice, in particular for facilitating patient stratification and therapeutic decisions.

8.7 The Natural History of SUDD

The knowledge of the outcomes of the disease is limited [48]. Three studies [49–51] evaluated the natural history of SUDD in terms of the occurrence of acute diverticulitis and its complication during a 5-year follow-up, whereas the most recent study [48] has evaluated, in addition, the symptom score and the quality-of-life (QoL) score using a visual analog scale (VAS) during a median time of 156 (91–171) months of follow-up.

Four studies reported the prevalence of acute diverticulitis in SUDD patients between 1.7% and 10.4% [48–51], and the diverticulitis risk in SUDD patients seems to become null after 10 years from the diagnosis of SUDD [48].

Regarding the recurrence/persistence of symptoms in patients with SUDD, the results are discordant. Comparato et al. [52], Carabotti et al. [53], and Tursi et al. [48] found that SUDD negatively affects patients' QoL due to persistence/recurrence of symptoms, and 91.3% patients [36] often require more than one course of treatment. On the contrary, Salem et al. [49] found that the majority of SUDD patients (97%) do not have mild symptoms after a median follow-up of 66 months.

8.8 Conclusions

A correct diagnosis of diverticular syndromes is challenging for clinicians. Patient's symptoms are nonspecific and may overlap with other gastroenterological conditions (e.g., IBS), for instance, in young women (<40 years), who also have gynecological disorders. The onset of symptoms in diverticular patients is controversial and may be due to excessive growth of bacteria, low inflammation, diet, obesity, and hereditary factors. SUDD is an important disease that affects patients significantly in the long term.

Conflict of Interest Statement The authors have no conflicts of interest to declare.

Funding Sources The authors have no sources of funding to declare.

Author Contributions C.M.S. drafted and revised the manuscript. D.LD. proposed the idea of the manuscript, suggested the structure of the text, revised the manuscript, and approved the final text. I.B. contributed to the writing of the manuscript and offered valuable suggestions.

References

1. Tursi A, Papagrigoriadis S. Review article: the current and evolving treatment of colonic diverticular disease. Aliment Pharmacol Ther. 2009;30:532–46.
2. Barroso AO, Quigley EMM. Diverticula and diverticulitis: time for a reappraisal. Gastroenterol Hepatol (N Y). 2015;11(10):680–8.

3. Peery AF. Colonic diverticula and diverticular disease: ten facts a clinician should know. N C Med J. 2016;77(3):220–2.
4. Weizman AV, Nguyen GC. Diverticular disease: epidemiology and management. Can J Gastroenterol. 2011;25(7):385–9.
5. Etzioni DA, Mack TM, Beart RW Jr, Kaiser AM. Diverticulitis in the United States: 1998-2005: changing patterns of disease and treatment. Ann Surg. 2009;249(2):210–7.
6. Tursi A, Brandimarte G, Di Mario F, et al. International consensus on diverticulosis and diverticular disease. Statements from the 3rd international symposium on diverticular disease. J Gastrointestin Liver Dis. 2019;28(suppl. 4):57–66.
7. Strate LL, Modi R, Cohen E, Spiegel BM. Diverticular disease as a chronic illness: evolving epidemiologic and clinical insights. Am J Gastroenterol. 2012;107(10):1486–93.
8. Tursi A, Papa A, Danese S. Review article: the pathophysiology and medical management of diverticulosis and diverticular disease of the colon. Aliment Pharmacol Ther. 2015;42(6):664–84.
9. Trifan A, Gheorghe C, Marica Sabo C, Diculescu M, Nedelcu L, Singeap AM, et al. Diagnosis and treatment of colonic diverticular disease: position paper of the Romanian Society of Gastroenterology and Hepatology. J Gastrointestin Liver Dis. 2018;27(4):449–57.
10. Rezapour M, Ali S, Stollman N. Diverticular disease: an update on pathogenesis and management. Gut Liver. 2018;12(2):125–32.
11. Shahedi K, Fuller G, Bolus R, et al. Long-term risk of acute diverticulitis among patients with incidental diverticulosis found during colonoscopy. Clin Gastroenterol Hepatol. 2013;11(12):1609–13.
12. Bhucket TP, Stollman NH. Diverticular disease of the colon. In: Feldman M, Friedman LS, Brandt LJ, editors. Sleisenger and Fordtran's gastrointestinal and liver disease: pathophysiology, diagnosis, management, vol. 2. 10th ed. Philadelphia: Elsevier; 2014. p. 1–15.
13. Carabotti M, Annibale B. Treatment of diverticular disease: an update on latest evidence and clinical implications. Drugs Context. 2018;7:212526.
14. Annibale B, Lahner E, Maconi G, Usai P, Marchi S, Bassotti G, Barbara G, Cuomo R. Clinical features of symptomatic uncomplicated diverticular disease: a multicenter Italian survey. Int J Color Dis. 2012;27(9):1151–9.
15. Yamada E, Inamori M, Uchida E, et al. Association between the location of diverticular disease and the irritable bowel syndrome: a multicenter study in Japan. Am J Gastroenterol. 2014;109:1900–5.
16. Clemens CH, Samsom M, Roelofs J, van Berge Henegouwen GP, Smout AJ. Colorectal visceral perception in diverticular disease. Gut. 2004;53:717–22.
17. Cuomo R, Barbara G, Andreozzi P, Bassotti G, Casetti T, Grassini M, et al. Symptom patterns can distinguish diverticular disease from irritable bowel syndrome. Eur J Clin Investig. 2013;43:1147–55.
18. Jung HK, Choung RS, Locke GR 3rd, Schleck CD, Zinsmeister AR, Talley NJ. Diarrhea-predominant irritable bowel syndrome is associated with diverticular disease: a population-based study. Am J Gastroenterol. 2010;105(3):652–61.
19. Scarpignato C, Barbara G, Lanas A, Strate LL. Management of colonic diverticular disease in the third millennium: highlights from asymposium held during the united European gastroenterology week 2017. Ther Adv Gastroenterol. 2018;11:1–21.
20. Costedio MM, Coates MD, Danielson AB, Buttolph TR 3rd, Blaszyk HJ, Mawe GM, Hyman NH. Serotonin signaling in diverticular disease. J Gastrointest Surg. 2008;12(8):1439–45.
21. Tursi A. Diverticulosis today: unfashionable and still under-researched. Ther Adv Gastroenterol. 2016;9(2):213–28.
22. Barbaro MR, Cremon C, Fuschi D, Scaioli E, Veneziano A, Marasco G, Festi D, Stanghellini V, Barbara G. Nerve fiber overgrowth in patients with symptomatic diverticular disease. Neurogastroenterol Motil. 2019;31(9):e13575.
23. Simpson J, Scholefield JH, Spiller RC. Origin of symptoms in diverticular disease. Br J Surg. 2003;90:899–908.

24. Barbara G, et al. Gut microbiota, metabolome and immune signatures in patients with uncomplicated diverticular disease. Gut. 2016:1–10.
25. Tursi A, Mastromarino P, Capobianco D, Elisei W, Miccheli A, Capuani G, Tomassini A, Campagna G, Picchio M, Giorgetti G, Fabiocchi F, Brandimarte G. Assessment of fecal microbiota and fecal metabolome in symptomatic uncomplicated diverticular disease of the colon. J Clin Gastroenterol. 2016;50(Suppl 1):S9–S12.
26. Laghi L, Mastromarino P, Elisei W, Capobianco D, Zhu CL, Picchio M, Giorgetti G, Brandimarte G, Tursi A. Impact of treatments on fecal microbiota and fecal metabolome in symptomatic uncomplicated diverticular disease of the colon: a pilot study. J Biol Regul Homeost Agents. 2018;32(5):1421–32.
27. Tursi A, Brandimarte G, Elisei W, Giorgetti GM, Inchingolo CD, Aiello F. Faecal calprotectin in colonic diverticular disease: a casecontrol study. Int J Color Dis. 2009;24:49–55.
28. Tursi A, Elisei W, Picchio M, Giorgetti GM, Brandimarte G. Moderate to severe and prolonged left lower-abdominal pain is the best symptom characterizing symptomatic uncomplicated diverticular disease of the colon: a comparison with fecal calprotectin in clinical setting. J Clin Gastroenterol. 2015;49(3):218–21.
29. Humes DJ, Simpson J, Smith J, Sutton P, Zaitoun A, Bush D, Bennett A, Scholefield JH, Spiller RC. Visceral hypersensitivity in symptomatic diverticular disease and the role of neuropeptides and low grade inflammation. Neurogastroenterol Motil. 2012;24(4):318–e163.
30. Tursi A, Elisei W, Brandimarte G, Giorgetti GM, Inchingolo CD, Nenna R, et al. Mucosal tumour necrosis factor-alpha in diverticular disease of the colon is overexpressed with disease severity. Color Dis. 2012;14:e258–63.
31. Tursi A, Elisei W, Brandimarte G, Giorgetti GM, Inchingolo CD, Nenna R, Picchio M, Giorgio F, Ierardi E. Mucosal expression of basic fibroblastic growth factor, Syndecan 1 and tumor necrosis factor-alpha in diverticular disease of the colon: a case-control study. Neurogastroenterol Motil. 2012;24(9):836–e396.
32. Aldoori WH, Giovannucci EL, Rimm EB, Wing AL, Trichopoulos DV, Willett WC. A prospective study of diet and the risk of symptomatic diverticular disease in men. Am J Clin Nutr. 1994;60(5):757–64.
33. Crowe FL, Appleby PN, Allen NE, Key TJ. Diet and risk of diverticular disease in Oxford cohort of European prospective investigation into cancer and nutrition (EPIC):prospective study of British vegetarians and non-vegetarians. BMJ. 2011;343:d4131.
34. Nagata N, Niikura R, Shimbo T, et al. Alcohol and smoking affect risk of uncomplicated colonic diverticulosis in Japan. PLoS One. 2013;8:e81137.
35. Song J, Kim Y, Lee J, Ok K, Ryu S, Lee J, et al. Clinical characteristics of colonic diverticulosis in Korea: a prospective study. Korean J Intern Med. 2010;25:140–6.
36. Strate LL, Liu YL, Aldoori WH, et al. Obesity increases the risks of diverticulitis and diverticular bleeding. Gastroenterology. 2009;136:115–22.
37. Kopylov U, Ben-Horin S, Lahat A, et al. Obesity, metabolic syndrome and the risk of development of colonic diverticulosis. Digestion. 2012;86:201–5.
38. Barbara G, Grover M, Bercik P, et al. Rome foundation working team report on post-infection irritable bowel syndrome. Gastroenterology. 2019;156:46–58.
39. Cohen E, Fuller G, Bolus R, et al. Increased risk for irritable bowel syndrome after acute diverticulitis. Clin Gastroenterol Hepatol. 2013;11(12):1614–9.
40. Kvasnovsky CL, Adams K, Papagrigoriadis S. Diverticular disease as a chronic gastrointestinal condition: experience from a specialist clinic. Eur J Gastroenterol Hepatol. 2015;27(4):442–8.
41. Egger B, Peter MK, Candinas D. Persistent symptoms after elective sigmoid resection for diverticulitis. Dis Colon Rectum. 2008;51(7):1044–8.
42. Levack MM, Savitt LR, Berger DL, et al. Sigmoidectomy syndrome? Patients' perspectives on the functional outcomes following surgery for diverticulitis. Dis Colon Rectum. 2012;55(1):10–7.
43. Tursi A, Elisei W, Franceschi M, Picchio M, Di Mario F, Brandimarte G. The prevalence of symptomatic uncomplicated diverticular disease could be lower than expected: a single-center

colonoscopy-based cohort study. Eur J Gastroenterol Hepatol. 2021;33(1S Suppl 1):e478–83. https://doi.org/10.1097/MEG.0000000000002142. Online ahead of print. PMID: 33867449
44. Turco F, Andreozzi P, Palumbo I, et al. Bacterial stimuli activate nitric oxide colonic mucosal production in diverticular disease. Protective effects of L. casei DG (lactobacillus paracasei CNCM I-1572). United European. Gastroenterol J. 2017;5(5):715–24.
45. Lahat A, Necula D, Yavzori M, et al. Prolonged recurrent abdominal pain is associated with ongoing underlying mucosal inflammation in patients who had an episode of acute complicated diverticulitis. J Clin Gastroenterol. 2019;53(5):e178–85.
46. Zidar N. Why do we have to look deep to understand diverticulitis? Am J Gastroenterol. 2019;114(8):1347–8.
47. Lahat A, Fidder HH, Ben-Horin S. Development and validation of a diverticular clinical score for symptomatic uncomplicated diverticular disease after acute diverticulitis in a prospective patient cohort. Ther Adv Gastroenterol. 2020;13:1756284820913210.
48. Tursi A, Franceschi M, Elisei W, Picchio M, Di Mario F, Brandimarte G. The natural history of symptomatic uncomplicated diverticular disease: a long-term follow-up study. Ann Gastroenterol. 2021;34(2):208–13.
49. Salem TA, Molloy RG, O'Dwyer PJ. Prospective, five-year followup study of patients with symptomatic uncomplicated diverticular disease. Dis Colon Rectum. 2007;50:1460–4.
50. Gatta L, Di Mario F, Curlo M, et al. Long-term treatment with mesalazine in patients with symptomatic uncomplicated diverticular disease. Intern Emerg Med. 2012;7:133–7.
51. Järbrink-Sehgal ME, Rassam L, Jasim A, et al. Diverticulosis, symptoms and colonic inflammation: a population-based colonoscopy study. Am J Gastroenterol. 2019;114:500–10.
52. Comparato G, Fanigliulo L, Aragona G, et al. Quality of life in uncomplicated symptomatic diverticular disease: is it another good reason for treatment? Dig Dis. 2007;25:252–9.
53. Carabotti M, Cuomo R, Barbara G, Pace F, Andreozzi P, Cremon C, Annibale B. Demographic and clinical features distinguish subgroups of diverticular disease patients: results from an Italian nationwide registry. United European Gastroenterol J. 2018;6(6):926–34.

Acute Diverticulitis

9

Angel Lanas and Giovanni Latella

9.1 Introduction

Acute diverticulitis can be both uncomplicated and complicated. Uncomplicated diverticulitis is characterized by the presence of localized colonic inflammation with or without small abscess formation confined to the colonic wall. Complicated diverticulitis is characterized by the presence of abscess, fistula, obstruction, or free perforation. Fistulas and obstruction are early or late complications of diverticulitis [1]. The localization of diverticulitis (left colon or right colon) impacts both the clinical presentation and the differential diagnosis with other pathologies. Acute diverticulitis of the left colon (mainly sigmoid) prevails in Western countries, whereas diverticulitis of the right colon prevails in Asian populations, which, in 70% of cases, mimics acute appendicitis.

Several modifiable (overweight/obesity, low fiber intake, high fat and red meat intake, smoking, reduced physical activity, medications) and nonmodifiable (age, sex, genetics) risk factors have been associated with an increased risk of diverticulitis and complicated diverticulitis [2].

Notably, diverticulitis is the most severe form of diverticular disease. Recent studies have shown that acute diverticulitis occurs in less than 5% of patients with diverticulosis [3]. In the USA, diverticulitis is the seventh most frequent

A. Lanas (✉)
Service of Digestive Diseases, University Clinic Hospital, University of Zaragoza. CIBERehd. IIS Aragón, Zaragoza, Spain
e-mail: angel.lanas@gmail.com

G. Latella
Gastroenterology, Hepatology and Nutrition Division, Department of Life, Health and Environmental Sciences, University of L'Aquila, L'Aquila, Italy
e-mail: giolatel@tin.it

© The Author(s), under exclusive license to Springer Nature Switzerland AG 2022
A. Tursi et al. (eds.), *Colonic Diverticular Disease*,
https://doi.org/10.1007/978-3-030-93761-4_9

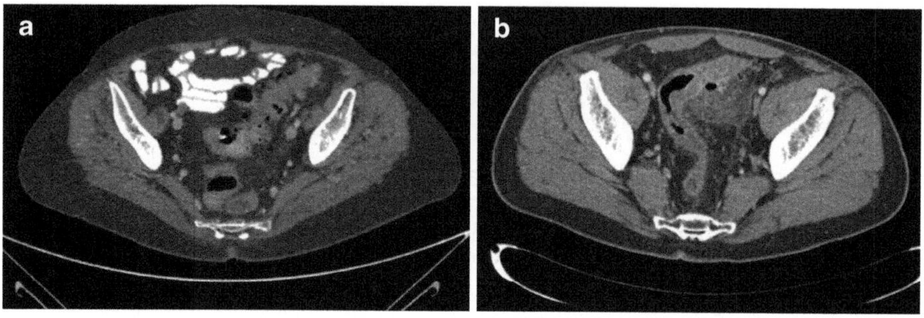

Fig. 9.1 (**a**) CT image of acute uncomplicated diverticulitis with evidence of multiple sigmoid diverticula and marked increase in wall thickness, reaching 13–15 mm. (**b**) CT image of complicated acute diverticulitis with voluminous abscess/phlegmon adjacent to the sigmoid, following perforation of the diverticulum. Abscess is about 6 cm, with marked inhomogeneity of the adipose tissue and with air inside. Courtesy of Prof. Francesca Maccioni, Sapienza University of Rome

gastrointestinal diagnosis from hospital admissions [4]. Complications of diverticulitis can occur in approximately 12–25% of patients with diverticulitis [5].

The initial suspicion of acute diverticulitis is based on clinical history and physical examination, although its final and confirmatory diagnosis requires an objective test, which is usually a CT scan and/or an ultrasonography test (Fig. 9.1) [6, 7]. The classical clinical presentation of acute diverticulitis includes a combination of abdominal pain and fever. Pain is often located in the left lower quadrant of the abdomen, is acute at onset, and is persistent. The location of pain may be different in cases of redundant sigmoid or in the Asiatic population where the diverticula are more often located in the right colon. Fever and chills are also frequent. These symptoms are often accompanied by leukocytosis. Other symptoms can also be present and these include nausea, vomiting, and diarrhea or even constipation, but, when other symptoms such as dysuria or diffuse abdominal pain are present, they indicate the presence of complicated acute diverticulitis. Abdominal tenderness in the left lower abdominal quadrant is common and can be associated with involuntary muscular contractions as the consequence of peritoneal inflammation [8] (Table 9.1). If pain allows, a gross and painful sigmoid colon can be palpable. Auscultation of the abdomen may show decreased intestinal movement, but there is no rule. Rectal examination can be painful, especially if there is occupation of the cul-de-sac [1].

However, there are differences in the clinical presentation of acute diverticulitis depending on a number of aspects that deserve to be taken into account, including the severity and location of the inflamed diverticula, the age of the patient, and the degree of the immune response of the patient, which can often be modulated by the use of different drugs such as corticosteroids or immunosuppressive drugs or biological agents. In most patients, acute diverticulitis is mild, responds well to medical treatment, and usually does not recur. However, in up to 30% of patients, the disease may recur, and up to 25% of the patients might suffer from complications such as abscess formation, fistula, or free perforation [1].

Table 9.1 Clinical characteristics of acute diverticulitis

Type of patient	Common Clinical Features
Uncomplicated diverticulitis	Abdominal pain, usually not intense, located most frequently in the inferior left abdominal quadrant (Western countries) or in the inferior right abdominal quadrant (Eastern countries). Mild fever and leukocytosis. No need for hospitalization in most cases
Complicated Diverticulitis	Abdominal pain located most frequently in the inferior left abdominal quadrant (Western countries) or in the inferior right abdominal quadrant (eastern countries) (often misdiagnosed as acute appendicitis). Abdominal pain can be intense with rebound and tenderness if peritonitis is present. Other symptoms, such as nausea, vomiting, diarrhea, abdominal distension, etc., can also be present. Fever and leukocytosis. Hospitalization required. Surgical intervention often required
Acute diverticulitis in the elderly	Pain, fever, and leukocytosis are milder than in younger patients. Higher rate of comorbidities and higher risk of developing complications and death
Acute diverticulitis in young patients	Pain, fever, and leukocytosis can be more prominent than in older patients, but it is unclear whether this is followed by a higher rate of complicated diverticulitis. Higher rate of recurrence
Acute diverticulitis in immunocompromised patients	Symptoms of acute diverticulitis in immunocompromised patients are subtler than in immunocompetent patients. Higher rates of complicated acute diverticulitis
Acute diverticulitis in the right colon	Often misdiagnosed as acute appendicitis. Patients are younger, more likely to be male, taller, with a lower body mass index, and less advanced modified Hinchey stages than patients with acute diverticulitis of the left colon

The combination of clinical and laboratory findings can allow not only to differentiate uncomplicated from complicated diverticulitis but also to predict the occurrence of complicated disease.

The severity of acute diverticulitis can be graded based on the modified Hinchey classification, which depends on clinical features combined with objective tests (Table 9.2). Here, we revise the different clinical features of acute diverticulitis based on the severity of presentation and in patients with different baseline conditions.

9.2 Uncomplicated Acute Diverticulitis

Most cases (75%) of acute diverticulitis can be considered uncomplicated since the inflammatory process is limited to the wall of the colon. These patients often have mild or medium symptoms limited to pain, usually in the left lower abdominal quadrant, and mild or absent fever and leukocytosis. These cases are usually classified as Hinchey 0 or Ia (Table) since the radiological test shows that the inflammatory process takes place in the colonic wall or not beyond the pericolic fat at the most (Fig. 9.1) [3, 9]. Today, these patients are usually not hospitalized and are treated as outpatients. One study [10] compared the clinical features of patients with

Table 9.2 Acute diverticulitis and clinical features according to modified Hinchey classification. Modified from reference 3

Stage		Clinical Category	Common Clinical Features
0	Mild diverticulitis, diverticula with colonic wall thickening on CT	Uncomplicated	Mild pain located, most frequently, in the inferior left abdominal quadrant. Mild fever and leukocytosis or often not present. No need for hospitalization
Ia	Colonic wall thickening inflammatory phlegmon in the pericolic fat	Uncomplicated	Mild pain located, most frequently, in the inferior left abdominal quadrant Mild fever and leukocytosis. Abdominal tenderness. No need for hospitalization unless there are risk factors (e.g., immunocompromised patients)
Ib	Pericolic/mesenteric abscess proximal to the primary inflammatory process	Complicated	Pain located, most frequently, in the inferior left abdominal quadrant. Abdominal tenderness. Fever and leukocytosis. Hospitalization usually required
II	Intra-abdominal abscess distant from the primary process; pelvic or retroperitoneal abscess	Complicated	Abdominal pain that can be present beyond the left inferior abdominal quadrant. Other symptoms may be present. Fever and leukocytosis. Hospitalization required
III	Generalized purulent peritonitis	Complicated	Diffuse abdominal pain with rebound, high fever and marked leukocytosis. Other symptoms, such as nausea or vomiting and abdominal distension, are usually present. Hospitalization and urgent surgical action required
IV	Generalized fecal peritonitis	Complicated	Diffuse abdominal pain with rebound, high fever and marked leukocytosis. Other symptoms, such as nausea or vomiting and abdominal distension, are present. Hospitalization and urgent surgical action required

acute diverticulitis who were hospitalized with those of patients who were seen at the emergency department and not hospitalized. Patients who were hospitalized were younger and had more frequent abdominal pain not limited to the lower abdomen, nausea and vomiting, diarrhea, constipation, oral temperature > 37.5 °C, leukocytosis >7700 mm^3, band cells >700 mm^3, and the triad (abdominal pain, fever, and leukocytosis) > 11,000 mm^3. Similar findings were observed in other studies. In a retrospective cohort study of 1749 patients [11], presenting clinical features and computed tomography findings were analyzed. Inpatients were older, had more comorbidities, had no history of past diverticulitis, and were more often underweight/normal weight than those not hospitalized. The typical acute diverticulitis triad (abdominal pain + fever + leukocytosis) was rarely seen (5.2%) in outpatients or those (10.7%) only attended at the emergency department compared with the 38.6% observed in hospitalized patients. In a multivariable analysis, females had a lower risk for the presence of the triad features but increased odds of vomiting. Older patients had decreased odds of fever, but patients with ≥1 comorbidity had increased risk of presenting the typical triad of acute diverticulitis.

Another study evaluated the clinical features of patients who were treated for abdominal pain, which were significantly associated with a final diagnosis of acute diverticulitis [12]. From a cohort of 1021 patients, 112 eventually had a diagnosis of acute diverticulitis. There were three clear clinical features defining the presence of diverticulitis: direct tenderness only in the left lower quadrant, the absence of vomiting, and a C-reactive protein level > 50 mg/L.

9.3 Complicated Acute Diverticulitis

Around 8–35% of patients with acute diverticulitis can be included in the term "complicated acute diverticulitis" [13, 14]. Within the modified Hinchey classification (Table), these cases are Ib–IV and include the development of pericolic or mesenteric abscess in the proximity of the inflammatory process (Ib), intra-abdominal and distal to the colon abscess, including those of the pelvic or retroperitoneal location (II), and diffuse purulent (III) or fecal peritonitis (IV).

The development of pericolic or intramesenteric abscess is relatively frequent and is the consequence of perforation of the colonic diverticula, which is usually controlled (Fig. 9.1). In fact, one study of patients clinically diagnosed as uncomplicated diverticulitis that underwent elective surgery after an acute episode found that almost half (47.8%) of them had abscess during surgical or pathological examination [15]. Clinical features that suggest the presence of abscesses during the course of an acute diverticulitis event include the presence of an abdominal painful mass and the presence of persistent fever and leukocytosis, despite the administration of an appropriate antibiotic therapy. A confirmatory CT scan or an ultrasonography will guide the appropriate therapy, which will rapidly reduce the symptoms and signs described above.

Although uncommon, acute diverticulitis can induce diffuse purulent or fecal peritonitis due to free perforation, and this is a surgical emergency. Early detection of peritonitis is critical and should be suspected in patients with important diffuse abdominal pain, abdominal muscular defense, and positive Blumberg's sign, although these signs may not be highly apparent in the elderly and in immunocompromised patients. In these cases, confirmatory CT scans or simple radiological examinations of the abdomen may detect free air [1].

Partial or, more rarely, a complete obstruction of the colon may occur in an acute diverticulitis event due to a reduction of the luminal diameter of the colon because of the pericolic inflammatory process or abscesses. In these cases, patients will present abdominal distension, nausea, vomiting, and intermittent abdominal pain as the consequence of increased intestinal movements. The clinical picture usually improves rapidly with treatment of the baseline cause. However, after the acute event, some patients may develop a colonic chronic stricture with severe constipation, abdominal distension, and pain, which will require either endoscopic or surgical treatment.

Finally, another complication of acute diverticulitis is the development of fistula connecting the colonic lumen with the adjacent organs. The organs affected more frequently are the urinary bladder (65%), especially in men, and the vagina (25%) in women [13, 16–18]. The presence of fecal material in urine, or more often hematuria or pneumaturia together with persistent urine infection, should alert the presence of this complication. The presence of spontaneous vaginal flatus and infections should prompt the investigation of the presence of colovaginal fistula. Other less common fistulas are coloenteric fistula or fistulas connecting the colon with the uterus or the abdominal wall.

9.4 Acute Diverticulitis in the Elderly and in Young Patients

The prevalence of diverticulosis increases with age, and, therefore the occurrence of acute diverticulitis may affect patients with advanced age. It is believed that acute diverticulitis occurs more frequently in the elderly than in younger patients, although this has been challenged in recent years [19]. Advanced age is usually accompanied by a lower capacity of response and a higher prevalence of comorbidities, which should result in a higher risk of developing more serious acute diverticulitis. However, pain, fever, and leukocytosis in the elderly are usually subtler than in younger patients with acute diverticulitis, which can make the diagnosis difficult, but, in general, acute diverticulitis in the elderly is mild, but the risk of dying is higher if complications arise. One study [20] aimed to compare the clinical outcomes of acute diverticulitis in patients older with patients younger than 80 years of age. Patients >80 years had less fever (21.4 vs. 35.2%; $p < 0.001$) and abdominal pain (47.8 vs. 65.6%; $p < 0.001$) than did younger patients but higher rates of digestive tract bleeding (31.5 vs. 12.3%; $p < 0.001$) and fatigue (12.7 vs. 7.1%; $p = 0.004$). Length of hospital stay, rates of major complications, and mortality were higher for patients >80 years.

Colon diverticula are more frequent in elderly patients who, for cardiovascular or musculoskeletal pathologies, frequently take acetylsalicylic acid and/or nonsteroidal anti-inflammatory agents (NSAIDs). Such drugs represent a risk factor for diverticulitis and for the perforation of diverticula as they inhibit the cyclooxygenase enzyme and reduce prostaglandin synthesis in the gut [21, 22]. Prostaglandins have important protective effects on the colonic mucosal barrier. Therefore, to reduce the complications of colonic diverticula, it is necessary to prescribe with caution NSAIDs and/or acetylsalicylic acid in patients with colonic diverticular disease.

The incidence of acute diverticulitis in patients under 50 years of age has clearly been increasing in recent years. The reasons for this increase are not clear, but they are likely to reflect a combination of changing lifestyle influences and more accurate diagnosis [2]. Young patients with acute diverticulitis have been considered to follow a more aggressive course than older patients and to have more prominent symptoms of the characteristic diverticulitis triad (pain, fever, and leukocytosis), but data are scarce to confirm this assertion. A recent meta-analysis [23] has compared outcomes in patients with acute diverticulitis younger and older than 50 years of age. In all, 8 studies were included in the analysis with a total of 4.751 patients younger and 18.328 older than 50 years of age. The study concluded that there were not many differences between these two groups of age, although younger patients have a higher risk of having recurrences and a bit higher risk (7.3 vs. 4.9%) of developing complicated acute diverticulitis requiring surgery.

Another meta-analysis including 12 studies with 4982 patients under the age of 50 confirmed that acute diverticulitis was no more severe and aggressive in young patients than in elderly patients [24]. Most young patients were males (RR 1.70, 95% CI 1.31–2.21), without a tendency toward a more complicated disease at admission (RR 0.95, 95% CI 0.46–1.97). Although there was no significant difference in the rate of surgery during hospitalization (RR 0.69, 95% CI 0.46–1.06), young patients underwent more elective surgeries (RR 2.39, 95% CI 1.82–3.15). No mortality was recorded among young patients. The disease recurrence rate was significantly higher than that for elderly patients (RR 1.70, 95% CI 1.31–2.21).

Finally, one small study [25] of 76 patients under the age of 40 who developed an episode of acute diverticulitis showed that 30.2% of them had fever (>38 °C) and 68.4% had leukocytosis (≥11,000/mm [3]). It was of interest to see that the majority of these young patients (63.1%) were obese and 38.1% patients had complications, with perforation (62%) being the most common. The authors concluded that high fever and obesity were predictors of complications in this range of age. However, another earlier study, [26] from the Kaiser Permanente Los Angeles Medical Center, analyzed a small subset of patients ≤40 years of age and considered that their data did not support a "virulent" label in the young who develop an acute diverticulitis event.

9.5 Acute Diverticulitis in Immunocompromised Patients

Immunosuppression could increase the complication rate in patients with acute diverticulitis. Well-documented groups of immunocompromised patients comprise transplantation patients, in whom many prospective studies have been conducted.

Symptoms of acute diverticulitis in immunocompromised patients are subtler than those in immunocompetent patients. This implies the need to have a higher level of suspicion in this type of patients when referring to mild symptoms in the abdomen. A delay in the diagnosis may have serious consequences. Acute diverticulitis in these patients is not more frequent, but the development of complications has been described more frequently [27]. Immunocompromised patients include those who have undergone an organ transplant or those receiving immunosuppressive drugs for other reasons, chronic corticosteroid patients, patients undergoing chemotherapy, or patients with AIDs [28]. A systematic review of complicated acute diverticulitis in 11,966 post-transplant patients showed that the overall incidence of complicated diverticulitis ranged from 0.1% to 3.5% and that more often they developed a complicated disease course [29]. Still, most patients can be managed conservatively, but they require a more aggressive initial approach [27]. When they require urgent surgery, they also have worse outcomes including a higher mortality when compared with immunocompetent patients [30], and that is why it has been advised that immunocompromised patients must undergo elective surgery after the first episode of acute diverticulitis [31].

Although immunosuppression in a transplant patient is therapeutic and adjustable, immune deficiency in an AIDS patient is inimical and uncontrolled. In earlier studies, no evidence for any increased susceptibility to diverticulitis in HIV-positive patients was reported [32]. A recent study has reported the results of 2375 patients with HIV infection hospitalized for diverticulitis and 160,391 patients without HIV infection hospitalized for diverticulitis from 2007 to 2011 [33]. Patients with HIV infection were younger and more likely to be male and non-white. After multivariate analysis, patients with diverticulitis and HIV infection had a significantly increased in-hospital mortality rate (odds ratio (OR) 3.94, (95% confidence interval (95% CI), 1.52–10.20) and a lower rate of surgical intervention (OR 0.74, 95% CI 0.57–0.95). From 2003 to 2011, there was a linear increasing trend in the prevalence of HIV infection among patients hospitalized for diverticulitis ($P < 0.001$).

9.6 Acute Diverticulitis in the Right Colon

Although in Western countries diverticula are more frequently located in the sigmoid and left colon, they can be present in any part of the colon, and, in fact, diverticula in the right colon are more prevalent in Asiatic populations. In any case, the diagnosis of acute diverticulitis in the right colon must be considered in the differential diagnosis of any patient presenting sudden abdominal symptoms in the right colon, especially with the typical triad of pain, fever, and leukocytosis. In this case, the differential diagnosis must be performed with other pathologies that mimic diverticulitis of the right colon such as acute appendicitis. Some clinical aspects must be considered in favor of an episode of acute diverticulitis. These include the presence of a previous history of diverticular disease in the right colon, Asian ethnicity, younger age (40–45 years), and the absence, or less prominent presence, of nausea and vomiting, [34–37]. Clinical examination reveals an inflammatory mass in the right lower quadrant in 30% of cases; diffuse peritonitis, large abscesses, and fistulae are rare. A CT scan, in addition to acute appendicitis, allows the differential diagnosis with other pathologies that mimic diverticulitis of the right colon including Meckel's diverticulitis, Crohn's disease, infectious colitis of the right colon (such as Yersinia), typhlitis, ileocecal tuberculosis, omental infarction, omental appendicitis, and abscesses or tumors of the psoas.

A recent study [38] has compared the clinical features of right-side with those of left-side acute diverticulitis. Patients with acute diverticulitis of the right colon were younger, more likely to be male, taller, had a lower body mass index, and less advanced modified Hinchey stages. Although it seems that the proportion of left acute colonic diverticulitis seems to be increasing in some Asiatic populations, such as the Japanese [39], the different clinical features between right and left colonic diverticulitis seem to be similar to those describe above.

References

1. Tursi A, Scarpignato C, Strate LL, Lanas A, Kruis W, Lahat A, et al. Colonic diverticular disease. Nat Rev Dis Primers. 2020;6(1):20.
2. Turner GA, O'Grady MJ, Purcell RV, Frizelle FA. Acute diverticulitis in young patients: a review of the changing epidemiology and etiology. Dig Dis Sci. 2021; https://doi.org/10.1007/s10620-021-06956-w. Epub ahead of print
3. Swanson SM, Strate LL. Acute Colonic Diverticulitis. Ann Intern Med. 2018;168(9):ITC65–80.
4. Peery AF, Crockett SD, Barritt AS, Dellon ES, Eluri S, Gangarosa LM, et al. Burden of gastrointestinal, liver, and pancreatic diseases in the United States. Gastroenterology. 2015;149(7):1731–1741.e3.
5. Bharucha AE, Parthasarathy G, Ditah I, Fletcher JG, Ewelukwa O, Pendlimari R, et al. Temporal Trends in the Incidence and Natural History of Diverticulitis: A Population-Based Study. Am J Gastroenterol. 2015 Nov;110(11):1589–96.
6. Hammond NA, Nikolaidis P, Miller FH. Left lower-quadrant pain: guidelines from the American College of Radiology appropriateness criteria. Am Fam Physician. 2010;82:766–70.
7. Rafferty J, Shellito P, Hyman NH. Standards Committee of the American Society of colon and Rectal surgeons. Practice parameters for sigmoid diverticulitis. Dis Colon Rectum. 2006;49:939–44.
8. Jacobs DO. Diverticulitis. N Engl J Med. 2007;357:2057–66.
9. Pesce A, Barchitta M, Agodi A, Salerno M, La Greca G, Magro G, Latteri S, Puleo S. Comparison of clinical and pathological findings of patients undergoing elective colectomy for uncomplicated diverticulitis. Sci Rep. 2020;10(1):8854. https://doi.org/10.1038/s41598-020-65727-1. PMID: 32483125; PMCID: PMC7264214
10. Longstreth GF, Iyer RL, Chu LH, Chen W, Yen LS, Hodgkins P, Kawatkar AA. Acute diverticulitis: demographic, clinical and laboratory features associated with computed tomography findings in 741 patients. Aliment Pharmacol Ther. 2012;36(9):886–94. https://doi.org/10.1111/apt.12047. PMID: 22967027
11. Iyer R, Longstreth GF, Chu LH, Chen W, Yen L, Hodgkins P, Kawatkar AA. Acute colonic diverticulitis: diagnostic evidence, demographic and clinical features in three practice settings. J Gastrointestin Liver Dis. 2014;23(4):379–86. https://doi.org/10.15403/jgld.2014.1121.234.acdd.
12. Laméris W, van Randen A, van Gulik TM, Busch OR, Winkelhagen J, Bossuyt PM, Stoker J, Boermeester MA. A clinical decision rule to establish the diagnosis of acute diverticulitis at the emergency department. Dis Colon Rectum. 2010;53(6):896–904. https://doi.org/10.1007/DCR.0b013e3181d98d86.
13. Strate LL, Morris AM. Epidemiology, pathophysiology, and treatment of diverticulitis. Gastroenterology. 2019;156(5):1282–1298.e1. https://doi.org/10.1053/j.gastro.2018.12.033. Epub 2019 Jan 17. PMID: 30660732; PMCID: PMC6716971.
14. Cirocchi R, Popivanov G, Corsi A, Amato A, Nascimbeni R, Cuomo R, Annibale B, Konaktchieva M, Binda GA. The trends of complicated acute colonic diverticulitis-a systematic review of the National Administrative Databases. Medicina (Kaunas). 2019;55(11):744. https://doi.org/10.3390/medicina55110744. PMID: 31744067; PMCID: PMC6915450
15. Mari GM, Crippa J, Borroni G, Cocozza E, Roscio F, Scandroglio I, Origi M, Ferrari G, Forgione A, Riggio V, Pugliese R, Costanzi ATM, Maggioni D. On behalf of the AIMS academy clinical research network. Symptomatic uncomplicated diverticular disease and incidence of unexpected abscess during Sigmoidectomy: a multicenter prospective observational study.

Dig Surg. 2020;37(3):199–204. https://doi.org/10.1159/000500084. Epub 2019 May 22. PMID: 31117071
16. Woods RJ, Lavery IC, Fazio VW, Jagelman DG, Weakley FL. Internal fistulas in diverticular disease. Dis Colon Rectum. 1988;31(8):591–6. https://doi.org/10.1007/BF02556792.
17. McBeath RB, Schiff M Jr, Allen V, Bottaccini MR, Miller JI, Ehreth JT. A 12-year experience with enterovesical fistulas. Urology. 1994;44(5):661–5. https://doi.org/10.1016/s0090-4295(94)80200-9.
18. Humes DJ, West J. Role of acute diverticulitis in the development of complicated colonic diverticular disease and 1-year mortality after diagnosis in the UK: population-based cohort study. Gut. 2012;61(1):95–100. https://doi.org/10.1136/gut.2011.238808. Epub 2011 May 6
19. Zaidi E, Daly B. CT and clinical features of acute diverticulitis in an urban U.S. population: rising frequency in young, obese adults. AJR Am J Roentgenol. 2006;187(3):689–94. https://doi.org/10.2214/AJR.05.0033. PMID: 16928931
20. Covino M, Rosa F, Ojetti V, Quero G, Fiorillo C, Sganga G, Gasbarrini A, Franceschi F, Alfieri S. Acute diverticulitis in elderly patients: does age really matter? Dig Dis. 2021;39(1):33–41. https://doi.org/10.1159/000509049. Epub 2020 Jun 2. PMID: 32485716
21. Tan JPL, Barazanchi AWH, Singh PP, Hill AG, Maccormick AD. Predictors of acute diverticulitis severity: a systematic review. Int J Surg. 2016;26:43–521.
22. Kvasnovsky CL, Papagrigoriadis S, Bjarnason I. Increased diverticular complications with nonsteroidal anti-inflammatory drugs and other medications: a systematic review and meta-analysis. Color Dis. 2014;16(6):O189–96.
23. van de Wall BJ, Poerink JA, Draaisma WA, Reitsma JB, Consten EC, Broeders IA. Diverticulitis in young versus elderly patients: a meta-analysis. Scand J Gastroenterol. 2013;48(6):643–51. https://doi.org/10.3109/00365521.2012.758765. Epub 2013 Jan 21
24. Katz LH, Guy DD, Lahat A, Gafter-Gvili A, Bar-Meir S. Diverticulitis in the young is not more aggressive than in the elderly, but it tends to recur more often: systematic review and meta-analysis. J Gastroenterol Hepatol. 2013;28:1274–81.
25. Shah AM, Malhotra A, Patel B, Spira R, DePasquale JR, Baddoura W. Acute diverticulitis in the young: a 5-year retrospective study of risk factors, clinical presentation and complications. Color Dis. 2011;13(10):1158–61. https://doi.org/10.1111/j.1463-1318.2010.02372.x. Epub 2010 Jul 14
26. Schweitzer J, Casillas RA, Collins JC. Acute diverticulitis in the young adult is not "virulent.". Am Surg. 2002;68(12):1044–7. PMID: 12516805
27. Serrano González J, Lucena de la Poza JL, García R, de León L, García Schiever JG, Farhangmehr Setayeshi N, Calvo Espino P, Sánchez Movilla A. Sánchez Turrión V. diverticulitis in immunodeficient patients: our experience in the management of high-risk patients. Rev Esp Enferm Dig. 2020;112(1):47–52. https://doi.org/10.17235/reed.2019.6281/2019. PMID: 31830795
28. Hwang SS, Cannom RR, Abbas MA, Etzioni D. Diverticulitis in transplant patients and patients on chronic corticosteroid therapy: a systematic review. Dis Colon Rectum. 2010;53(12):1699–707. https://doi.org/10.1007/DCR.0b013e3181f5643c. PMID: 21178867
29. Oor JE, Atema JJ, Boermeester MA, Vrouenraets BC, Ünlü Ç. A systematic review of complicated diverticulitis in post-transplant patients. J Gastrointest Surg. 2014;18(11):2038–46. https://doi.org/10.1007/s11605-014-2593-2. Epub 2014 Aug 16
30. Reshef A, Stocchi L, Kiran RP, Flechner S, Budev M, Quintini C, Remzi FH. Case-matched comparison of perioperative outcomes after surgical treatment of sigmoid diverticulitis in solid organ transplant recipients versus immunocompetent patients. Color Dis. 2012;14(12):1546–52. https://doi.org/10.1111/j.1463-1318.2012.03077.x. PMID: 22564266
31. Biondo S, Borao JL, Kreisler E, Golda T, Millan M, Frago R, Fraccalvieri D, Guardiola J, Jaurrieta E. Recurrence and virulence of colonic diverticulitis in immunocompromised patients. Am J Surg. 2012;204(2):172–9. https://doi.org/10.1016/j.amjsurg.2011.09.027. Epub 2012 Mar 23
32. Sachar DB. Diverticulitis in immunosuppressed patients. J Clin Gastroenterol. 2008;42:1154–5.

33. Cronley K, Wenzke J, Hussan H, Vasquez AM, Hinton A, El-Dika S, Conwell DL, Krishna SG, Stanich PP. Diverticulitis in HIV-infected patients within the United States. HIV Med. 2016;17(3):216–21. https://doi.org/10.1111/hiv.12304.
34. Lê P, Blondon H, Billey C. Right colon diverticulitis. J Chir (Paris). 2004;141(1):11–20. https://doi.org/10.1016/s0021-7697(04)95288-x. PMID: 15029058 Review. French
35. Fortuny JV, Buchs NC, Morel P, Ris F. Right-sided colonic diverticular disease: quo vadis? Rev med Suisse. 2014;10(435):1325–30. PMID: 25051594 review. French
36. Ferrara F, Bollo J, Vanni LV, Targarona EM. Diagnosis and management of right colonic diverticular disease: a review. Cir Esp. 2016;94(10):553–9. https://doi.org/10.1016/j.ciresp.2016.08.008. Epub 2016 Nov 5. PMID: 27823760
37. Imaeda H, Hibi T. The burden of diverticular disease and its complications: West versus east. Inflamm Intest Dis. 2018;3(2):61–8. https://doi.org/10.1159/000492178. Epub 2018 Aug 7. PMID: 30733949
38. Lee KY, Lee J, Park YY, Kim Y, Oh ST. Difference in clinical features between right- and left-sided acute colonic diverticulitis. Sci Rep. 2020;10(1):3754. https://doi.org/10.1038/s41598-020-60397-5. PMID: 32111862; PMCID: PMC7048749
39. Mizuki A, Tatemichi M, Nakazawa A, Tsukada N, Nagata H, Kanai T. Changes in the clinical features and long-term outcomes of colonic diverticulitis in japanese patients. Intern Med. 2017;56(22):2971–7. https://doi.org/10.2169/internalmedicine.7710-16. Epub 2017 Oct 11. PMID: 29021428; PMCID: PMC5725849

Diverticular Bleeding

10

Marcello Picchio and Eiji Yamada

10.1 Introduction

Colonic diverticular bleeding (CDB) is the most common cause of lower gastrointestinal hemorrhage. A recent large population-based study reported an incidence of 14/100,000 inhabitants per year, although the diagnosis is mostly presumptive in the presence of colonic diverticula without any other detected source of bleeding [1]. Approximately 70–80% of diverticular bleedings stop spontaneously, but rebleeding occurs in up to 38% of patients [2]. In an older population, CDB can lead to significant morbidity, especially in those with hemodynamic instability and comorbid conditions, such as hypertension, diabetes mellitus, chronic obstructive pulmonary disease, chronic renal insufficiency, and coronary artery disease [3]. In spite of continuous improvement in both diagnostic and therapeutic approaches, CDB management remains challenging, due to the persisting low rate of bleeding site identification and a relatively high rate of rebleeding after achieving hemostasis.

10.2 Pathogenesis and Risk Factors

The pathogenesis of diverticular bleeding is not completely understood, but one common theory is that it originates over time because of repetitive injury to the *vasa recta* as they pass through the muscular layer to drape over the dome of the

M. Picchio (✉)
Division of General Surgery, "P. Colombo" Hospital, ASL Roma 6, Velletri (Roma), Italy
e-mail: marcello.picchio.63@alice.it

E. Yamada
Gastroenterology Division, National Hospital Organization Yokohama Medical Center, Yokohama-shi, Kanagawa, Japan
e-mail: eiji_age_h_oceanblue@yahoo.co.jp

© The Author(s), under exclusive license to Springer Nature Switzerland AG 2022

A. Tursi et al. (eds.), *Colonic Diverticular Disease*,
https://doi.org/10.1007/978-3-030-93761-4_10

diverticulum [4]. Older age was found to be related to an increased incidence of CDB [5, 6]. A possible explanation is that arteriosclerosis, which commonly accompanies aging, weakens the arterial wall of the vasa recta, thus predisposing them to traumatic rupture.

Data regarding the use of concurrent drugs and risk of developing CDB have been widely reported in the literature. Two systematic reviews with meta-analysis showed increased odds of bleeding from use of aspirin and other nonsteroidal anti-inflammatory drugs [7, 8]. More recently, use of antiplatelets, but not anticoagulants, has been reported to be associated with increased risk of bleeding [9].

10.3 Diagnosis

CDB usually presents with acute-onset painless hematochezia [10]. Patients may rarely present with mild abdominal cramping or the urge to defecate. The stool may be bright red to dark maroon in color [11]. If hematochezia is abundant, nasogastric lavage should be performed to exclude an upper gastrointestinal source [12].

At initial clinical assessment, vital signs such as state of consciousness, blood pressure, and heart rate should be evaluated to assess the hemodynamic status of the patient.

Contemporarily, thorough medication history, with particular attention to anticoagulants, antiplatelets, and nonsteroidal anti-inflammatory drugs (NSAIDs), it is important to predict the risk of rebleeding and for management, as well as the presence of comorbidities, such as chronic kidney disease, cirrhosis, hypertension, and diabetes [13, 14].

Blood tests (e.g., hemoglobin, hematocrit, prothrombin time international normalized ratio, blood urea nitrogen, and creatinine) are useful to determine the indication for admission, intensive care, and timing of tests. In particular, in patients with severe hematochezia, the ratio of blood urea nitrogen and creatinine was found to be useful in the differential diagnosis of upper gastrointestinal tract bleeding. According to a meta-analysis, upper gastrointestinal tract bleeding is likely with a ratio ≥ 30 [15].

Colonoscopy, CT, angiography, and abdominal US are commonly used to diagnose CDB. CDB diagnosis has evolved during the last decade with the constant use of CT helical angiography. In patients with CDB, contrast-enhanced CT is advised before colonoscopy because identifying the source of bleeding prior to surgery may result in a less-invasive urgent colonoscopy and more effective hemostasis [16] (Fig. 10.1).

Colonoscopy, unlike CT angiography and other noninvasive diagnostic tools, enables treatment directly after diagnosis. Considering both the diagnostic and therapeutic outcomes of colonoscopy, its use is associated with lower medical costs [17].

CBD is difficult to diagnose by abdominal ultrasound; however, it may be an effective screening method for lower gastrointestinal bleeding because it does not require bowel preparation and is not associated with radiation exposure [18].

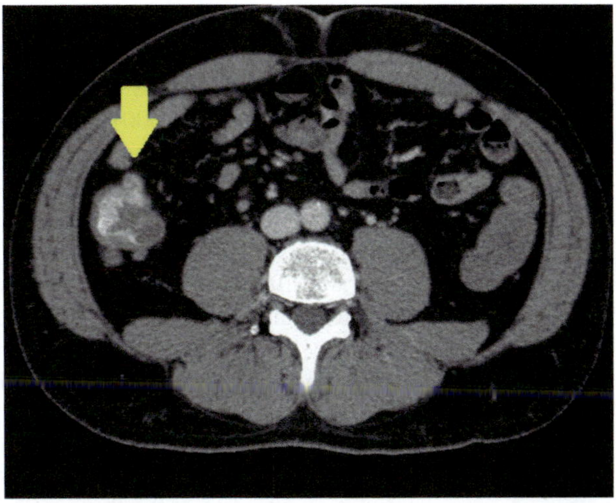

Fig. 10.1 (**a**) *Enhanced computed tomography image showing extravasation in the ascending colon* (arrow)

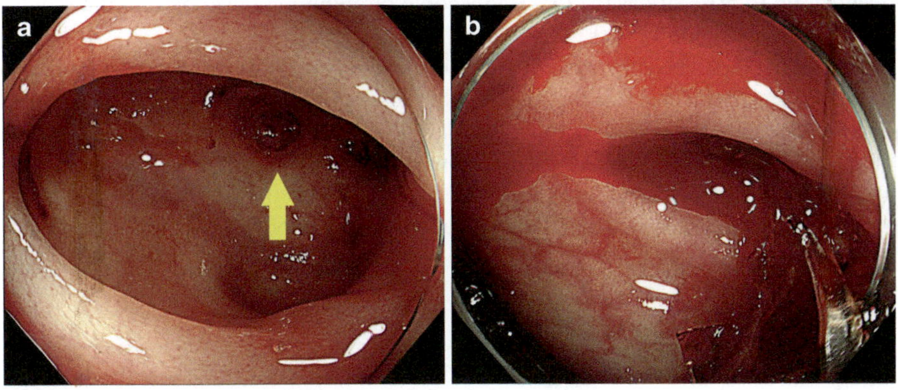

Fig. 10.2 (**a**) *Nonbleeding visible vessel at the base* of a *diverticulum* (arrow). (**b**) Active bleeding during endoscopic hemostasis

10.4 Treatment

The management of CDB has evolved in the last 10 years with the introduction of interventional endoscopy and angiographic treatment.

10.4.1 Endoscopic Hemostasis

Endoscopic treatment is indicated when the following stigmata of hemorrhage are detected: active bleeding, nonbleeding visible vessels, and adherent clot underlying them [19] (Fig. 10.2a, b).

With many options to achieve endoscopic hemostasis, it is first important to determine the appropriate method.

One option to achieve endoscopic hemostasis includes a four-quadrant submucosal injection of dilute epinephrine (1:10000). Epinephrine injection therapy alone can show vasoconstrictive and mechanical effects, often providing only temporary cessation of hemorrhage with significant risk of early rebleeding within 30 days [20]. Therefore, epinephrine injection therapy should be used concurrently with other modalities [21, 22].

Endoscopic clipping is a diffuse method because it induces less tissue injury than other endoscopic modalities and enables continued treatment without withdrawal of the colonoscope. Clips may be directly applied on the visible source of bleeding or they may be used to close the opening of the bleeding diverticula. Direct clipping of the exposed vessel or erosions is more effective than clipping of the entire diverticular orifice [23]. However, because colonic diverticular bleeding often occurs at the base of the diverticulum, clipping hemostasis is often difficult to be achieved [24]. Primary hemostasis can be achieved in 83–100% of cases, but early rebleeding may occur in up to 50% of cases [25]. Endoscopic clipping may also be combined with epinephrine injection [26] (Fig. 10.3).

An over-the-scope clip system (Ovesco Endoscopy AG, Tübingen, Germany) has been designed for a full-thickness tight closure using saw-like teeth of a shark. It allows secure anchoring within the normal tissue surrounding the neck of the bleeding diverticulum (Fig. 10.4a–c). However, it is very expensive and cannot be applied on firm diverticula that cannot be sufficiently suctioned [27].

Endoscopic band ligation (EBL) can be a secure method, allowing a tight closure of the bleeding site.

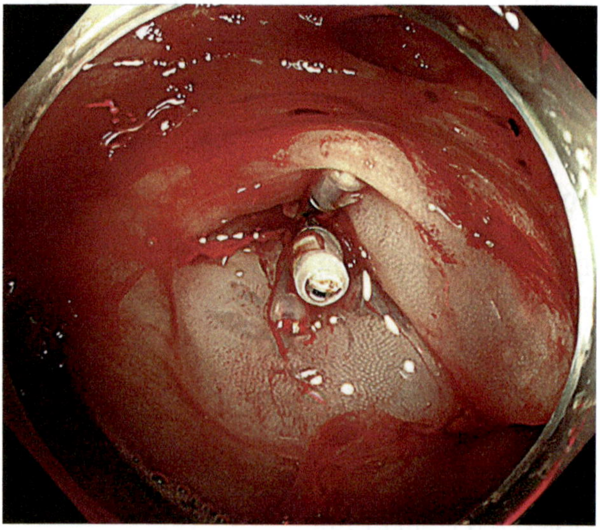

Fig. 10.3 Combination therapy with epinephrine injection and endoscopic clipping

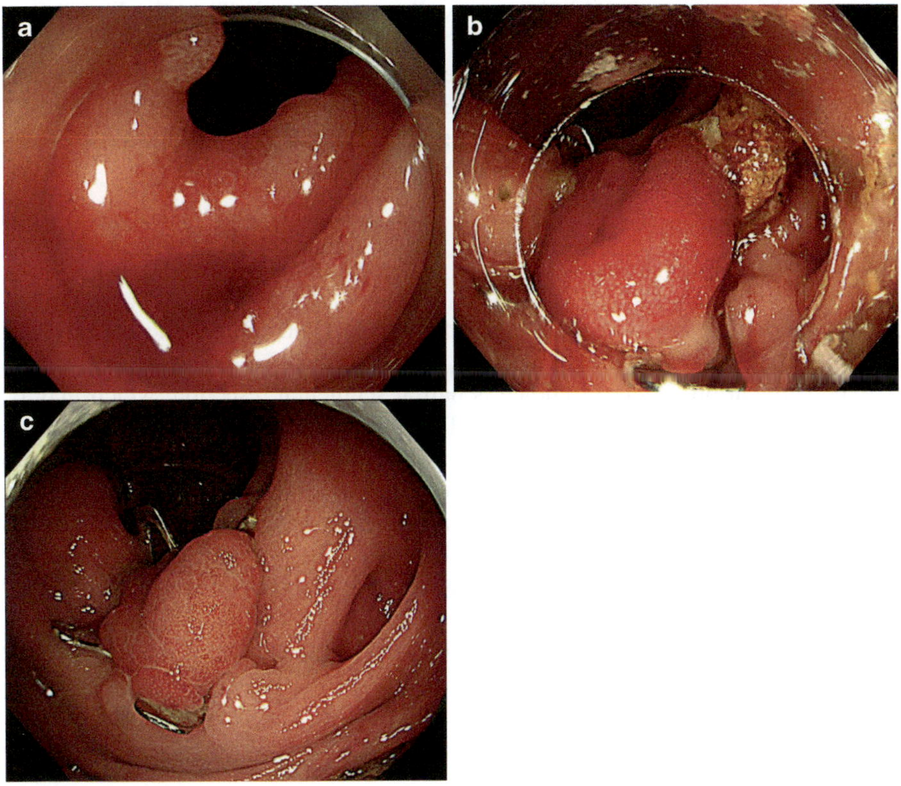

Fig. 10.4 (**a**, **b**) Use of an *OTSC* for *diverticular bleeding*. (**c**) Endoscopic hemostasis using an OTSC after a month

EBL has been proven to be more effective in decreasing rebleeding when compared with endoscopic clipping [28]. However, a delayed perforation might develop as a rare complication of EBL [29].

10.4.2 Arterial Embolization

Interventional radiology should be considered in patients with ongoing bleeding who do not respond adequately to hemodynamic resuscitation efforts and are, therefore, unlikely to tolerate bowel preparation and urgent colonoscopy [10]. Moreover, it may be used when endoscopic hemostasis fails or rebleeding occurs after endoscopic therapy [24].

A variety of materials can be used for embolization with no significant difference among them. The most frequently used materials are coils and polyvinyl alcohol particles. When performing arterial embolization, it is absolutely necessary to identify the site of bleeding on angiography and it should be performed as close to the source of bleeding as possible because collateralization distal to the ligament of Treitz is not adequate to avoid the risk of infarction.

The success rate of embolization is reported to be 70–90% [10, 30]. Intestinal ischemia is a complication specific to arterial embolization, occurring in up to 10% of patients [31, 32]. It is also important to pay attention to contrast-induced nephropathy and other side effects associated with contrast media.

10.4.3 Surgery

Emergency colectomy is recommended for severe CDB after unsuccessful endoscopic therapy or arterial embolization.

The surgical procedure of choice is partial segmental resection, which may be performed when the bleeding site is localized before surgery. A subtotal colectomy performed for nonlocalized lower gastrointestinal tract bleeding is associated with increased morbidity (37%) and mortality (11–33%), and it should be indicated only in patients with uncontrolled massive hemorrhage, when there are no alternatives [33]. The rebleeding rate in one study with a mean follow-up of 1 year was zero for subtotal colectomy, 14% for segmental resection with localization of bleeding, and 42% with segmental resection with nonlocalization of bleeding [34].

Elective resection should be considered in patients with recurrent diverticular bleeding.

References

1. Olafsson GD, Hreinsson JP, Björnsson ES. Incidence of diverticular bleeding: a population-based study. Scand J Gastroenterol. 2019;54:205–9. https://doi.org/10.1080/00365521.2019.1566494.
2. Raphaeli T, Menon R. Current treatment of lower gastrointestinal hemorrhage. Clin Colon Rectal Surg. 2012;25:219–27. https://doi.org/10.1055/s-0032-1329393.
3. Strate LL, Orav EJ, Syngal S. Early predictors of severity in acute lower intestinal tract bleeding. Arch Intern Med. 2003;163:838–43. https://doi.org/10.1001/archinte.163.7.838.
4. Meyers MA, Alonso DR, Gray GF, Baer JW. Pathogenesis of bleeding colonic diverticulosis. Gastroenterology. 1976;71:577–83.
5. Carabotti M, Morselli Labate AM, Cremon C, Cuomo R, Pace F, Andreozzi P, et al. REMAD group. Distinguishing features between patients with acute diverticulitis and diverticular bleeding: results from the REMAD registry. Dig Liver Dis. 2021;53:202–9. https://doi.org/10.1016/j.dld.2020.05.045.
6. Urabe M, Nishida T, Shimakoshi H, Shimoda A, Amano T, Sugimoto A, et al. Distinct clinical factors in hospitalized patients with diverticular bleeding and diverticulitis. Digestion. 2019;99:239–46. https://doi.org/10.1159/000491875.
7. Kvasnovsky CL, Papagrigoriadis S, Bjarnason I. Increased diverticular complications with nonsteriodal anti-inflammatory drugs and other medications: a systematic review and meta-analysis. Color Dis. 2014;16:O189–96. https://doi.org/10.1111/codi.12516.
8. Yuhara H, Corley DA, Nakahara F, Nakajima T, Koike J, Igarashi M, eta al. Aspirin and non-aspirin NSAIDs increase risk of colonic diverticular bleeding: a systematic review and meta-analysis. J Gastroenterol. 2014;49:992–1000. https://doi.org/10.1007/s00535-013-0905-z.

9. Nagata N, Niikura R, Aoki T, Shimbo T, Kishida Y, Sekine K, et al. Colonic diverticular hemorrhage associated with the use of nonsteroidal anti-inflammatory drugs, low-dose aspirin, antiplatelet drugs, and dual therapy. J Gastroenterol Hepatol. 2014;29:1786–93. https://doi.org/10.1111/jgh.12595.
10. Strate LL, Gralnek IM. ACG clinical guideline: Management of Patients with Acute Lower Gastrointestinal Bleeding. Am J Gastroenterol. 2016;111:459–74. https://doi.org/10.1038/ajg.2016.41.
11. Fine KD, Nelson AC, Ellington RT, Mossburg A. Comparison of the color of fecal blood with the anatomical location of gastrointestinal bleeding lesions: potential misdiagnosis using only flexible sigmoidoscopy for bright red blood per rectum. Am J Gastroenterol. 1999;94:3202–10. https://doi.org/10.1111/j.1572-0241.1999.01519.x.
12. Hwang JH, Fisher DA, Ben-Menachem T, Chandrasekhara V, Chathadi K, Decker GA, et al. Practice Committee of the American Society for gastrointestinal endoscopy. The role of endoscopy in the management of acute non-variceal upper GI bleeding. Gastrointest Endosc. 2012;75:1132–8. https://doi.org/10.1016/j.gie.2012.02.033.
13. Aoki T, Nagata N, Shimbo T, Niikura R, Sakurai T, Moriyasu S, et al. Development and validation of a risk scoring system for severe acute lower gastrointestinal bleeding. Clin Gastroenterol Hepatol. 2016;14:1562–70.e2. https://doi.org/10.1016/j.cgh.2016.05.042.
14. Das A, Ben-Menachem T, Cooper GS, Chak A, Sivak MV Jr, Gonet JA, et al. Prediction of outcome in acute lower-gastrointestinal haemorrhage based on an artificial neural network: internal and external validation of a predictive model. Lancet. 2003;362:1261–6. https://doi.org/10.1016/S0140-6736(03)14568-0.
15. Srygley FD, Gerardo CJ, Tran T, Fisher DA. Does this patient have a severe upper gastrointestinal bleed? JAMA. 2012;307:1072–9. https://doi.org/10.1001/jama.2012.253.
16. Nakatsu S, Yasuda H, Maehata T, Nomoto M, Ohinata N, Hosoya K, et al. Urgent computed tomography for determining the optimal timing of colonoscopy in patients with acute lower gastrointestinal bleeding. Intern Med. 2015;54:553–8. https://doi.org/10.2169/internalmedicine.54.2829.
17. Strate LL, Syngal S. Predictors of utilization of early colonoscopy vs. radiography for severe lower intestinal bleeding. Gastrointest Endosc. 2005;61:46–52. https://doi.org/10.1016/s0016-5107(04)02227-8.
18. Yamaguchi T, Manabe N, Hata J, Tanaka S, Haruma K, Chayama K. The usefulness of transabdominal ultrasound for the diagnosis of lower gastrointestinal bleeding. Aliment Pharmacol Ther. 2006;23:1267–72. https://doi.org/10.1111/j.1365-2036.2006.02883.x.
19. Nagata N, Ishii N, Manabe N, Tomizawa K, Urita Y, Funabiki T, et al. Guidelines for colonic diverticular bleeding and colonic diverticulitis: Japan gastroenterological association. Digestion. 2019;99(Suppl 1):1–26. https://doi.org/10.1159/000495282.
20. Bloomfeld RS, Rockey DC, Shetzline MA. Endoscopic therapy of acute diverticular hemorrhage. Am J Gastroenterol. 2001;96:2367–72. https://doi.org/10.1111/j.1572-0241.2001.04048.x.
21. Kaltenbach T, Watson R, Shah J, Friedland S, Sato T, Shergill A, et al. Colonoscopy with clipping is useful in the diagnosis and treatment of diverticular bleeding. Clin Gastroenterol Hepatol. 2012;10:131–7. https://doi.org/10.1016/j.cgh.2011.10.029.
22. Jensen DM, Machicado GA, Jutabha R, Kovacs TO. Urgent colonoscopy for the diagnosis and treatment of severe diverticular hemorrhage. N Engl J Med. 2000;342:78–82. https://doi.org/10.1056/NEJM200001133420202.
23. Kominami Y, Ohe H, Kobayashi S, Higashi R, Uchida D, Morimoto Y, et al. Classification of the bleeding pattern in colonic diverticulum is useful to predict the risk of bleeding or re-bleeding after endoscopic treatment. Nihon Shokakibyo Gakkai Zasshi. 2012;109:393–9. Japanese
24. Ishii N, Hirata N, Omata F, Itoh T, Uemura M, Matsuda M, et al. Location in the ascending colon is a predictor of refractory colonic diverticular hemorrhage after endoscopic clipping. Gastrointest Endosc. 2012;76:1175–81. https://doi.org/10.1016/j.gie.2012.07.040.

25. Kaise M, Nagata N, Ishii N, Omori J, Goto O, Iwakiri K. Epidemiology of colonic diverticula and recent advances in the management of colonic diverticular bleeding. Dig Endosc. 2020;32:240–50. https://doi.org/10.1111/den.13547.
26. Couto-Worner I, González-Conde B, Estévez-Prieto E, Alonso-Aguirre P. Colonic diverticular bleeding: urgent colonoscopy without purging and endoscopic treatment with epinephrine and hemoclips. Rev Esp Enferm Dig. 2013;105:495–8. https://doi.org/10.4321/s1130-01082013000800010.
27. Wedi E, von Renteln D, Jung C, Tchoumak I, Roth V, Gonzales S, et al. Treatment of acute colonic diverticular bleeding in high risk patients, using an over-the-scope clip: a case series. Endoscopy. 2016;48(S01):E383–5. https://doi.org/10.1055/s-0042-118168.
28. Nagata N, Niikura R, Ishii N, Kaise M, Omata F, Tominaga N, et al. Cumulative evidence for reducing recurrence of colonic diverticular bleeding using endoscopic clipping versus band ligation: systematic review and meta-analysis. J Gastroenterol Hepatol. 2021;36(7):1738–43. https://doi.org/10.1111/jgh.15370.
29. Sato Y, Yasuda H, Fukuoka A, Kiyokawa H, Kato M, Yamashita M, et al. Delayed perforation after endoscopic band ligation for colonic diverticular hemorrhage. Clin J Gastroenterol. 2020;13:6–10. https://doi.org/10.1007/s12328-019-01027-0.
30. Gillespie CJ, Sutherland AD, Mossop PJ, Woods RJ, Keck JO, Heriot AG. Mesenteric embolization for lower gastrointestinal bleeding. Dis Colon Rectum. 2010;53:1258–64. https://doi.org/10.1007/DCR.0b013e3181e10e90.
31. Maleux G, Roeflaer F, Heye S, Vandersmissen J, Vliegen AS, Demedts I, et al. Long-term outcome of transcatheter embolotherapy for acute lower gastrointestinal hemorrhage. Am J Gastroenterol. 2009;104:2042–6. https://doi.org/10.1038/ajg.2009.186.
32. Adusumilli S, Gosselink MP, Ctercteko G, Pathmanathan N, El-Khoury T, Dutton P, et al. The efficacy of selective arterial embolization in the management of colonic bleeding. Tech Coloproctol. 2014;18:529–33. https://doi.org/10.1007/s10151-013-1088-6.
33. Mohammed Ilyas MI, Szilagy EJ. Management of diverticular bleeding: evaluation, stabilization, intervention, and recurrence of bleeding and indications for resection after control of bleeding. Clin Colon Rectal Surg. 2018;31:243–50. https://doi.org/10.1055/s-0037-1607963.
34. Parkes BM, Obeid FN, Sorensen VJ, Horst HM, Fath JJ. The management of massive lower gastrointestinal bleeding. Am Surg. 1993;59:676–8.

Segmental Colitis Associated with Diverticulosis

11

Silvio Danese and Adi Lahat

11.1 Introduction

Segmental colitis associated with diverticulosis (SCAD) is a defined pathological entity characterized by an inflammatory process engaging the inter-diverticular mucosa of the colonic segment involved. The rectum and the right colon are spared from inflammation [1].

Limitation of the mucosal lesion to the diverticular segment is the most important diagnostic criterion for SCAD (rectal sparing). Rectal and descending colon biopsies are required to distinguish SCAD from inflammatory bowel disease (IBD) [1].

The disease is relatively rare, with a prevalence of 0.25–1.4% in the general population and 1.15–11.4% amongst diverticular disease (DD) patients. The mean age at diagnosis is early to mid-60s, with a slightly higher male preponderance [2–4]. The pathogenesis is multifactorial and includes genetic susceptibility, alternation in the bowel microbiome, local ischemia, mucosal prolapse, and recurrent acute diverticulitis attacks [5–8].

The clinical presentation as well as the endoscopic and histological appearance vary among four major subtypes and resemble IBD.

SCAD type A (Fig. 11.1) is endoscopically characterized by red patches involving the colonic folds and diverticular sparing with neutrophil and lymphocyte

S. Danese (✉)
Gastroenterology and Endoscopy, IRCCS Ospedale "San Raffaele", "Vita-Salute San Raffaele" University, Milan, Italy
e-mail: sdanese@hotmail.com

A. Lahat
Department of Gastroenterology, Chaim Sheba Medical Center, Tel Hashomer, Ramat Gan 52651, and Sackler Medical School, Tel Aviv University, Tel Aviv, Israel
e-mail: zokadi@gmail.com

© The Author(s), under exclusive license to Springer Nature Switzerland AG 2022
A. Tursi et al. (eds.), *Colonic Diverticular Disease*,
https://doi.org/10.1007/978-3-030-93761-4_11

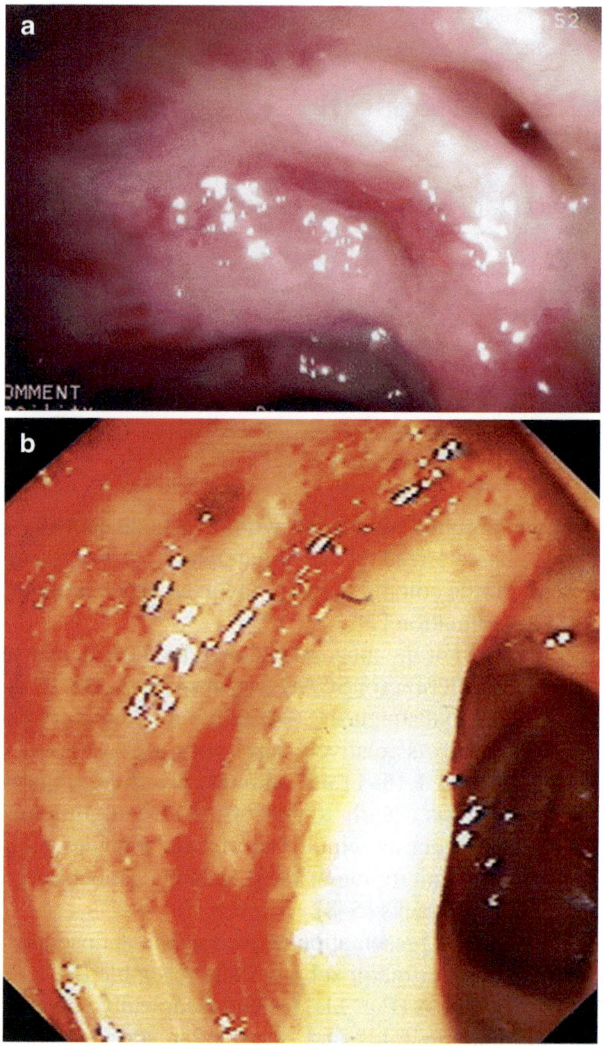

Fig. 11.1 (**a**, **b**) SCAD type A. Red stains involve the colonic folds, and the diverticular orifices are spared. (Tursi A, Elisei W et al. Segmental colitis associated with diverticulosis: a 5-year follow-up. Int J Colorectal Dis. 2012 Feb;27(2):179–85)

infiltrates limited to the crypt epithelium histologically. SCAD types B and D are both characterized by ulcerative colitis (UC)-like changes endoscopically and histologically, with erosions and hyperemic areas in the affected mucosa.

While in SCAD type B (Fig. 11.2), inflammation is milder, type D correlates with severe disease, and the inflammation includes diffuse ulceration and narrowing of the bowel lumen [6–10]. (Fig. 11.3). In these severe cases, the differential diagnosis of ulcerative colitis (UC) is based on rectal sparing in SCAD compared to prominent rectal inflammation in UC.

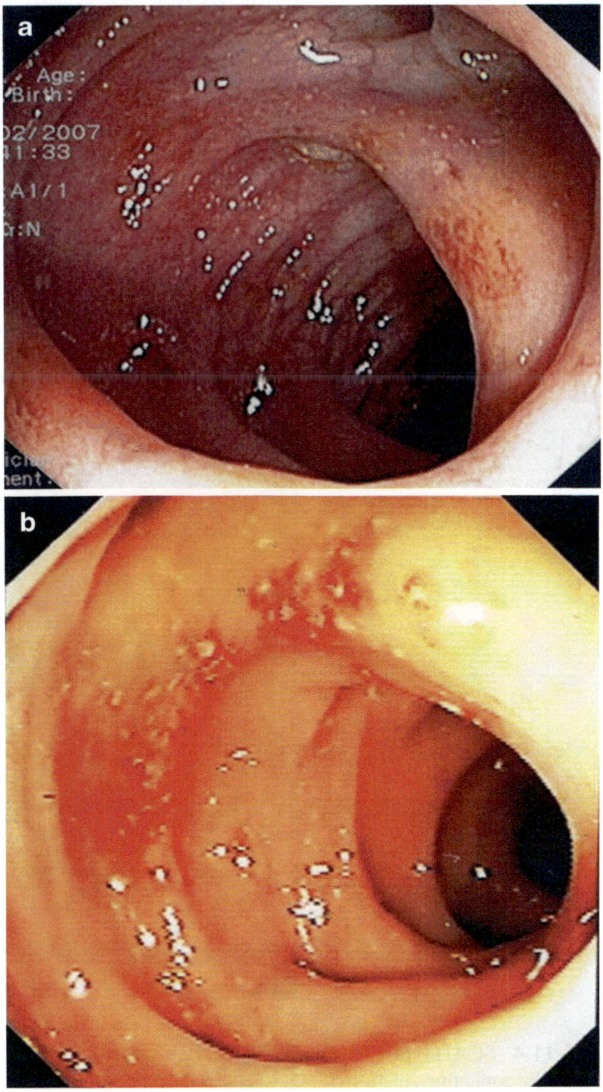

Fig. 11.2 (**a**, **b**) SCAD type B. Erosions and hyperemia affecting the colonic folds while the diverticular orifices are spared

Histological changes in both subtypes (B and D), similar to UC, involve crypt distortion and crypt abscesses [6–10].

SCAD type C is characterized by Crohn's disease-like changes, with isolated aphthous ulcers and transmural inflammatory changes (Fig. 11.4) [6–10].

Table 11.1 presents the typical endoscopic and histological presentations of all different SCAD subtypes.

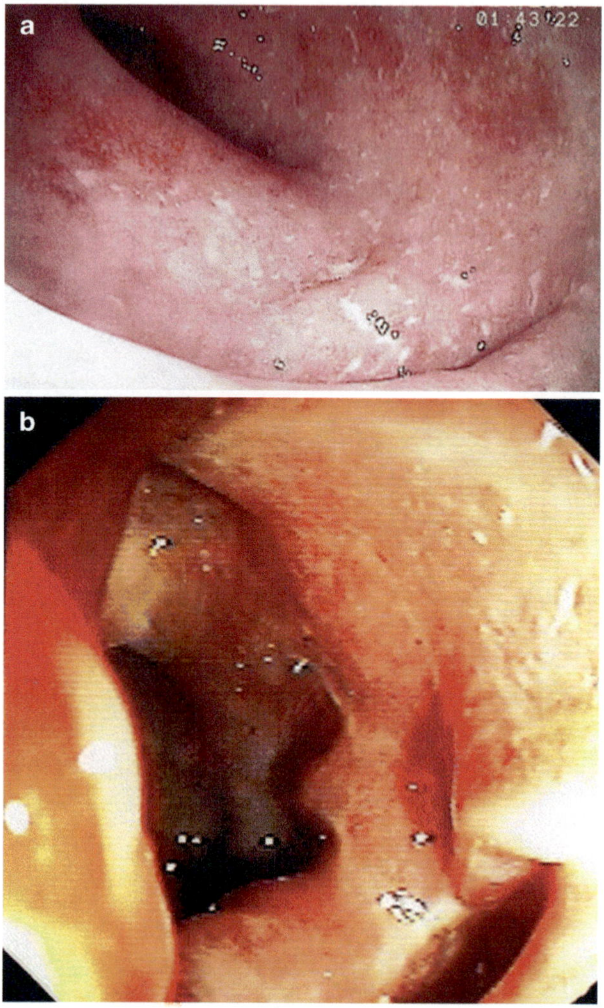

Fig. 11.3 SCAD type D. Diffuse mucosal inflammation affecting the entire diverticular area

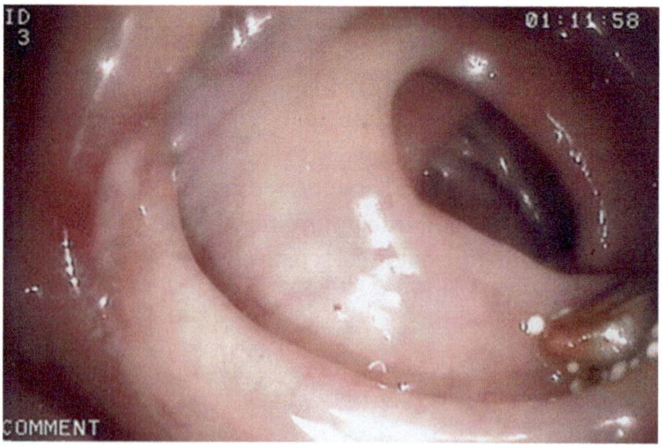

Fig. 11.4 SCAD type C. Endoscopic presentation is characterized by aphthous ulcers surrounded by a normal-looking mucosa

Table 11.1 SCAD subtypes: endoscopic and histological features. (From: Schembri J, Bonello J et al. Segmental colitis associated with diverticulosis: is it the coexistence of colonic diverticulosis and inflammatory bowel disease? Ann Gastroenterol. 2017;30(3):257–261)

Feature	Type			
	A	B	C	D
Pattern	Crescentic fold	Mild-to-moderate UC-like	CD-like	Severe UC-like
Macroscopic appearance	Red round lesions 0.5–1.5 cm at top of mucosal folds	Diffuse loss of vascular pattern, edema, hyperemia and pinpoint erosions	Isolated aphthous ulcers	As in B but more severe with diffuse ulceration and reduced caliber of lumen
Histological appearance	No architectural crypt distortion	Crypt distortion present together with Chronic changes in lamina propria	Highest variability. Transmucosal inflammation with microfissures	Crypt distortion present together with chronic changes in lamina propria
Cellular changes	Neutrophil and lymphocyte infiltrates limited to crypt epithelium	Crypt abscesses and goblet cell depletion	Lymphoid follicles and non-specific infiltrates	Crypt abscesses and goblet cell depletion
Diverticular sparing	Yes	Yes	Yes	Yes

CD Crohn's disease, *SCAD* segmental colitis associated with diverticulosis, *UC* ulcerative colitis

11.2 Clinical Presentation and Laboratory Markers

Similar to that of IBD, the clinical presentation of SCAD usually involves chronic diarrhea, abdominal pain, or rectal bleeding [11]. SCAD type may dictate symptoms, and while type A SCAD is usually presented with diarrhea, types B and D may present as rectal bleeding. However, unlike most IBD presentations, systemic symptoms such as fever, high white blood cell (WBC) count, and weight loss are rare. Furthermore, the disease course is usually milder than that of IBD, and, in many cases, patients experience full recovery after initial presentation with no further symptomatic relapses [12].

Disease type affects the prognosis, and while type A and type C SCAD may fully recover even without any specific medical treatment, types B and D, which resemble UC with more robust mucosal inflammation, have a higher risk of symptom recurrence and usually require treatment [10]. In rare cases, the disease might even progress to involve more colonic segments and become a full-blown UC [13, 14].

Laboratory studies in SCAD are usually normal, with a normal WBC count and negative serological markers such as perinuclear antineutrophil cytoplasmic antibodies (pANCAs) [15] or anti-*Saccharomyces cerevisiae* antibodies (ASCAs) [16], which are often positive in IBD. However, fecal calprotectin, which indicates migration of neutrophils to the bowel mucosa and by that functions as a marker of intestinal inflammation [17], is usually elevated [18].

11.3 Treatment

Treatment options are derived mainly from the clinical presentations and are built as a step-up ladder. Thus, first-line treatment is composed of antibiotic treatment – usually ciprofloxacin and metronidazole – for variable time periods depending on clinical improvement. Second-line therapy for nonresponders or remitters includes 5-ASA – first at a loading dose of up to 4 g per day, with dose reduction according to clinical response [19]. Another treatment option offered by Tursi et al. [20] suggests treatment with a combination of beclomethasone dipropionate (BDP) and the probiotic VSL#3 for 4 weeks, with the option of using 5-ASA for maintenance of remission [10]. Severe cases who do not respond to the initial treatment might require steroid treatment, with the use of steroid-sparing agents for maintenance of remission.

Data in the literature are scarce and mainly consist of only a few case reports.

As in IBD, the accepted steroid-sparing medications are azathioprine, 6-MP [10], and biological therapy – mainly anti-TNF-α agents such as infliximab and adalimumab [21, 22]. Notably, TNF-α was shown to be overexpressed in SCAD [23] and downregulated after successful treatment [24].

With regard to the current recommendations for IBD treatment in the elderly, considering potential side effects [25] and the fact that most SCAD patients are usually in that age group, we recommend considering an anti-TNF-α agent or vedolizumab (although not backed up by the current literature) rather that thiopurines as steroid-sparing treatment. Surgery is reserved for severe unresponsive cases [25]. Treatment duration might vary depending on the clinical presentation and response and can last for several weeks or months [26]. A schematic summary of a step-up treatment algorithm is shown in Fig. 11.5.

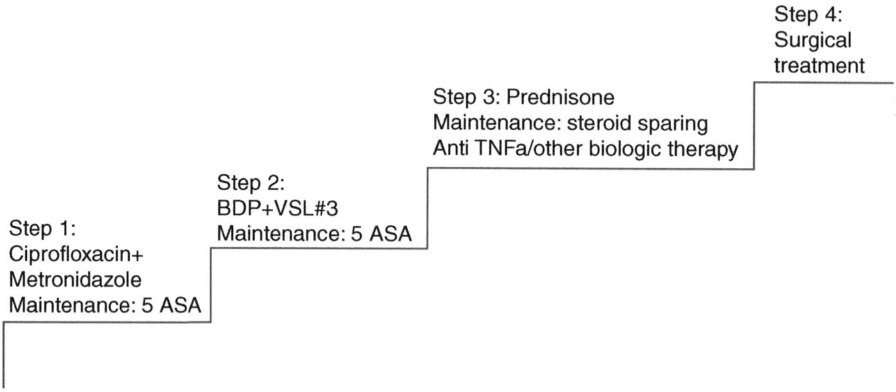

Fig. 11.5 Schematic of a step-up therapeutic algorithm. * BDP: beclomethasone dipropionate # 5-ASA: 5-aminosalicylic acid

11.4 Conclusions

SCAD is a relatively rare complication of diverticular disease, which resembles IBD clinically, endoscopically, and histologically. The differential diagnosis of IBD might be difficult and mainly consists of anamnestic data and disease location – inflammation that exclusively affects the diverticular area of the colon. SCAD has four defined clinical subtypes, determined according to specific endoscopic and histological features. The disease is usually mild with a favorable prognosis. Treatment is based on a step-up design, and only rare refractory cases compel surgical treatment.

References

1. Cuomo R, Barbara G, Pace F, et al. Italian consensus conference for colonic diverticulosis and diverticular disease. United European Gastroenterol J. 2014;2(5):413–42.
2. Tursi A. Segmental colitis associated with diverticulosis: complication of diverticular disease or autonomous entity? Dig Dis Sci. 2011;56(1):27–34.
3. Imperiali G, Meucci G, Alvisi C, et al. Segmental colitis associated with diverticula: a prospective study. Gruppo di Studio per le Malattie Infiammatorie Intestinali (GSMII). Am J Gastroenterol. 2000;95(4):1014–6.
4. Mann NS, Hoda KK. Segmental colitis associated with diverticulosis: systematic evaluation of 486 cases with meta-analysis. Hepato-Gastroenterology. 2012;59(119):2119–2.
5. Ludeman L, Shepherd NA. What is diverticular colitis? Pathology. 2002;34:568.
6. Gore S, Shepherd NA, Wilkinson SP. Endoscopic crescentic fold disease of the sigmoid colon: the clinical and histopathological spectrum of a distinctive endoscopic appearance. Int J Color Dis. 1992;7:76–81.
7. Shepherd NA. Diverticular disease and chronic idiopathic inflammatory bowel disease: associations and masquerades. Gut. 1996;38:801–2.
8. Schembri J, Bonello J, et al. Segmental colitis associated with diverticulosis: is it the coexistence of colonic diverticulosis and inflammatory bowel disease? Ann Gastroenterol. 2017;30(3):257–61.
9. Tursi A, Elisei W, et al. Segmental colitis associated with diverticulosis: a 5-year follow-up. Int J Color Dis. 2012;27(2):179–85.
10. Harpaz N, Sachar DB. Segmental colitis associated with diverticular disease and other IBD look-alikes. J Clin Gastroenterol. 2006;40(Suppl 3):S132–5.
11. Freeman HJ. Natural history and long-term clinical behavior of segmental colitis associated with diverticulosis (SCAD syndrome). Dig Dis Sci. 2008;53:2452–7.
12. Hokama A, Kinjo F, Tomiyama R, et al. Progression of diverticular colitis to ulcerative colitis. Inflamm Bowel Dis. 2005;11:618.
13. Maeshiro T, Hokama A, Kinjo T, Fujita J. Diverticular colitis of the ascending colon preceding the onset of ulcerative colitis. BMJ Case Rep. 2014;2014:bcr2014204361.
14. Freeman HJ. Atypical perinuclear antineutrophil cytoplasmic antibodies in patients with Crohn's disease. Can J Gastroenterol. 1997;11:689–93.
15. Torres J, Petralia F, Sato T, et al. Serum biomarkers identify patients who will develop inflammatory bowel diseases up to 5 years before diagnosis. Gastroenterology. 2020;159(1):96–104.
16. Konikoff MR, Denson LA. Role of fecal calprotectin as a biomarker of intestinal inflammation in inflammatory bowel disease. Inflamm Bowel Dis. 2006;12(6):524–34.
17. Tursi A, Elisei W, Giorgetti G, Aiello F, Brandimarte G. Role of fecal calprotectin in the diagnosis and treatment of segmental colitis associated with diverticulosis. Minerva Gastroenterol Dietol. 2011;57:247–55.

18. Rampton DS. Diverticular colitis: diagnosis and management. Color Dis. 2001;3:149–53.
19. Tursi A, Brandimarte G, Giorgetti GM, Elisei W. Beclomethasone dipropionate plus VSL#3 for the treatment of mild to moderate diverticular colitis: an open, pilot study. J Clin Gastroenterol. 2005;39:644–5.
20. Hassan C, Zullo A, Ierardi E, et al. Tumour necrosis factor alpha downregulation and therapeutic response to infliximab in a case of segmental colitis associated with diverticula. Gut. 2006;55(4):589–90.
21. Ierardi E, Meucci G, Hassan C, et al. Tumour necrosis factor alpha in segmental colitis associated with diverticula. Dig Dis Sci. 2008;53(07):1865–8.
22. Tursi A, Nenna R, Danese S. Therapeutic response to adalimumab in a case of steroid dependent segmental colitis associated with diverticulosis. Am J Gastroenterol. 2021;116:1760–1.
23. Tursi A, Elisei W, Brandimarte G, et al. Tumour necrosis factor-alpha expression in segmental colitis associated with diverticulosis down-regulates after treatment. J Gastrointestin Liver Dis. 2011;20(04):365–70.
24. John ES, Katz K, Saxena M, et al. Management of Inflammatory Bowel Disease in the elderly. Curr Treat Options Gastroenterol. 2016;14(3):285–304.
25. Imperiali G, Terpin MM, Meucci G, Ferrara A, Minoli G. Segmental colitis associated with diverticula: a 7-year follow-up study. Endoscopy. 2006;38:610–2.
26. Kucejko RJ, Poggio JL. Considerations and changes in the evaluation, management, and outcomes in the Management of Diverticular Disease: the diagnosis, pathology, and treatment of diverticular colitis. Clin Colon Rectal Surg. 2018;31(4):221–5.

Part IV

Diagnosis

Biomarkers

12

Debora Compare, Kok-Ann Gwee, and Gerardo Nardone

12.1 Introduction

The diagnosis of diverticular disease (DD) continues to be a challenge due to the broad spectrum of disease presentation and its overlap with other abdominal conditions mimicking its clinical picture.

Indeed, up to 75% of patients with colonic diverticulosis remain completely asymptomatic throughout their lives, whereas approximately 25% of individuals with diverticulosis develop symptomatic uncomplicated diverticular disease (SUDD), and an even smaller proportion develop acute diverticulitis (AD) [1]. About 12% of patients presenting with AD will have a complication, including perforation, abscess, or fistula, and 20% of patients will have at least one recurrent episode. Finally, fewer than 5% of patients with diverticulosis will experience diverticular hemorrhage [1].

Patients with SUDD may develop unspecific chronic gastrointestinal symptoms (abdominal pain, bloating, or changes in bowel habits), resembling those of irritable bowel symptom (IBS), and patients with diverticulosis rarely develop segmental colitis that closely resembles or even overlaps with inflammatory bowel disease (IBD) [2]. Consequently, clinical evaluation of DD alone results in a wrong diagnosis in 34–68% of the cases, which means delayed or inadequate treatment, unnecessary investigations, avoidable and prolonged hospital stay, and increased costs [3].

D. Compare · G. Nardone (✉)
Gastroenterology Unit, Department of Clinical Medicine & Surgery, University Federico II of Naples, Naples, Italy
e-mail: debora.compare@unina.it; nardone@unina.it

K.-A. Gwee
Gleneagles Hospital, Singapore, Singapore
e-mail: slbclinic@gmail.com

© The Author(s), under exclusive license to Springer Nature Switzerland AG 2022

A. Tursi et al. (eds.), *Colonic Diverticular Disease*,
https://doi.org/10.1007/978-3-030-93761-4_12

The use of imaging techniques may help clinicians in the daily management of these patients. In clinical practice, ultrasonography (US) is usually the first-line diagnostic tool for patients with abdominal complaints. However, although US criteria for AD are well-established, there are no standardized criteria for SUDD diagnosis [4]. Conventional abdominal computed tomography (CT) plays a crucial role in evaluating patients with the suspicion of AD, and, due to its wide availability and high accuracy in diagnosing acute disease, it is considered the preferred front-line radiological test worldwide [5]. Nevertheless, abdominal US is examiner-dependent, and CT is expensive and potentially harmful. In recent years, novel techniques have been proposed for the diagnosis of DD. Computed tomography colonography (CTC) is strongly advisable in cases in which colonoscopy is incomplete, has failed, or is unfeasible, but it is contraindicated in acute abdominal conditions, such as AD, because of the high risk of complications [6]. Magnetic resonance imaging (MRI) has significant potential as a radiation-free imaging test for AD, but results from this technique remain inconclusive in terms of their ability to provide clinical direction [7].

Looking at the drawbacks of clinical evaluation and imaging techniques, the availability of biomarkers would be strongly advisable for better management of DD.

The history of the term "biomarker" dates back to the 1950s when it was first included in the English language [8]. In the 1970s, the term was used to indicate the presence of material of biological origin. However, it then took nearly another two decades for The National Institute of Health Biomarkers Definitions Working Group to officially recognize the term 'biomarker' in 1998 [8]. Before long, the term began to be widely used and correlated with the clinical course of the disease [9]. Currently, according to the World Health Organization (WHO), biomarkers are defined as "almost any measurement reflecting an interaction between a biological system and a potential hazard, which may be chemical, physical, or biological. The measured response may be functional and physiological, biochemical at the cellular level, or molecular interaction" [10]. Therefore, biomarkers may allow the diagnosis, classification, staging, outcome, and prognosis of a disease and also evaluate response to therapy. Ideal biomarkers should be accurate, reproducible, noninvasive, and cost-saving.

Nowadays, serum, fecal, and genetic biomarkers and gut microbiota signatures seem to have a promising role in helping clinicians in the diagnosis, staging, and follow-up of DD.

Here, we analyze data about the use of biomarkers in the setting of DD and provide insight into how these data might improve clinical practice.

12.2 Serum Biomarkers

The inflammatory process is the main player in the pathophysiology of DD. Thus, proinflammatory markers, such as C-reactive protein (CRP), erythrocyte sedimentation rate (ESR), and white blood cell (WBC) count, might have a role as biomarkers of DD.

Serum levels of CRP have been largely investigated in patients with DD. In a large study, including 124 patients with AD and 163 patients without AD, CRP

>50 mg/L had an OR of 3.78 in predicting AD occurrence, and, in a multivariate analysis, it was the only independent predictor of AD [3]. In addition, in 21 patients with uncomplicated AD, CRP was the most sensitive marker of mild-to-moderate histological damage, as it was increased in 4/10 (40%) patients scoring 0 or 1 in the neutrophilic infiltrate, that is, the absence of mild active inflammation ($p = 0.005$) [11]. Recently, in a large prospective cohort of 46,418 men, among whom 1110 cases of incident AD were observed during a 28-year follow-up, the authors have found that plasma levels of inflammatory markers were associated with incident AD with the multivariable-adjusted relative risk being 1.85 for CRP (95% CI 1.04–3.30) and 2.04 for IL-6 (95% CI 1.09–3.84) [12].

Beyond the difficulties in making a clinical diagnosis of AD, it is necessary to keep in mind that the discriminating power of the different variables alone is generally low. A nomogram based on age, a previous episode of AD, tenderness in the lower left abdomen both as a complaint and at physical examination, aggravation of pain on bowel movements, CRP >50 mg/L, and the absence of vomiting increased the diagnostic accuracy up to 86% [3].

Acute diverticulitis can appear uncomplicated or complicated. Uncomplicated AD is characterized by thickening of the colon wall and pericolic inflammatory changes, whereas complicated disease also includes abscess, peritonitis, obstruction, and/or fistula. The clinical management of AD depends on disease severity and the presence of complications. While selected patients with uncomplicated AD can be safely managed without antibiotics, patients with complicated AD must be necessarily treated with antibiotics and often require surgical intervention. Thus, the early identification of a complicated disease is critical to provide clinical direction.

In a total of 50 consecutive patients affected by AD of the colon, 11 of whom with a complicated disease, all the inflammatory markers, including CRP, fibrinogen, β2-globulin, α1-acid glycoprotein, and WBC count, were significantly higher than those in uncomplicated AD [11, 13]. Interestingly, in 350 patients who presented with symptoms of AD and underwent CT imaging on admission, CRP >150 mg/L and old age were independent risk factors for complicated AD, and CRP >200 mg/L had a positive predictive value of 90% and a negative predictive value of 59% for complicated AD [14]. Similarly, serum levels of CRP > 200 mg/L on admission had a specificity of 93% for perforation in AD patients, [15] whereas serum levels of CRP = 175 mg/L were the optimal threshold for diagnosing complicated AD with a positive predictive value of 36%, a negative predictive value of 92%, a sensitivity of 61%, and a specificity of 82% [16]. In a retrospective study on 374 patients with uncomplicated AD and 167 patients with complicated AD, CRP was significantly different between the complicated and uncomplicated disease ($p < 0.0001$) [17]. Indeed, patients with a CRP higher than 100 mg/L had a positive predictive value of 59% for having complicated AD, which increased to 71% for a CRP higher than 200 mg/L, whereas a CRP less than 5 mg/L had a negative predictive value of 91% [17]. However, in the same study, CRP failed to identify patients needing surgery [17]. On the contrary, in another study, CRP was significantly higher in patients who required urgent surgery than in those who did not (mean CRP 171.8 mg/L vs. 101.5 mg/L, respectively, $p < 0.001$) [15]. These findings strongly suggest that a CT examination should be promptly conducted in patients with such increased CRP levels and antibiotics must be started as soon as possible.

A few studies also evaluated the role of ESR in DD, which showed a lower specificity and sensitivity compared with those of CRP in the assessment of diverticulitis, mainly related to its long half-life and consequent prolonged latency period, and influenced by anemia and smoking [18].

CRP levels together with WBC count might be useful in predicting AD severity.

Back in 1996, Ambrosetti et al., in 423 patients with a first attack of AD, found that a leukocyte left shift >550 (absolute number) was one of the five parameters statistically predictive of medical failure [19]. Similarly, another study found that in 39 patients with uncomplicated AD and in 11 patients with complicated AD, the WBC count was able to discriminate between the two conditions better than other inflammatory markers [11, 13]. Moreover, an additional study found that a reduction in the WBC count on day 2 from admission was predictive of an early discharge [20]. However, the best cutoff value of the WBC count useful for identifying a complicated disease is far from being stated. A cutoff of a WBC count >12,000/mL was not able to predict a requirement for surgical versus medical treatment for AD, [19] and a cutoff of a WBC count >10,000/mL failed to predict complicated AD [14]. More recently, Kechagias et al. have shown that a WBC count >15,000/mL was associated with complicated AD, but they did not assess the diagnostic value or perform a multivariate analysis [21]. Finally, Kumarasinghe et al. found that patients with a WBC count >15,000/mL had a positive predictive value of 57% for having complicated AD, which increased to 86% for a WBC count >19,000/mL [17]. On the contrary, Käser et al. failed to demonstrate a correlation between an elevated WBC count and perforations, [15] and van de Wall et al. found that the diagnostic value of the WBC count had a poor AUC of only 0.58 in predicting perforation [16].

The neutrophil-to-lymphocyte ratio (NLR) is a novel biomarker that has been studied in AD. Reynolds et al. compared the accuracy of NLR, CRP, WBC count, neutrophil count, and white cell-to-lymphocyte ratio (WLR) for predicting radiological or surgical intervention in 101 patients with AD. The NLR had the greatest accuracy of the five biomarkers in predicting the need for intervention with an AUC of 0.79 ($p < 0.0001$). The optimal cutoff point for NLR was 5.34 ($J = 0.45$) [22].

Among patients with uncomplicated AD, the risk of progression to complicated AD is about 5%. According to the recent Clinical Practice Update on Medical Management of Colonic Diverticulitis from the American Gastroenterological Association, the risk factors for progression include baseline classification III or IV of the American Society of Anesthesiologists Physical Status, duration of symptoms longer than 5 days before presentation, the presence of vomiting, CRP > 140 mg/L, and a baseline WBC count >15,000/mL [23].

Several other serum biomarkers have been evaluated in patients with DD. Fibrinogen, β2-globulin, and α1-acid glycoprotein were found to be significantly higher in patients with complicated AD than in those with uncomplicated AD [11, 13]. Interleukin-6 and lipopolysaccharide-binding protein (LBP) were unable to distinguish between patients with AD with perforation and those without; however, sigmoid stenosis was predicted by LBP at admission (AUC of 0.88) [24]. Urea

>9 mmol/L and increased creatinine levels were associated with a lower rate of complicated diverticulitis, but the diagnostic significance of those markers was not assessed [19]. High levels of serum procalcitonin, a marker of bacterial infection, differentiated (sensitivity 80%, specificity 91%) complicated from uncomplicated AD when combined with CT scans [25]. Moreover, serum vitamin D levels have been shown to be associated with the severity of endoscopic mucosal alterations in diverticular disease [1].

12.3 Fecal Calprotectin

Fecal calprotectin (FC) is a cytoplasmic protein released by neutrophils, monocytes, and macrophages to the extracellular environment during an inflammatory response or necrosis. The presence of calprotectin in feces correlates with neutrophil migration toward the gastrointestinal tract, and its levels seem to be unaffected by causes of inflammation beyond the intestinal ones as for other systemic inflammatory markers [26].

FC can be measured using a commercially available enzyme-linked immunosorbent assay (ELISA), and it is stable in feces for several days after excretion [27].

The presence of an inflammatory infiltrate has been described in the colonic mucosa of patients affected by DD with respect to healthy controls [28]. Although the role of FC in distinguishing between IBD and IBS and as a sensitive marker of disease activity in IBD has been extensively explored, data on the clinical utility of FC in colonic DD are still limited [29, 30].

In a case–control study, Tursi et al. compared FC levels of 48 patients with DD (16 with asymptomatic DD, 16 with SUDD, and 16 with uncomplicated AD), 16 with IBS, and 16 healthy controls. The authors found significantly higher FC levels in patients with SUDD ($p < 0.005$) and uncomplicated AD ($p < 0.0005$) than in those with asymptomatic DD, healthy controls, or IBS. Moreover, FC levels significantly correlated with inflammatory infiltrates ($p < 0.0005$) and decreased after an 8-week treatment with mesalamine and rifaximin in DD ($p < 0.0005$) [28]. Recently, Tursi et al. have performed a post hoc analysis of the Diverticular Inflammation and Complication Assessment (DICA) prospective study, in 24 patients equally subdivided between the DICA 2 and DICA 3 score, in whom previous standard treatments (mesalamine and/or rifaximin) failed to control the symptoms. The median (IQR) FC level was 244.5 (171.5–322.0) μg/g at baseline. After budesonide MMX™ for 4 weeks, followed by mesalamine for 5 months, FC levels decreased to 51.0 (IQR, 35.5–61.5) μg/g ($p < 0.001$) at a 6-month follow-up [31].

These findings suggest that a positive FC seems to be useful not only for detecting colonic inflammation and assessing DD severity but also for monitoring therapeutic response.

Even more intriguing would be the role of FC in distinguishing SUDD from IBS. The latter point is crucial since SUDD and IBS share many symptoms, with a consequent risk of either overtreating or undertreating patients suffering from incorrectly classified abdominal pain. Some clinical criteria have been developed to differentiate these two entities, in particular, left lower abdominal pain has been considered the main symptom characterizing SUDD, but it has not yet been validated [32].

In a prospective study on 72 patients with recurrent abdominal pain and colon diverticulosis, the authors found that both left lower abdominal pain and FC score can differentiate true SUDD patients from those harboring diverticula fulfilling the IBS criteria [33].

Finally, FC could be a useful biomarker for predicting DD severity and complications. In a prospective cohort study analyzing 54 patients with previous uncomplicated AD, the same authors also found that diverticulitis recurrence was strictly related to the presence of an abnormal FC test during follow-up [34]. A further review study found that FC >60 μg/g was correlated with acute complications of DD [35].

Recently, in a pilot study, Murray et al. have demonstrated a moderate correlation between FC levels and the visceral adipose tissue ($\rho = 0.3$, $p = 0.05$) in patients with diverticulosis. This result reinforced the concept of the adipose tissue's proinflammatory effect that could predispose to diverticulosis complications [36].

Thus, even if FC assessment suffers from some limitations (intraindividual biological variations, reduced sensitivity in aqueous feces, nonsteroidal anti-inflammatory drug-induced enteropathy, proton pump inhibitor use, and neoplasms of the gastrointestinal tract), and the best cutoff values for AD and complicated AD have yet to be defined, it represents a highly promising tool for managing DD [37–40].

12.4 Genetic Biomarkers

The prevalent incidence of DD in Western countries and industrialized areas supported the hypothesis that diet and lifestyle are determinants of its pathogenesis. However, colonic distribution of diverticula, generally left-sided in the Western world and right-sided in the Asian regions, and familial predisposition suggest the importance of factors other than the environment in the development of DD [41]. Epidemiological twin data suggest genetic factors as additional players in the pathogenesis of DD. A Danish study, involving 923 twins with DD, found a heritability of 53% [42]. In a large Swedish study, 2296 out of 104,452 twins had a diagnosis of DD. The OR of developing the disease, given that one's co-twin was affected, was 7.15 (95% CI 4.82–10.61) for monozygotic and 3.20 (95% CI 2.21–4.63) for same-gender dizygotic twins [43].

Moreover, in line with a genetic hypothesis of DD, several genetic diseases involving neuromuscular and collagen disorders such as Ehlers–Danlos, Williams–Beuren, and Coffin–Lowry syndromes and autosomal dominant polycystic kidney disease show a strong predisposition toward diverticula formation [44, 45].

Finally, epidemiological studies on moving populations showed no change in DD incidence and distribution despite the new environmental factors [46].

Based on these premises, the previous year's research focused on the correlation between genetic variants and DD.

A genome-wide association study (GWAS) of DD (27,444 cases; 382,284 controls) performed using data from the UK Biobank and tested for replication in the Michigan Genomics Initiative (2572 cases; 28,649 controls) found 42 loci associated with DD, 39 of which were novel. A genome-wide association analysis of the 42 variants showed a common etiology of DD with obesity and hernia [47]. A similar study from the Iceland Biobank, analyzing 32.4 million sequence variants, identified associations of *ARHGAP15* and *COLQ* variants with uncomplicated DD and *FAM155A* variant with AD [48].

Recently, using the same UK Biobank, a GWAS analysis has been performed on 31,964 cases and 419,135 controls of European descent. Associations were replicated in a European sample of 3893 cases and 2829 diverticula-free controls and evaluated for risk contribution to diverticulitis and uncomplicated diverticulosis [49]. In all, 48 loci, 12 of which were novel, with genome-wide significance, were identified. The most significant novel risk variant in the replication analysis was rs9960286, located near CTAGE1 (p 0.002). Four loci showed stronger effects for diverticulitis, namely, PHGR1 (OR 1.32, 95% CI 1.12–1.56), FAM155A-2 (OR 1.21, 95% CI 1.04–1.42), CALCB (OR 1.17, 95% CI 1.03–1.33), and S100A10 (OR 1.17, 95% CI 1.03–1.33) [49].

The associations between ARHGAP15 (rs4662344), COLQ (rs7609897), and FAM155A (rs67153654), reported in the Icelandic GWAS by applying weighted thresholds and confirmed in the North-American [47] and European [49] GWASs, were evaluated in 1332 patients (634 men) who underwent colonoscopy. The variant in *FAM155A* was associated with diverticulitis, but not with diverticulosis, in Caucasians, whereas the variant in *ARHGAP15* might be associated with both diverticulosis and diverticulitis [50].

Diverticular disease is associated with enteric neuropathology and alterations of the Ret/GDNF pathway that are modulated by Phox2b [51]. The expression of Phox2b, analyzed in colonic surgical samples, was altered in 20 patients with AD with respect to 20 adult controls [51].

Genetic variants may also be associated with the outcome of DD, i.e., recurrence of acute attacks, and with the severity of the disease. In a retrospective study including 404 patients with CT-confirmed AD episodes, RNA-seq was conducted on full-thickness colonic tissues of 10 multifocal diverticulitis (MFD) and 11 unifocal diverticulitis (UFD), and 69 genes that were differentially expressed between MFD and UFD patients were identified [52]. In MFD, there was a significant downregulation of genes that were associated with immune response pathways. Thus, MFD appears to be a more severe subset of diverticulitis with a unique immune-associated transcriptomic profile [52]. Finally, in 21 sporadic surgical AD patients and 5 individuals from a single family with surgically managed AD, compared with 3 separate groups of healthy, Crohn's disease, and ulcerative colitis control patients, the SNP rs7848647 in the *TNFSF15* gene, previously identified as playing a role in diseases affecting the gastrointestinal tract, was significantly associated with surgical AD ($p = 0.0003$) versus all control groups studied [53].

A genetic substrate of DD has been postulated through GWASs, revealing a correlation between genetic variants and the DD phenotype; however, confirmation by a more detailed genetic mapping is required before drawing definite associations, useful in clinical practice.

12.5 Gut Microbiota Signatures

The entire gastrointestinal tract, particularly the large bowel, is inhabited by a multitude of microorganisms, namely, the gut microbiota. Therefore, being a part of the colonic ecosystem, it is reasonable to hypothesize that alterations in the gut microbiota and the related inflammatory response may be implicated in colonic diseases in general, particularly in DD development and complications. However, despite this premise, thus far, there are only limited data linking bacterial dysbiosis to DD pathogenesis.

Analyzing the mucosal microbiota of sigmoid biopsies of subjects undergoing screening colonoscopy, Jones et al. found little association between mucosal microbiota profile and number and location of diverticula among 309 cases and 226 controls [54]. The comparisons of bacterial abundances across all taxonomic levels showed differences for the *Proteobacteria* phylum ($p = 0.038$) and the *Comamonadaceae* family ($p = 0.035$). The authors suggested that the mucosal-adherent microbiota community composition is unlikely to play a substantial role in the development of diverticulosis [54].

A metagenomic gene-targeted approach, evaluating gut microbiota composition among SUDD, IBS, and IBD patients and healthy controls, found that among phyla, Biplot PC2/PC3 and the dendrogram plot showed major differences in samples from IBS and IBD, whereas SUDD patients resembled the microbiota composition of healthy controls, but not for *Bacteroides fragilis* [55].

An analysis of the gut microbiota found that in a diseased tissue and an adjacent unaffected tissue of the sigmoid colon chronically affected by diverticulitis, *Pseudomonas* and *Basidiomycota* OTUs were enriched in the adjacent unaffected tissue, whereas *Microbacteriaceae* and *Ascomycota* were enriched in the diseased tissue [56].

A comparison of fecal samples from 31 patients with left-sided uncomplicated AD and 25 controls by a high-throughput polymerase chain reaction on DNA isolates revealed a higher diversity for *Proteobacteria* ($p < 0.00002$) and all phyla combined ($p = 0.002$) in AD with respect to controls. The most discriminative species derived largely from the *Enterobacteriaceae* family [57].

The family of *Enterobacteriaceae*, including *Escherichia coli*, is a common component of the gut microbiota. Increased levels of *Enterobacteriaceae* were linked to IBD in humans. The analysis of mucosa samples from 16 patients with DD and 35 controls without any diverticula showed a higher amount of *Enterobacteriaceae* in patients with DD than in those without DD ($p = 0.043$) [58].

In contrast, Tursi et al., by analyzing the microbiota composition in stool samples from 15 patients with SUDD, 13 with asymptomatic diverticulosis, and 16 healthy controls, did not find a significant difference among the 3 groups in *Bacteroides – Prevotella, Clostridium coccoides – Bifidobacterium,* and *Lactobacillus – Escherichia coli.* Only levels of *Akkermansia muciniphila* were significantly increased in asymptomatic diverticulosis and SUDD ($p = 0.019$) [59].

Finally, the gut microbiome and metabolome were analyzed in stool samples of patients with diverticulosis, SUDD, and healthy controls [60]. Compared with controls, patients with diverticula, regardless of symptoms, had a depletion of *Clostridium cluster IV*; *Clostridium cluster IX, Fusobacterium,* and *Lactobacillaceae* were reduced in SUDD than in asymptomatic patients.

A negative correlation was found between *Clostridium cluster IV* and *Akkermansia.* In addition, the analysis of urinary and fecal metabolome profiles showed an increase of hippurate and kynurenine pathways, which were able to discriminate between diverticular subgroups and controls [60].

In support of this hypothesis, patients with different gastrointestinal diseases including IBD, IBS, and DD reported a clinical benefit from treatment with rifaximin, a nonsystemic drug that employs a eubiotic effect on the gut microbiota [61]. Patients who improved post rifaximin treatment showed a significant microbial alpha diversity increase ($p = 0.271$) and a *Fecalibacterium* abundance increase (log2FC 1.959, $p = 0.042$) with respect to patients who did not improve. *Roseburia* abundance decreased in both groups, whereas *Ruminococcus* decreased only in patients who clinically improved [61].

Thus, taken together, these findings, although preliminary, suggest that gut microbiota signatures could allow assessing DD presence and severity and monitor response to treatment.

12.6 Conclusions

Diverticular disease and its complications continue to be a worldwide burden on health-care systems and a challenge for clinicians due to the broad spectrum of disease presentation and its overlap with other abdominal conditions that, sometimes, may result in a wrong diagnosis.

The use of imaging techniques may help clinicians, but their availability, operator dependence, potential harms for some and low accuracy for others, and high costs may differentially impact their use in clinical practice. Therefore, the availability of biomarkers would be strongly advisable for a better clinical management of DD.

Although biomarkers have not been extensively investigated in DD, the current data show that they may be helpful in substantiating clinical suspicion and assessing disease severity and monitoring. Serum CRP is the most extensively studied, and high levels are most consistently associated with being predictive of AD severity. Fecal calprotectin seems to be a promising tool, particularly for differentiating between IBS and SUDD and for monitoring response to therapy.

In addition, even if we need large studies before drawing definite conclusions, GWAS analyses revealed a correlation between genetic variants and the

DD phenotype, and mounting evidence suggests that gut microbiota signatures could allow assessing DD presence and severity and monitor response to treatment.

References

1. Tursi A, Scarpignato C, Strate LL, Lanas A, Kruis W, Lahat A, et al. Colonic diverticular disease. Nat Rev Dis Prim. 2020;6(1):1–23.
2. Strate LL, Modi R, Cohen E, Spiegel BMR. Diverticular disease as a chronic illness: evolving epidemiologic and clinical insights. Am J Gastroenterol. 2012;107(10):1486–93.
3. Andeweg CS, Knobben L, Hendriks JCM, Bleichrodt RP, Van Goor H. How to diagnose acute left-sided colonic diverticulitis: proposal for a clinical scoring system. Ann Surg. 2011;253(5):940–6.
4. Ripollés T, Sebastián-Tomás JC, Martínez-Pérez MJ, Manrique A, Gómez-Abril SA, Torres-Sanchez T. Ultrasound can differentiate complicated and noncomplicated acute colonic diverticulitis: a prospective comparative study with computed tomography. Abdom Radiol (NY). 2021;46(8):3826–34. https://doi.org/10.1007/s00261-021-03060-5. Epub ahead of print
5. Minordi LM, Larosa L, Berte G, Pecere S, Manfredi R. CT of the acute colonic diverticulitis: a pictorial essay. Diagnostic Interv Radiol. 2020;26(6):546–51.
6. Flor N, Maconi G, Cornalba G, Pickhardt PJ. The current role of radiologic and endoscopic imaging in the diagnosis and follow-up of colonic diverticular disease. Am J Roentgenol. 2016;207(1):15–24.
7. Jerjen F, Zaidi T, Chan S, Sharma A, Mudliar R, Soomro K, et al. Magnetic resonance imaging for the diagnosis and management of acute colonic diverticulitis: a review of current and future use. J Med Radiat Sci. 2021;68:310–9.
8. Aronson JK, Ferner RE. Biomarkers-a general review. Curr Protoc Pharmacol. 2017;76:9.23.1–9.23.17.
9. Mayeux R. Biomarkers: potential uses and limitations. NeuroRx. 2004;1(2):182–8.
10. Strimbu K, Tavel JA. What are biomarkers? Curr Opin HIV AIDS. 2010;5(6):463–6.
11. Tursi A, Elisei W, Brandimarte G, Giorgetti GM, Aiello F. Predictive value of serologic markers of degree of histologic damage in acute uncomplicated colonic diverticulitis. J Clin Gastroenterol. 2010;44(10):702–6.
12. Ma W, Jovani M, Nguyen LH, Tabung FK, Song M, Liu PH, et al. Association between inflammatory diets, circulating markers of inflammation, and risk of diverticulitis. Clin Gastroenterol Hepatol. 2020;18(10):2279–2286.e3.
13. Tursi A, Brandimarte G, Giorgetti GM, Elisei W, Maiorano M, Aiello F. The clinical picture of uncomplicated versus complicated diverticulitis of the colon. Dig Dis Sci. 2008;53(9):2474–9.
14. Mäkelä JT, Klintrup K, Takala H, Rautio T. The role of C-reactive protein in prediction of the severity of acute diverticulitis in an emergency unit. Scand J Gastroenterol. 2015;50(5):536–41.
15. Käser SA, Fankhauser G, Glauser PM, Toia D, Maurer CA. Diagnostic value of inflammation markers in predicting perforation in acute sigmoid diverticulitis. World J Surg. 2010;34(11):2717–22.
16. van de Wall BJM, Draaisma WA, van der Kaaij RT, Consten ECJ, Wiezer MJ, Broeders IAMJ. The value of inflammation markers and body temperature in acute diverticulitis. Color Dis. 2013;15(5):621–6.
17. Kumarasinghe D, Zahid A, O'Grady G, Leow T, Sheriff T, Ctercteko G, et al. The use of biochemical markers in complicated and uncomplicated acute diverticulitis. Int Surg. 2018; https://doi.org/10.9738/INTSURG-D-16-00241.1.
18. Gallo A, Ianiro G, Montalto M, Cammarota G. The role of biomarkers in diverticular disease. J Clin Gastroenterol. 2016;50:S26–8.

19. Ambrosetti P, Morel P. Acute left colonic diverticulitis: indications for operation and predictive parameters of early and late medical treatment failure: a prospective non-randomized study of 423 patients. Dig Surg. 1996;13(4–5):349–52.
20. Evans J. Does a 48-hour rule predict outcomes in patients with acute sigmoid diverticulitis? J Gastrointest Surg. 2008;12(3):577–82.
21. Kechagias A, Rautio T, Kechagias G, Mäkelä J. The role of C-reactive protein in the prediction of the clinical severity of acute diverticulitis. Am Surg. 2014;80(4):391–5.
22. Reynolds IS, Heaney RM, Khan W, Khan IZ, Waldron R, Barry K. The utility of neutrophil to lymphocyte ratio as a predictor of intervention in acute diverticulitis. Dig Surg. 2017;34(3):227–32.
23. Peery AF, Shaukat A, Strate LL. AGA clinical practice update on medical Management of Colonic Diverticulitis: expert review. Gastroenterology. 2021;160(3):906–911.e1.
24. Tan JPL, Barazanchi AWH, Singh PP, Hill AG, Maccormick AD. Predictors of acute diverticulitis severity: a systematic review. Int J Surg. 2016;26:43–52.
25. Jeger V, Pop R, Forudastan F, Barras JP, Zuber M, Piso RJ. Is there a role for procalcitonin in differentiating uncomplicated and complicated diverticulitis in order to reduce antibiotic therapy? A prospective diagnostic cohort study. Swiss Med Wkly. 2017;147(4748):w14555.
26. Montalto M, Gallo A, Santoro L, D'Onofrio F, Landolfi R, Gasbarrini A. Role of fecal calprotectin in gastrointestinal disorders. Eur Rev Med Pharmacol Sci. 2013;17(12):1569–82.
27. Costa F, Mumolo MG, Bellini M, Romano MR, Ceccarelli L, Arpe P, et al. Role of faecal calprotectin as non-invasive marker of intestinal inflammation. Dig Liver Dis. 2003;35(9):642–7.
28. Tursi A, Brandimarte G, Elisei W, Giorgetti GM, Inchingolo CD, Aiello F. Faecal calprotectin in colonic diverticular disease: a case-control study. Int J Color Dis. 2009;24(1):49–55.
29. Mari A, Baker FA, Mahamid M, Yacoob A, Sbeit W, Khoury T. Clinical utility of fecal calprotectin: potential applications beyond inflammatory bowel disease for the primary care physician. Ann Gastroenterol. 2019;32(5):425–30.
30. Reenaers C, Bossuyt P, Hindryckx P, Vanpoucke H, Cremer A, Baert F. Expert opinion for use of faecal calprotectin in diagnosis and monitoring of inflammatory bowel disease in daily clinical practice. United European Gastroenterol J. 2018;6:1117–25.
31. Tursi A, Cassieri C, Colucci R, Elisei W, Picchio M, Brandimarte G. Budesonide MMX™ is effective in patients having persistent symptoms and raised fecal calprotectin following treatments for diverticular disease. J Gastrointest Liver Dis. 2019;28:45–7.
32. Spiller R. Is it diverticular disease or is it irritable bowel syndrome? Dig Dis. 2012;30(1):64–9.
33. Tursi A, Elisei W, Picchio M, Giorgetti GM, Brandimarte G. Moderate to severe and prolonged left lower-abdominal pain is the best symptom characterizing symptomatic uncomplicated diverticular disease of the colon: a comparison with fecal calprotectin in clinical setting. J Clin Gastroenterol. 2015;49(3):218–21.
34. Tursi A, Elisei W, Picchio M, Brandimarte G. Increased faecal calprotectin predicts recurrence of colonic diverticulitis. Int J Color Dis. 2014;29(8):931–5.
35. Tursi A. Biomarkers in diverticular diseases of the colon. Dig Dis. 2012;30(1):12–8.
36. Murray KA, Hoad CL, Garratt J, Kaviani M, Marciani L, Smith JK, et al. A pilot study of visceral fat and its association with adipokines, stool calprotectin and symptoms in patients with diverticulosis. Green J, editor. PLoS One. 2019;14(5):e0216528.
37. Vestergaard TA, Nielsen SL, Dahlerup JF, Hornung N. Fecal calprotectin: assessment of a rapid test. Scand J Clin Lab Invest. 2008;68(4):343–7.
38. Tibble JA, Sigthorsson G, Foster R, Scott D, Fagerhol MK, Roseth A, et al. High prevalence of NSAID enteropathy as shown by a simple faecal test. Gut. 1999;45(3):362–6.
39. Johne B, Kronborg O, Tøn HI, Kristinsson J, Fuglerud P. A new fecal calprotectin test for colorectal neoplasia: clinical results and comparison with previous method. Scand J Gastroenterol. 2001;36(3):291–6.
40. Lundgren D, Eklöf V, Palmqvist R, Hultdin J, Karling P. Proton pump inhibitor use is associated with elevated faecal calprotectin levels. A cross-sectional study on subjects referred for colonoscopy. Scand J Gastroenterol. 2019;54(2):152–7.

41. Maguire LH. Genetic risk factors for diverticular disease-emerging evidence. J Gastrointest Surg. 2020;24(10):2314–7.
42. Strate LL, Erichsen R, Baron JA, Mortensen J, Pedersen JK, Riis AH, et al. Heritability and familial aggregation of diverticular disease: a population-based study of twins and siblings. Gastroenterology. 2013;144(4):736–742.e1.
43. Granlund J, Svensson T, Olén O, Hjern F, Pedersen NL, Magnusson PKE, et al. The genetic influence on diverticular disease - a twin study. Aliment Pharmacol Ther. 2012;35(9):1103–7.
44. Broad JB, Wu Z, Clark TG, Musson D, Jaung R, Arroll B, et al. Diverticulosis and nine connective tissue disorders: epidemiological support for an association. Connect Tissue Res. 2019;60(4):389–98.
45. Duarte-Chavez R, Stoltzfus J, Yellapu V, Martins N, Nanda S, Longo S, et al. Colonic diverticular disease in autosomal dominant polycystic kidney disease: is there really an association? A nationwide analysis. Int J Color Dis. 2021;36(1):83–91.
46. Reichert MC, Lammert F. The genetic epidemiology of diverticulosis and diverticular disease: emerging evidence. United Eur Gastroenterol J. 2015;3(5):409–18.
47. Maguire LH, Handelman SK, Du X, Chen Y, Pers TH, Speliotes EK. Genome-wide association analyses identify 39 new susceptibility loci for diverticular disease. Nat Genet. 2018;50(10):1359–65.
48. Sigurdsson S, Alexandersson KF, Sulem P, Feenstra B, Gudmundsdottir S, Halldorsson GH, et al. Sequence variants in ARHGAP15, COLQ and FAM155A associate with diverticular disease and diverticulitis. Nat Commun. 2017;8:1–7.
49. Schafmayer C, Harrison JW, Buch S, Lange C, Reichert MC, Hofer P, et al. Genome-wide association analysis of diverticular disease points towards neuromuscular, connective tissue and epithelial pathomechanisms. Gut. 2019;68(5):854–65.
50. Reichert MC, Kupcinskas J, Schulz A, Schramm C, Weber SN, Krawczyk M, et al. Common variation in FAM155A is associated with diverticulitis but not diverticulosis. Sci Rep. 2020;10(1):1–6.
51. Cossais F, Lange C, Barrenschee M, Möding M, Ebsen M, Vogel I, et al. Altered enteric expression of the homeobox transcription factor Phox2b in patients with diverticular disease. United Eur Gastroenterol J. 2019;7(3):349–57.
52. Kline BP, Schieffer KM, Choi CS, Connelly T, Chen J, Harris L, et al. Multifocal versus conventional unifocal diverticulitis: a comparison of clinical and transcriptomic characteristics. Dig Dis Sci. 2019;64(11):3143–51.
53. Connelly TM, Berg AS, Hegarty JP, Deiling S, Brinton D, Poritz LS, et al. The TNFSF15 gene single nucleotide polymorphism rs7848647 is associated with surgical diverticulitis. Ann Surg. 2014;259(6):1132–7.
54. Jones RB, Fodor AA, Peery AF, Tsilimigras MCB, Winglee K, McCoy A, et al. An aberrant microbiota is not strongly associated with incidental colonic diverticulosis. Sci Rep. 2018;8(1):4951.
55. Lopetuso LR, Petito V, Graziani C, Schiavoni E, Paroni Sterbini F, Poscia A, et al. Gut microbiota in health, diverticular disease, irritable bowel syndrome, and inflammatory bowel diseases: time for microbial marker of gastrointestinal disorders. Dig Dis. 2017;36(1):56–65.
56. Schieffer KM, Sabey K, Wright JR, Toole DR, Drucker R, Tokarev V, et al. The microbial ecosystem distinguishes chronically diseased tissue from adjacent tissue in the sigmoid colon of chronic, recurrent diverticulitis patients. Sci Rep. 2017;7(1):1–10.
57. Daniels L, Budding AE, de Korte N, Eck A, Bogaards JA, Stockmann HB, et al. Fecal microbiome analysis as a diagnostic test for diverticulitis. Eur J Clin Microbiol Infect Dis. 2014;33(11):1927–36.
58. Linninge C, Roth B, Erlanson-Albertsson C, Molin G, Toth E, Ohlsson B. Abundance of Enterobacteriaceae in the colon mucosa in diverticular disease. World J Gastrointest Pathophysiol. 2018;9(1):18–27.
59. Tursi A, Mastromarino P, Capobianco D, Elisei W, Miccheli A, Capuani G, et al. Assessment of fecal microbiota and fecal metabolome in symptomatic uncomplicated diverticular disease of the colon. J Clin Gastroenterol. 2016;50:S9–12.

60. Barbara G, Scaioli E, Barbaro MR, Biagi E, Laghi L, Cremon C, et al. Gut microbiota, metabolome and immune signatures in patients with uncomplicated diverticular disease. Gut. 2017;66(7):1252–61.
61. Ponziani FR, Scaldaferri F, de Siena M, Mangiola F, Matteo MV, Pecere S, et al. Increased Faecalibacterium abundance is associated with clinical improvement in patients receiving rifaximin treatment. Benef Microbes. 2020;11(6):519–25.

Ultrasonography

13

Giovanni Maconi and Alois Hollerweger

13.1 Introduction

Diverticular disease of the colon is a common clinical condition in industrialized countries. It is believed to be a disease of the elderly or middle-aged classes, but recent studies and our routine clinical practice have shown that its incidence is increasing among younger populations [1, 2]. The evolving epidemiology of colonic diverticulosis and that of diverticular disease, a term encompassing the presence of diverticula with symptoms and conditions such as colitis, hematochezia, and/or acute diverticulitis and its chronic complications, account for the increasing burden of ambulatory visits, diagnostic procedures, and hospital admissions for this condition [3]. On account of the growing demand for clinical investigations and the need to rationalize diagnostic workup for acute and chronic abdominal symptoms, intestinal ultrasound (IUS) has been introduced and suggested as a valid diagnostic tool for patients with diverticular disease (Table 13.1). While cross-sectional imaging like US and CT are the methods of choice in acute colonic diverticulitis, endoscopic and radiological procedures have gained acceptance for the remaining spectrum of diverticular disease. Colonoscopy as well as CT and CT colonography are frequently used to evaluate hematochezia and acute bleeding to diagnose chronic complications of diverticular disease and to confirm or exclude malignancy and other concomitant conditions.

G. Maconi (✉)
Gastroenterology Unit, Department of Biomedical and Clinical Sciences, "Luigi Sacco" University Hospital, University of Milan, Milan, Italy
e-mail: giovanni.maconi@unimi.it

A. Hollerweger
Department of Radiology, Hospital Barmherzige Brüder, Salzburg, Austria
e-mail: alois.hollerweger@aon.at

© The Author(s), under exclusive license to Springer Nature Switzerland AG 2022
A. Tursi et al. (eds.), *Colonic Diverticular Disease*,
https://doi.org/10.1007/978-3-030-93761-4_13

Table 13.1 Pros and cons of intestinal ultrasound in diverticular disease of the colon

Pros
– Intestinal ultrasound is a ready-to-use, prompt, noninvasive, and accurate diagnostic investigation for patients with suspected acute diverticulitis
– Intestinal ultrasound is a dynamic investigation that could also be performed at bedside, especially to assess well-defined and localized abdominal pain, such as that caused by acute diverticulitis
– Intestinal ultrasound allows excellent correlation between clinical symptoms and sonographic features
– Intestinal ultrasound is a radiation-free and inexpensive diagnostic tool, useful for short- and long-term monitoring of patients with acute diverticulitis
– As abdominal ultrasound is frequently requested for patients with abdominal complaints, the sonographic assessment of the colon can be of help in detecting sigmoid diverticula in patients with uncomplicated symptomatic diverticular disease.
Cons
– In acute complicated diverticulitis, intestinal ultrasound may provide a less panoramic view compared with CT scan
– Intestinal ultrasound may have limited diagnostic accuracy in obese and oversized patients and may more frequently produce inconclusive results in acute diverticulitis of the rectosigmoid junction and deep pelvic sigmoid loops, overlaid by intestinal gas
– The diagnostic accuracy, and especially the sensitivity, of intestinal ultrasound may be negatively affected by limited operator experience

All such examinations assist us in tailoring the best treatment for our patients, help us predict potential outcomes, and also help decide on follow-up requirements. In this regard, IUS has been shown to have valuable clinical applications complemented by the use of CT scanning and colonoscopy to make it more widely utilized.

Among diagnostic examinations, IUS has several advantages. It is a noninvasive test that is ready and quick to use. In fact, IUS is a natural extension of physical examination. It can help us guide therapy and improve patient outcomes. A clinical encounter in which bedside ultrasonography is used often results in increased patient satisfaction [4]. It has no radiation exposure and no sedation is required. Its repeatability and accuracy have been widely studied and proven to be satisfactory for the diagnosis of a number of bowel conditions, from bowel obstruction, to appendicitis, to inflammatory bowel disease [5–8].

In the following paragraphs, we will discuss the role of IUS in diverticular disease of the colon, particularly in the setting of diverticulitis, in detecting this condition and its complications, both at onset and in follow-up, as well as in showing its potential clinical applications.

13.2 Intestinal Ultrasonography in Colonic Diverticulosis

The term "colonic diverticulosis" simply refers to the presence of diverticula, regardless of symptomatology. It is a common condition in the Western world, with a prevalence of about 10% in the third decade of life and >70% over 80 years [9]. In Western countries, it is most commonly found in the sigmoid and descending colon,

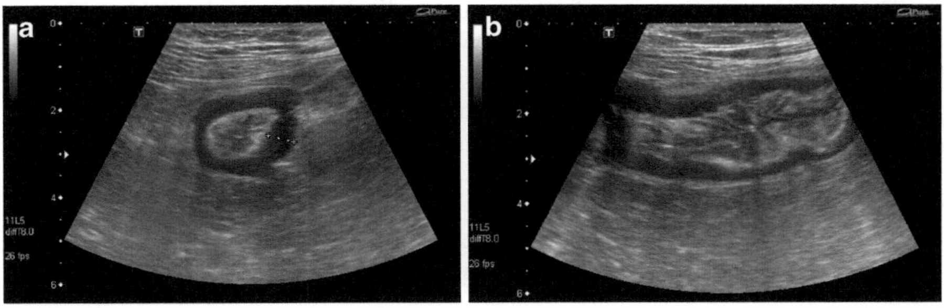

Fig. 13.1 Transversal (**a**) and longitudinal (**b**) scans of the sigmoid colon, showing increased thickening of the muscularis propria (external hypoechoic layer), frequently observed in patients with diverticulosis

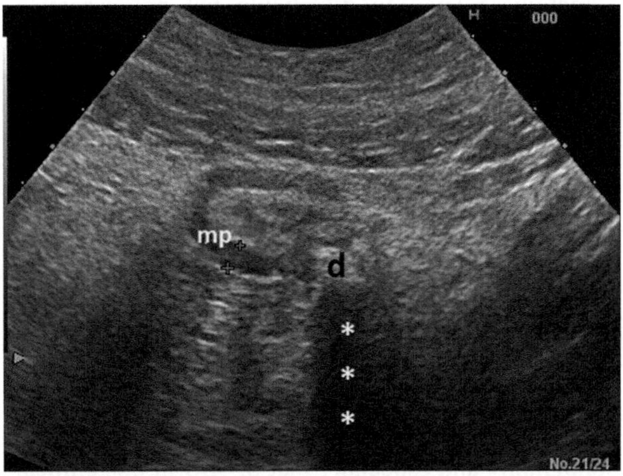

Fig. 13.2 Diverticulum (d) of the sigmoid colon, detected by IUS as protuberance of the colonic wall, externally to the proper muscular layer (mp), and frequently associated with air artifact with posterior acoustic shadowing (asterisks) due to the presence of a fecolith and/or gas within the diverticulum

where it may be associated with thickening of the muscularis propria, mainly of the circular smooth muscle, otherwise known as myochosis. This thickening produces increased stiffness and luminal narrowing that can easily be seen by IUS (Fig. 13.1). The above-mentioned features occur less frequently in right-sided diverticula, much more common in patients from Asia, and are harder to observe by ultrasound, unless there is presence of acute inflammation.

Diagnostic sonographic findings for diverticula include the presence of protuberances arising from the colonic wall, externally to the proper muscular layer, associated with air artifact and/or acoustic shadowing due to the presence of a fecolith into the diverticulum [6, 10] (Fig. 13.2). A number of studies have shown IUS to have a sensitivity and specificity >85% for the detection of uncomplicated left-sided colonic diverticulosis, using colonoscopy as the reference standard [10]. As mentioned, unlike the colonic wall that is often thickened, the noninflamed diverticular wall may not be easily demonstrated.

The sonographic detection of asymptomatic diverticula, which might occur incidentally during IUS, radiographic examinations, or colonoscopy, does not have an evidence-based clinical impact on patient outcomes and therefore does not necessarily require any treatment or dietary restriction. Similarly, there is no clear indication for IUS screening of patients with a strong family history of colonic diverticulosis.

13.3 Ultrasonography in Diverticular Disease of the Colon

Diverticular disease of the colon refers to a clinically relevant and symptomatic condition that includes acute diverticulitis, its complications, and chronic sequelae. As reported elsewhere in this book, diverticular disease of the colon can be subdivided into symptomatic uncomplicated diverticular disease (SUDD) and acute or chronic diverticulitis [11, 12]. SUDD is characterized by persistent abdominal symptoms related to diverticula but not associated with acute inflammation. Diverticulitis, on the other hand, is associated with macroscopic diverticular inflammation with or without the presence of related complications. Diverticular disease of the colon also includes segmental colitis associated with diverticula (SCAD or DAC) and diverticular bleeding, the diagnosis and management of which is mainly determined by endoscopic findings [11, 12].

13.3.1 Symptomatic Uncomplicated Diverticular Disease

The role of IUS, as well as of other imaging tools, in SUDD, is still largely uninvestigated. Abdominal ultrasound is frequently used as the first-line diagnostic investigation in patients with chronic or recurrent abdominal complaints and changes in bowel habits [13, 14]. However, the usefulness of transcutaneous abdominal ultrasonography and especially that of IUS in this clinical context, in particular for the detection of diverticular disease or functional bowel disorders, has yet to be well investigated [15]. However, IUS has a pivotal role in the differential diagnosis and the early diagnostic workup of abdominal complaints, as it has been shown to be highly effective in detecting intestinal inflammatory disorders, such as Crohn's disease and ulcerative colitis [7]. It could therefore be argued that this modality can be applied to differentiate between functional and organic disorders, especially in young patients without alarm symptoms, who do not necessarily require invasive investigations of the colon, as well as in symptomatic patients with low risk of organic disease (e.g., a recent negative colonoscopy and/or negative fecal occult blood test).

In fact, in a clinical context where polyps or cancer are unlikely, IUS can be performed as the first investigation to explore the source of symptoms. It offers the advantage of visualizing extraintestinal organs and the possibility of assessing the site of pain in real time, thus allowing a correlation between symptoms and intestinal and extraintestinal findings.

Currently, there are no standardized ultrasonographic criteria for the diagnosis of SUDD. Subtle features, such as mild thickening of the colonic or diverticular wall, may be postulated. In particular, thickening of the muscularis propria of the colonic wall has been found to be of some pathogenetic and diagnostic value for SUDD and irritable bowel syndrome [16, 17]. Pain caused by compression of the affected area, which may be produced during ultrasonographic assessment, could also be used as a diagnostic criterion.

13.3.2 Acute Diverticulitis

IUS is now considered a front-line imaging test for diagnosing acute diverticulitis. It is widely available and easily accessible within the emergency department; it is fast, low-cost, and noninvasive. In particular, it has excellent diagnostic accuracy in thin patients and may also be a reasonable consideration in young females, where radiation exposure is best avoided. The main and peculiar advantage of IUS is its ability to correlate imaging findings with the area of greatest tenderness in real time, thus providing useful information for differential diagnosis, such as in cases of epiploic appendagitis or omental infarction (Fig. 13.3).

IUS is an accurate diagnostic tool to assess acute diverticulitis, with an overall sensitivity and specificity greater than 90%. A meta-analysis and a systematic review have reported comparable accuracy of IUS and CT in the evaluation of acute diverticulitis [18, 19]. Therefore, it could be argued that as there is no statistically significant difference in the accuracy of IUS and CT in diagnosing acute colonic diverticulitis, both these techniques could be used as the initial diagnostic tool in patients with suspected acute diverticulitis.

A number of consensus statements of clinical guidelines that have incorporated IUS into an algorithm for the assessment of acute diverticular disease rely on the above-mentioned data [11, 20]. These guidelines state that, when performed by an expert examiner, IUS can be a highly effective technique and can be safely

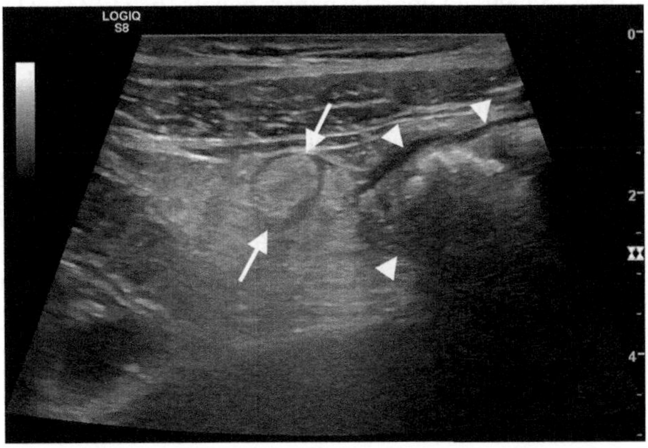

Fig. 13.3 Epiploic appendagitis observed at IUS as oval hyperechoic mass, with a hypoechoic rim (arrows), close to the sigmoid colon (arrow heads)

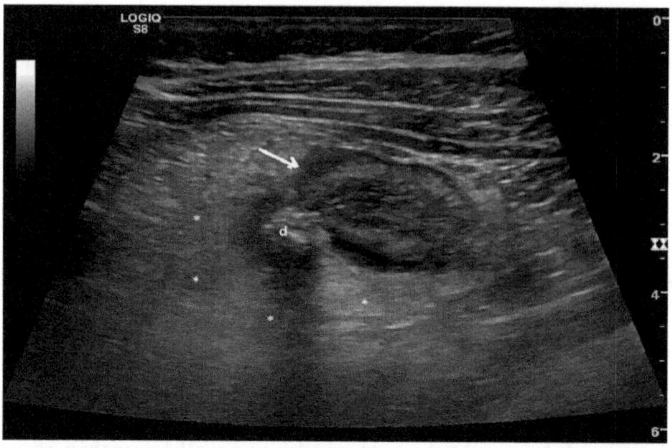

Fig. 13.4 Acute diverticulitis: short segmental bowel wall thickening (arrow), pericolic fat changes (asterisks), and the presence of an inflamed diverticulum (d)

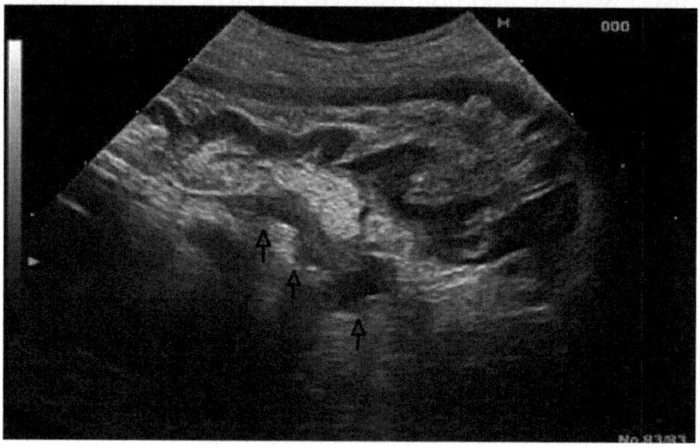

Fig. 13.5 Acute complicated diverticulitis. Small pericolic abscess (arrows), assessed as hypoechoic collection (here without gas within), adjacent to the colon, within the mesenteric fat

recommended as a preliminary test in a sequential diagnostic strategy in patients with suspected acute diverticulitis [11, 20]. Such a strategy recommends the use of CT scan in cases of negative or uncertain IUS results or to confirm severe complications of the disease.

Diagnostic sonographic criteria for acute diverticulitis have been well established and agreed upon by expert panels [6, 21–23]. They include at least two of the following: short segmental bowel wall thickening (>5 mm), pericolic fat changes, and the presence of an inflamed diverticulum (Fig. 13.4). The presence of the "dynamic sign" or intense pain evoked by graded compression at the site is another diagnostic feature. Hypoechoic pericolic changes may be associated with complicated diverticulitis. The presence of a pericolic abscess, a hypoechoic collection with or without gas, adjacent to the colon, within the mesenteric fat and more or less distant to the inflamed diverticulum, could accompany the above-mentioned findings in acute complicated diverticulitis (Fig. 13.5). In the latter, hypoechoic mesenteric strands or hyperechoic mesenteric fat (sometimes with gaseous artifacts) may suggest the presence of fistulas as complications of the inflamed diverticula (Fig. 13.6).

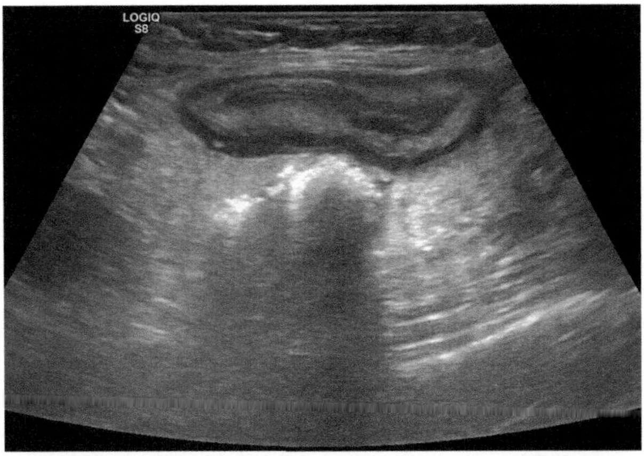

Fig. 13.6 Acute complicated diverticulitis. Hyperechoic mesenteric fat with gaseous artifacts, suggesting the presence of a perforation as complications of the inflamed diverticula

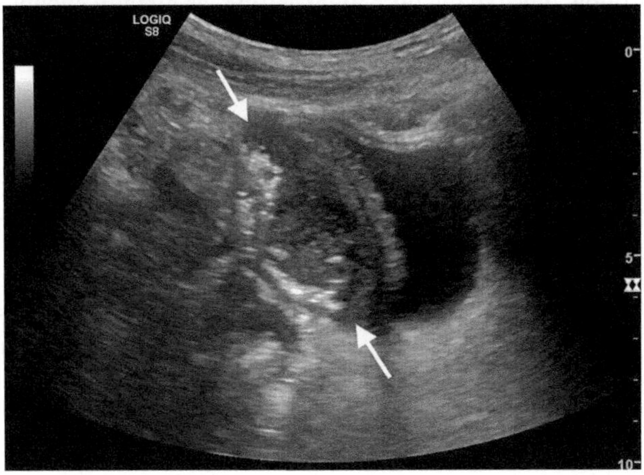

Fig. 13.7 Acute diverticulitis complicated with an abscess. The abscess (arrows) appears as large mixed hypoechoic and hyperechoic mass (due to gaseous artifacts) behind the urinary bladder

Contrast-enhanced ultrasound (CEUS) may be a useful imaging modality to discriminate the nature in hypoechoic lesions (whether inflammatory masses, phlegmons, or abscesses) and to better assess the severity of acute diverticulitis (Fig. 13.7). Increased flow within hypoechoic areas of inflammation can be used as a diagnostic criterion to discriminate fistulas and mesenteric phlegmons from localized perforation and abscesses [24, 25].

The relative disadvantages of IUS include the level of operator experience and difficulties in evaluating deep abdominal sites, particularly in obese patients. Operator experience may play a role in the accurate diagnosis [26], and the statements of the above-mentioned guidelines report that IUS may be the first choice for the diagnosis of acute diverticular disease provided a "qualified ultrasound examination" is performed, followed by CT in uncertain situations or complicated disease [11, 20].

In this regard, a Dutch study showed that the difference in sensitivity for detecting diverticulitis between unsupervised residents (who have already performed >500 exams) and supervised residents (with <500 exams) is substantial (former, more than 80%; latter, <60%), but their performance in terms of PPV was not significantly different [26]. This study confirms that the sonographer's experience is important and that a positive result in the hands of a nonexpert sonographer is unlikely to produce false-positive results.

However, an expert examiner is also the physician conscious of the limits of the technique, such as the suboptimal performance of transabdominal IUS in assessing deeper parts of the pelvis, particularly the rectosigmoid junction and the distal sigmoid colon, especially in obese patients and in the presence of overlaying gas [26].

Therefore, the appropriate and correct use of IUS as preliminary investigation in patients with suspected acute diverticulitis may be extremely useful to confirm the clinical hypothesis without the need of CT scan. This exam, however, must be performed anyway in case of inconclusive or negative results. Considering that most cases of acute diverticulitis observed in the emergency department are uncomplicated [27], the possibility to detect these conditions early by IUS and manage or follow these in the outpatient setting, as already shown in the literature, would be of benefit for patients and the health-care system.

13.3.3 Segmental Colitis Associated with Diverticulosis (SCAD) or Diverticular Disease-Associated Colitis (DAC)

This condition includes a spectrum of variable pathological entities characterized by chronic inflammation of the colonic mucosa adjacent to the diverticula. It usually does not involve the rectum or the right colon. Colonoscopy with biopsy for histopathology is necessary to obtain the diagnosis [11, 12]. Despite IUS is able to assess SCAD/DAC, its sonographic features are not yet well defined, and IUS accuracy as well as the diagnostic and clinical role in this condition to the best of our knowledge has never been explored so far. However, diverticula associated with inflammatory colitis, such as ulcerative colitis or infectious colitis, may show a mild thickening of the diverticular wall, associated with thickened colonic walls and usually a hypertrophy of the mesocolon (Fig. 13.8).

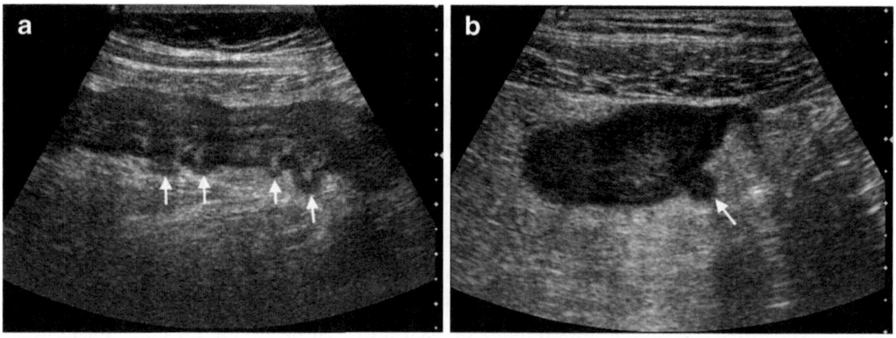

Fig. 13.8 Longitudinal (**a**) and transversal (**b**) scans of diverticula associated with inflammatory colitis (infectious colitis), showing a mild thickening and hypoechoic diverticular wall (arrows), associated with thickened colonic walls and hypertrophy of the mesocolon

13.4 Conclusions

There is a growing body of evidence that demonstrates the usefulness of IUS in the diagnosis and follow-up of patients with diverticular disease of the colon. The role of this modality in uncomplicated colonic diverticulosis remains largely uninvestigated. In the setting of acute diverticulitis, CT scanning and IUS have similar diagnostic accuracy for uncomplicated conditions. The accuracy of IUS, however, depends on patient features and operator experience. A good clinical approach may include IUS as a first line test, followed by CT if the results are nondiagnostic or inconclusive. In critically ill patients with obvious clinical evidence of sepsis, CT should be performed to rule out complications of acute diverticulitis.

References

1. Turner GA, O'Grady MJ, Purcell RV, Frizelle FA. Acute diverticulitis in young patients: a review of the changing epidemiology and etiology. Dig Dis Sci. 2021;31 https://doi.org/10.1007/s10620-021-06956-w. Epub ahead of print
2. Broad JB, Wu Z, Xie S, Bissett IP, Connolly MJ. Diverticular disease epidemiology: acute hospitalisations are growing fastest in young men. Tech Coloproctol. 2019;23:713–21.
3. O'Grady M, Turner G, Currie W, Yi M, Frizelle F, Purcell R. Acute diverticulitis: an ongoing economic burden on the health system. ANZ J Surg. 2020;90:2046–9.
4. Howard ZD, Noble VE, Marill KA, Sajed D, Rodrigues M, Bertuzzi B, Liteplo AS. Bedside ultrasound maximizes patient satisfaction. J Emerg Med. 2014;46:46–53.
5. Dietrich CF, Hollerweger A, Dirks K, Higginson A, Serra C, Calabrese E, e al. EFSUMB gastrointestinal ultrasound (GIUS) task force group: celiac sprue and other rare gastrointestinal diseases ultrasound features. Med Ultrason. 2019;21:299–315.
6. Dirks K, Calabrese E, Dietrich CF, Gilja OH, Hausken T, Higginson A, et al. EFSUMB position paper: recommendations for gastrointestinal ultrasound (GIUS) in acute appendicitis and diverticulitis. Ultraschall Med. 2019;40:163–75.
7. Maconi G, Nylund K, Ripolles T, Calabrese E, Dirks K, Dietrich CF, et al. EFSUMB recommendations and clinical guidelines for intestinal ultrasound (GIUS) in inflammatory bowel diseases. Ultraschall Med. 2018;39:304–17.
8. Hollerweger A, Maconi G, Ripolles T, Nylund K, Higginson A, Serra C, et al. Gastrointestinal ultrasound (GIUS) in intestinal emergencies - an EFSUMB position paper. Ultraschall Med. 2020;41:646–57.
9. Ferzoco LB, Raptopoulos V, Silen W. Acute diverticulitis. N Engl J Med. 1998;338:1521–6.
10. Hollerweger A, Macheiner P, Hübner E, Brunner W, Gritzmann N. Colonic diverticulosis: a comparison between sonography and endoscopy. Ultraschall Med. 2002;23:41–6.
11. Cuomo R, Barbara G, Pace F, Annese V, Bassotti G, Binda GA, et al. Italian consensus conference for colonic diverticulosis and diverticular disease. United European Gastroenterol J. 2014;2:413–42.
12. Tursi A, Brandimarte G, Di Mario F, Lanas A, Scarpignato C, Bafutto M, et al. International consensus on diverticulosis and diverticular disease. Statements from the 3rd international symposium on diverticular disease. J Gastrointestin Liver Dis. 2019;28(suppl. 4):57–66.
13. Soncini M, Stasi C, Usai Satta P, Milazzo G, Bianco M, Leandro G, et al. AIGO. IBS clinical management in Italy: the AIGO survey. Dig Liver Dis. 2019;51:782–9.
14. Francis CY, Duffy JN, Whorwell PJ, Martin DF. Does routine abdominal ultrasound enhance diagnostic accuracy in irritable bowel syndrome? Am J Gastroenterol. 1996;91:1348–50.

15. Maconi G, Hausken T, Dietrich CF, Pallotta N, Sporea I, Nurnberg D, et al. Gastrointestinal ultrasound in functional disorders of the gastrointestinal tract - EFSUMB consensus statement. Ultrasound Int Open. 2021;7(1):E14–24. https://doi.org/10.1055/a-1474-8013.
16. Mattii L, Ippolito C, Segnani C, Battolla B, Colucci R, Dolfi A, et al. Altered expression pattern of molecular factors involved in colonic smooth muscle functions: an immunohistochemical study in patients with diverticular disease. PLoS One. 2013;8(2):e57023.
17. Crade M, Pham V. Ultrasound examination of the sigmoid colon: possible new diagnostic tool for irritable bowel syndrome. Ultrasound Obstet Gynecol. 2006;27:206–9.
18. Lameris W, van Randen A, Bipat S, Bossuyt PM, Boermeester MA, Stoker J. Graded compression ultrasonography and computed tomography in acute colonic diverticulitis: meta-analysis of test accuracy. Eur Radiol. 2008;18:2498–511.
19. Liljegren G, Chabok A, Wickbom M, Smedh K, Nilsson K. Acute colonic diverticulitis: a systematic review of diagnostic accuracy. Color Dis. 2007;9:480–8.
20. Schreyer AG, Layer G. S2k guidlines for diverticular disease and diverticulitis: diagnosis, classification, and therapy for the radiologist. Rofo. 2015;187:676–84.
21. Wilson SR, Toi A. The value of sonography in the diagnosis of acute diverticulitis of the colon. Am J Roentgenol. 1990;154:1199–202.
22. Hollerweger A, Macheiner P, Rettenbacher T, Brunner W, Gritzmann N. Colonic diverticulitis: diagnostic value and appearance of inflamed diverticula-sonographic evaluation. Eur Radiol. 2001;11:1956.
23. Valentino M, Serra C, Ansaloni L, Mantovani G, Pavlica P, Barozzi L. Sonographic features of acute colonic diverticulitis. J Clin Ultrasound. 2009;37:457–63.
24. Girlich C, Schacherer D, Lamby P, Scherer MN, Schreyer AG, Jung EM. Innovations in contrast enhanced high resolution ultrasound improve sonographic imaging of the intestine. Clin Hemorheol Microcirc. 2010;45:207–15.
25. Braden B, Ignee A, Hocke M, Palmer RM, Dietrich C. Diagnostic value and clinical utility of contrast enhanced ultrasound in intestinal diseases. Dig Liver Dis. 2010;42:667.
26. Van Randen A, Laméris W, van Es HW, van Heesewijk HP, van Ramshorst B, Ten Hove W, et al. A comparison of the accuracy of ultrasound and computed tomography in common diagnoses causing acute abdominal pain. Eur Radiol. 2011;21:1535–45.
27. Kaiser AM, Jiang JK, Lake JP, Ault G, Artinyan A, Gonzalez-Ruiz C, et al. The management of complicated diverticulitis and the role of computed tomography. Am J Gastroenterol. 2005;100:910–7.

Radiology

14

Nicola Flor, Silvia Innamorati, and Perry Pickhardt

14.1 Acute Diverticulitis

The evaluation of patients with acute diverticulitis includes medical history, physical examination, and laboratory testing, but cross-sectional imaging often plays a pivotal role in verifying the diagnosis. In fact, clinical suspicion of acute diverticulitis alone is correct in only 40–65% [1, 2], especially in patients with no previous diagnosis of diverticulosis. Different radiological tests can be applied for the diagnosis of acute diverticulitis, including ultrasound, computed tomography (CT), and magnetic resonance (MR) imaging. CT colonography (CTC) and double-contrast barium enema (DCBE) are contraindicated in the setting of suspected acute diverticulitis.

Conventional CT has a high sensitivity and specificity in the diagnosis of acute diverticulitis [2] and is generally considered by most to be the preferred front-line radiological test for evaluating patients with suspected acute diverticulitis.

N. Flor (✉)
Unità Operativa di Radiodiagnostica, Ospedale Luigi Sacco, ASST Fatebenefratelli Sacco, Milan, Italy
e-mail: nicola.flor@unimi.it

S. Innamorati
Postgraduation School in Radiodiagnostic, Facoltà di Medicina e Chirurgia, Università degli Studi di Milano, Milan, Italy
e-mail: silvia.innamorati@unimi.it

P. Pickhardt
Department of Radiology, School of Medicine & Public Health, University of Wisconsin, Madison, WI, USA
e-mail: ppickhardt2@uwhealth.org

© The Author(s), under exclusive license to Springer Nature Switzerland AG 2022
A. Tursi et al. (eds.), *Colonic Diverticular Disease*,
https://doi.org/10.1007/978-3-030-93761-4_14

The strengths of CT examination include its reproducibility, operator independence, wide availability, and high accuracy for diagnosing acute disease [2, 3]. CT allows for a comprehensive evaluation, including the grading of severity and detection of complications that affect therapeutic management.

Two meta-analyses [2, 3] have reported that ultrasound may have comparable accuracy in the evaluation of acute diverticulitis, although these data may be somewhat biased, and certain European scientific societies guidelines [1, 4–6] propose ultrasound as the first-line examination. This test is safe, low-cost, widely available, and easily accessible within the emergency department. Another advantage of ultrasound is the ability to correlate imaging findings with the region of greatest tenderness in real time. The relative disadvantages of ultrasound include operator dependence, difficulties in evaluation of the distal sigmoid colon, especially in obese patients, and a lower accuracy for abscess identification. Moreover, a severity classification cannot be assessed by ultrasound [7].

Currently, MR imaging does not play an important role in the workup of patients with suspected acute diverticulitis, but it can be considered in selected cases, such as pregnant women. Although there are some advantages compared with other radiological tests (e.g., lack of ionizing radiation exposure and high intrinsic contrast resolution), MR availability in the emergency department is currently limited in most hospital settings. Moreover, to date, there is relatively little evidence regarding the accuracy of MR for acute diverticulitis, limited to small select patient cohorts [8, 9].

Both CTC and DCBE are contraindicated in patients with acute diverticulitis, adding no additional useful information to conventional CT evaluation for acute management. Since both examinations include active colonic distention with either room air or carbon dioxide, there is at least a theoretical concern for extension of the typical microperforation associated with acute diverticulitis to more frank perforation and peritonitis. DCBE in particular is an obsolete test and should be abandoned, regardless of the clinical scenario. This test has a lower accuracy than CTC and optical colonoscopy for colorectal evaluation [10], is associated with higher ionizing radiation exposure [11], and is less acceptable for patients [12]. On occasion, findings of unsuspected mild acute or subacute diverticulitis may be encountered at CTC in patients with only minimal or no apparent symptoms.

14.1.1 CT Protocol

There has been some controversy over the appropriate CT protocol regarding the use of oral, rectal, and intravenous contrast agents. In general, the use of intravenous contrast should be encouraged in cases of suspected complicated disease to confirm the severity of the event and better diagnose complications such as abscesses and fistulas.

In cases of massive diverticular bleeding, it may not be possible to identify the source by colonoscopy, and angiographic or surgical therapy may be necessary [13–15].

Given the delay associated with bowel preparation and the difficulty of endoscopic visualization in the setting of large-volume hemorrhage, CT angiography has seen an increasing role in the initial workup of acute lower GI bleeding [16–18]. CT provides more information regarding localization and potential structural causes for the bleeding.

Vice versa, some authors [19, 20] suggested that the unenhanced CT examination alone is an accurate and valuable tool for triaging patients older than 75 years, presenting to the emergency department with nontraumatic acute abdominal pain.

In our experience, neither an oral nor a rectal contrast is truly necessary, whereas visceral obesity and, in particular, a high amount of pericolic fat is beneficial in visualizing the typical findings (i.e., perifocal stranding; inflamed diverticula; abscesses) of this acute event.

14.1.2 Typical CT Findings and Severity Classifications

The diagnosis of acute diverticulitis can be directly made on the basis of localized bowel wall thickening that is centered on an inflamed diverticulum, with surrounding peridiverticular inflammation of pericolonic fat (Fig. 14.1). As diverticulitis is primarily an extraluminal disease, cross-sectional imaging holds a distinct advantage over luminal studies. Covered or free perforations can be rapidly and reliably diagnosed by the direct detection of air inclusions outside the intestinal lumen (Fig. 14.2), often associated with mesenteric fasciae thickening and free fluid. In case of severe disease, contrast-enhanced CT is an accurate test for diagnosing both parietal and peridiverticular abscesses (Fig. 14.3). When abscesses are present, CT is also useful for guiding abscess drainage, particularly in cases in which collections are small and located in regions difficult to assess [21].

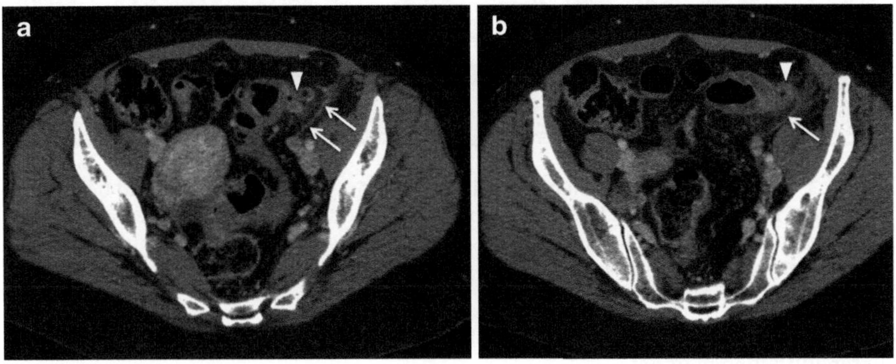

Fig. 14.1 Uncomplicated acute sigmoid diverticulitis in a 51-year-old woman with LLQ pain. (**a**) Unenhanced CT image showing inflamed sigmoid diverticula (arrow head) with extraluminal inflammatory changes surrounding the diverticula with thickening of the mesenteric fascia (arrows). (**b**) Contrast-enhanced CT image confirms uncomplicated acute sigmoid diverticulitis with an inflamed sigmoid diverticulum (arrow head), pericolonic fat stranding, and thickening of the mesenteric fascia (arrow); no abscess was present

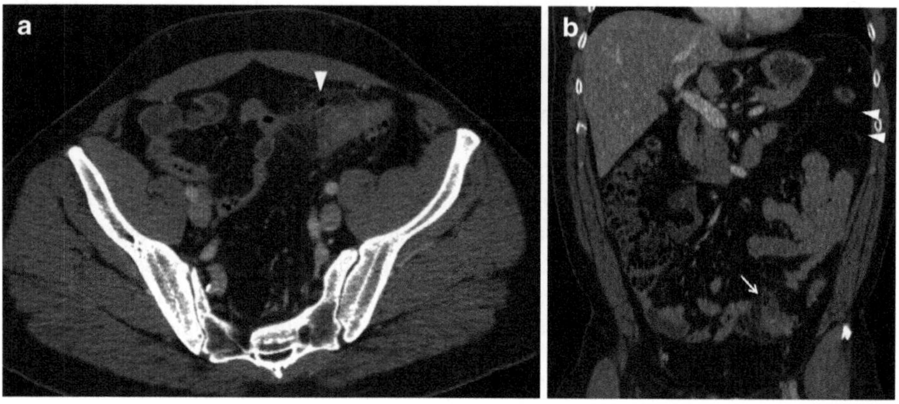

Fig. 14.2 Complicated acute sigmoid diverticulitis in a 50-year-old man with LLQ pain. (**a**) Contrast-enhanced axial CT image showing air inclusions outside the sigmoid colon lumen (arrow head) in a patient with sigmoid colon acute diverticulitis with evidence of extraluminal inflammatory changes surrounding the sigmoid diverticula. (**b**) Contrast-enhanced coronal CT image confirms complicated acute sigmoid diverticulitis with an inflamed sigmoid diverticulum (arrow), pericolonic fat stranding, and thickening of the mesenteric fascia (arrows); free perforations can be diagnosed by the direct detection of air inclusions outside the sigmoid colon and in the upper left quadrant (arrow heads)

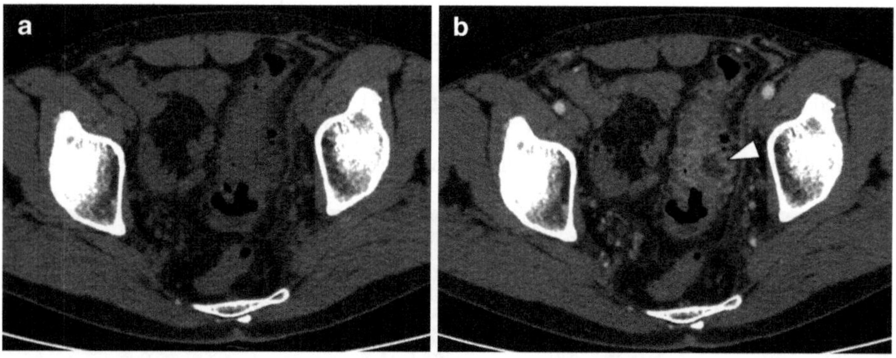

Fig. 14.3 Complicated acute sigmoid diverticulitis in a 56-year-old man diagnosed by contrast-enhanced CT examination. (**a**) Unenhanced axial CT image showing sigmoid diverticula with fat stranding and thickening of the mesenteric fascia. (**b**) Contrast-enhanced axial CT image showing intraparietal abscess (arrow head), not clearly visualizable at an unenhanced scan

CT evaluation is valuable for its appraisal of disease severity, which impacts therapeutic management.

There are many classifications of disease severity based on CT [6, 22–25] and none has been demonstrated to be clearly superior to the other. Among these, the modified version of the Hinchey classification has been used in several clinical trials and it is the most used in clinical practice.

This classification and that recently proposed by the WSES acute diverticulitis working group [25] strive to divide patients into two main categories, namely, uncomplicated and complicated acute diverticulitis.

In uncomplicated cases, the CT findings are generally limited to the phlegmonous reaction of the pericolonic fat tissue (Fig. 14.4a), whereas complicated features include peridiverticular abscess (Fig. 14.4b), significant pneumoperitoneum (Fig. 14.5), and diffuse peritonitis. Moreover, the CT grading of acute diverticulitis has prognostic significance in terms of disease recurrence after an initial episode of acute disease [26].

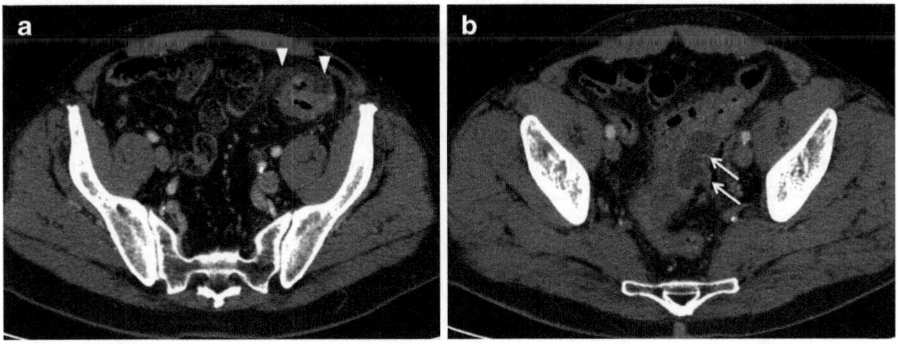

Fig. 14.4 Examples of uncomplicated and complicated acute diverticulitis. (**a**) Contrast-enhanced axial CT image in a 60-year-old man showing mild acute diverticulitis with an inflamed sigmoid diverticulum with fat stranding (arrow heads). (**b**) Contrast-enhanced axial CT image in a 48-year-old man showing complicated acute diverticulitis with a large peridiverticular abscess (arrows) adjacent to the sigmoid diverticula

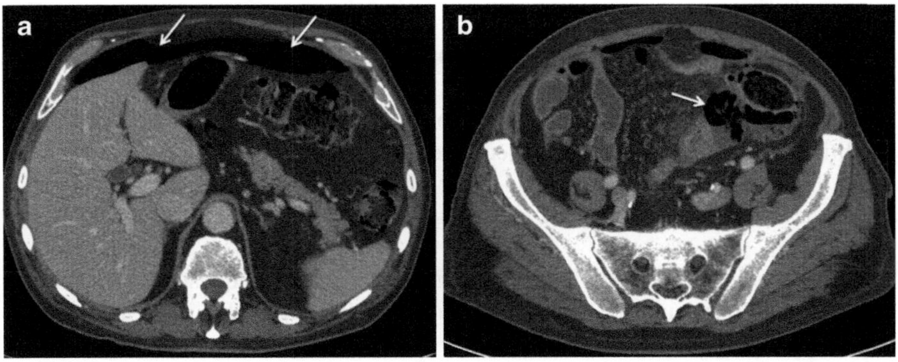

Fig. 14.5 Complicated acute sigmoid diverticulitis in a 73-year-old man with a large abscess and pneumoperitoneum due to perforation of an inflamed sigmoid diverticulum. Laparoscopic surgery confirmed sigmoid perforation in the presence of acute diverticulitis and purulent peritonitis-treated Hartmann sigmoid colon surgical resection. (**a**) Contrast-enhanced axial CT image showing significant pneumoperitoneum (arrows). (**b**) Contrast-enhanced axial CT image showing free air (arrow) adjacent to the inflamed sigmoid diverticula

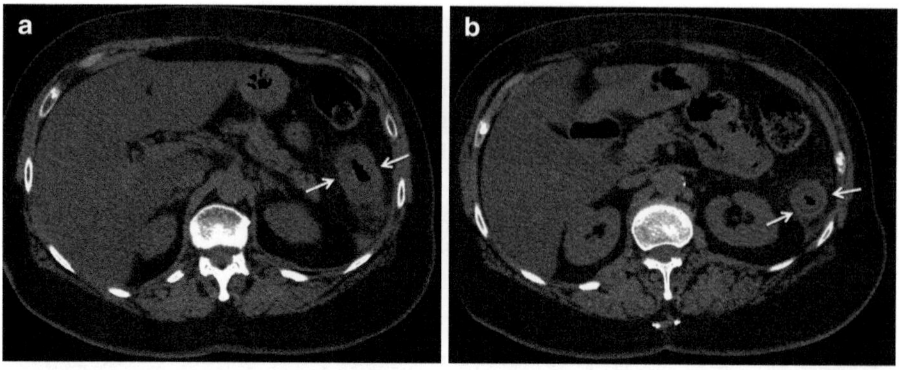

Fig. 14.6 Descending colon nonspecific acute colitis mimicking acute diverticulitis in a 77-year-old man with COVID-19 infection. (**a**) Unenhanced axial CT image showing circumferential descending colon wall thickening (arrows) with fat stranding and thickening of the left anterior renal fascia. (**b**) Unenhanced axial CT image showing circumferential distal descending colon wall thickening (arrows) with fat stranding and thickening of the left anterior renal fascia. No diverticula are present

14.1.3 Differential Diagnosis

In addition to being highly accurate for acute diverticulitis itself, CT is also the most accurate test for diagnosing alternative conditions [27, 28] (Fig. 14.6). Several studies have described characteristic CT features differentiating diverticular disease from CRC [29, 30], but, in some cases, findings overlap and the differential diagnosis remains challenging. In our opinion, this difficulty can explain data obtained from two large trials [31, 32], describing a higher 1-year CRC risk for patients recovering from an acute episode of diverticulitis.

14.2 Chronic Diverticular Disease

In contrast to acute diverticulitis, the role of imaging in the follow-up of acute diverticulitis is in evolution and still subject to debate.

In this setting, the evidence is in favor of computed tomography colonography (CTC) as a preferred radiological test, suggesting a complementary role of CTC and colonoscopy [33, 34].

Regardless of the specific scenario, radiologists are first requested to confirm the diagnosis of diverticular disease, ruling out other diseases and in particular a superimposed CRC.

CTC is able to depict the test number and site of diverticula [35], morphology of the diverticula necks (Fig. 14.7), less common disease-related findings such as focal or diffuse wall thickening (Fig. 14.8), and sigmoid colon stenosis (Fig. 14.9) [36–38], better than others. Moreover, CTC is highly accurate for diagnosing

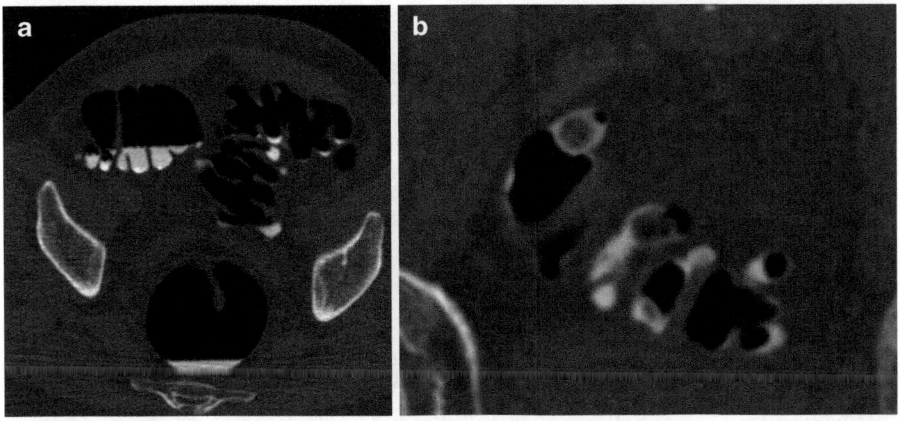

Fig. 14.7 Diagnosis of diverticulosis by CT colonography. (**a**, **b**) CTC axial images showing multiple sigmoid diverticula with small- and medium-sized necks

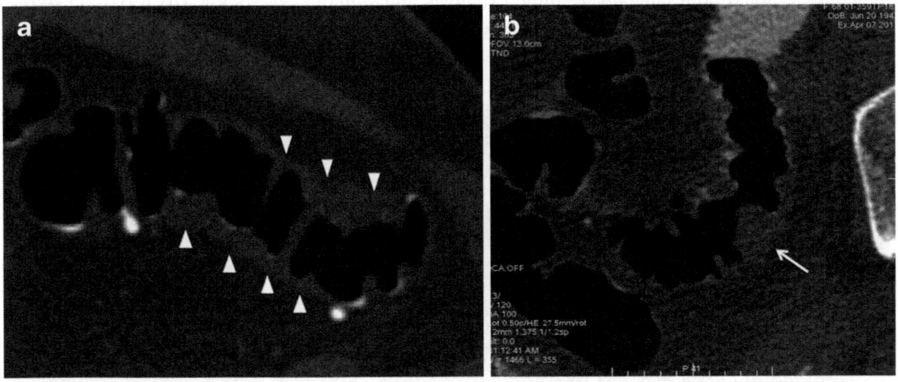

Fig. 14.8 Examples of wall thickening associated with sigmoid colon diverticula. (**a**) Axial CTC image showing mild sigmoid colon wall thickening (arrow heads) in the presence of sigmoid diverticula. These are typical findings of chronic diverticular disease. (**b**) Axial CTC image showing eccentric focal sigmoid colon wall thickening (arrow) in the presence of sigmoid diverticula. The benign nature of this finding has been confirmed at conventional colonoscopy

complications (abscesses and fistulas), which represent a validated indication for elective surgery; fistulas in particular could be overlooked by conventional abdominal CT performed at the time of an acute event (Fig. 14.10).

The advantage of CTC over colonoscopy in evaluating patients with diverticular disease relies on its minor invasiveness; even if diverticular disease is the first leading reason for a non-well-distended colonic tract at CTC [39], this test is always complete, different from colonoscopy. A high-quality CTC examination can be performed even in case of severe stenosis [34, 38], allowing adequate accuracy in diagnosing proximal colonic polyps and CRCs [40, 41].

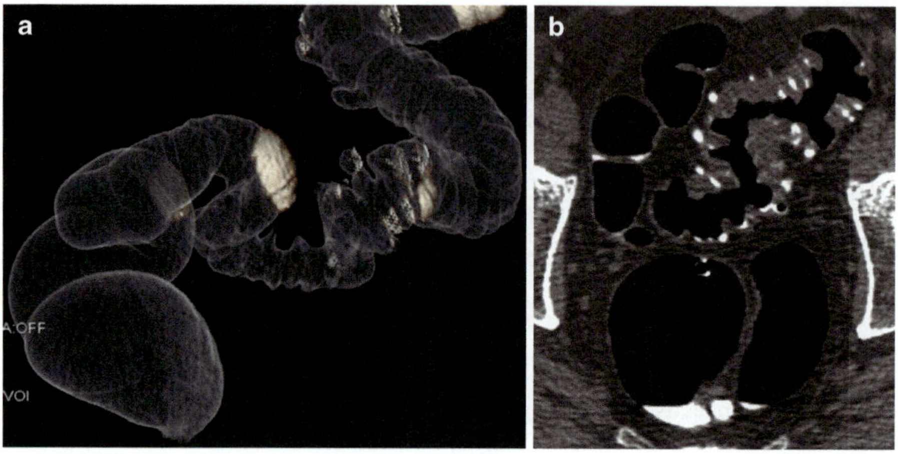

Fig. 14.9 A 49-year-old man with marked sigmoid colon wall thickening and lumen stenosis after recovering from acute diverticulitis. (**a**) Double-contrast barium enema like-view CTC image showing sigmoid colon with severe lumen stenosis and sigmoid diverticula. (**b**) Axial 2D supine CTC image showing marked sigmoid colon wall thickening with severe lumen stenosis, in the presence of sigmoid diverticula

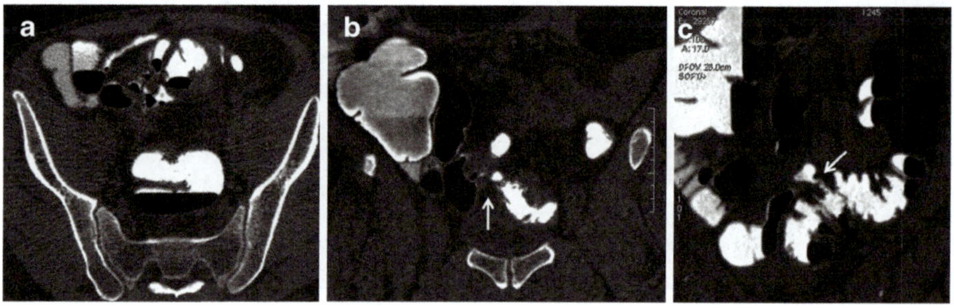

Fig. 14.10 A 49-year-old man with a double enteroenteric fistula in chronic diverticular inflammation. (**a**) Axial CTC image showing sigmoid colon wall thickening of both the distal ileum and the sigmoid colon with adjacent fat stranding. (**b**, **c**) Coronal CTC images demonstrating the two sigmoid colon–ileum fistulae (arrow) and sigmoid colon wall thickening. The patient underwent CTC elective surgery with confirmation of two sigmoid colon–ileum fistulae in chronic diverticular disease

This fact has a tremendous clinical impact if we consider the risk of advanced adenoma related to patients recovering from acute diverticulitis [42]. In particular, patients with severe stenosis caused by diverticular disease and responsive to an incomplete colonoscopy could have a significant delay in the diagnosis of proximal colon lesions (Fig. 14.11).

Even if the literature concerning the use of CTC in the follow-up of patients recovering from an episode of acute diverticulitis is not yet robust enough, no complications have been reported and in particular no cases of perforation have ever been described [34, 43].

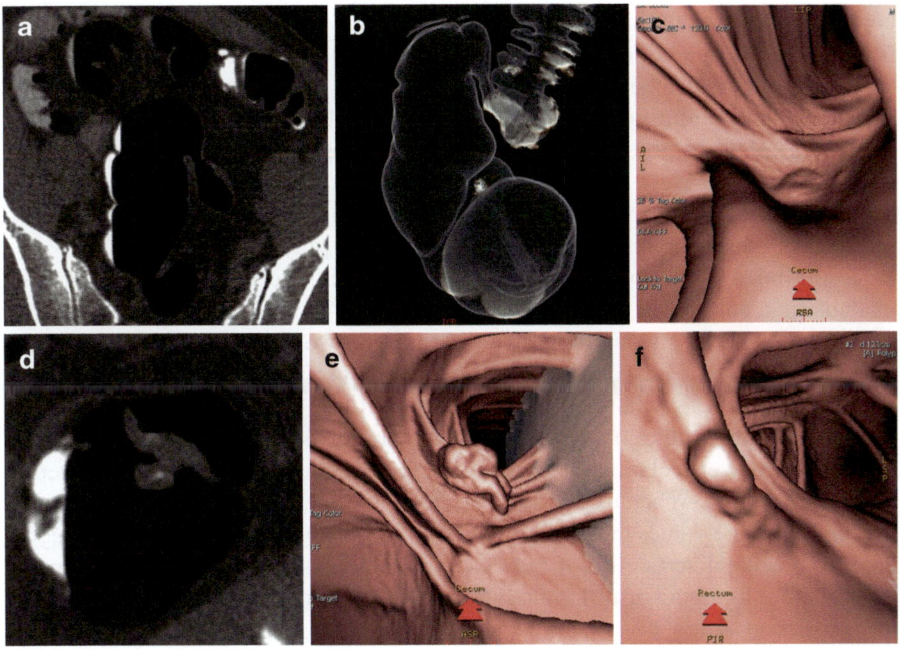

Fig. 14.11 Positive CTC examination in a 57-year-old-man recovering from acute diverticulitis, with incomplete colonoscopy. (**a**, **b**) 2D axial CTC image (A) and 3D colon map (B) showing severe luminal narrowing associated with diverticula at the distal sigmoid colon, explaining the incomplete colonoscopy. (**c**) 3D endoluminal CTC view showing a nonpolypoid lesion in the transverse colon. (**d**, **e**) Axial 2D (D) and 3D endoluminal (E) CTC views showing a 20 mm pedunculated polyp in the ascending colon. (**f**) 3D endoluminal (H) CTC view showing a 7 mm sessile polyp in the transverse colon. The patient underwent subtotal colectomy; the pathology confirmed the presence of three right colon lesions revealing as tubular adenoma. In particular, the larger one contained high-grade dysplasia

For patients recovering from an episode of acute diverticulitis, CTC should be carried out at least 3 or 4 months after the acute event to reduce both the risk of perforation and because of the likelihood of a residual acute inflammatory component.

14.2.1 CTC Protocol

It may be advisable to slightly modify the standard CTC protocol in the setting of a known complicated diverticular disease. For example, it can be useful to perform the CTC examination with an IV contrast in the presence of severe wall thickening and luminal stenosis, when the differential diagnosis between diverticular disease and CRC is more relevant. Another scenario generally requiring an IV contrast is when there is potential concern for a diverticular complication such as abscesses or fistulas. Evaluation with soft tissue windowing improves the assessment for these complications over the standard CTC polyp window. In patients with severe diverticular disease, an additional third scan in the right lateral decubitus position (after supine and prone) can be valuable for confirming the severity of both luminal stenosis and wall thickening, avoiding errors caused by colon spasms [43–45]. To achieve the best distention of the sigmoid colon, which is most commonly involved in diverticular disease, the right lateral decubitus position is generally obtained for gravitational reasons. Moreover, a lateral decubitus position is much more comfortable and feasible for obese and otherwise debilitated patients [45].

To optimize distention of the entire colon, which is critical for a high-quality examination, automated carbon dioxide insufflation is preferred [46]. In addition, a spasmolytic agent may help optimize distention as well. Taylor et al. [47] demonstrated significantly improved distention using hyoscine butylbromide as a hypotonic drug in CTC, given that it is especially useful in patients with diverticulosis. Carbon dioxide insufflation with an automatic device is preferable when evaluating patients with diverticular disease because of the continuous low pressure and reproducible distention. When using room air, the risk of perforation is increased due to the high-pressure values that can be achieved. If the patient has only recently recovered from acute diverticulitis, it may be reasonable to scan the entire abdomen and pelvis before initiating insufflation. If the pre-insufflation scan shows signs suggesting persistent acute diverticulitis, active colonic distention should be aborted (Fig. 14.12).

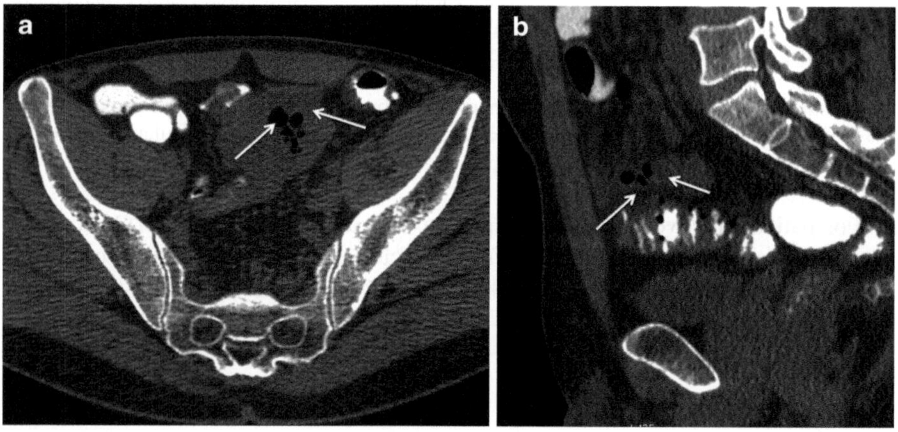

Fig. 14.12 Unsuspected persistent complication from diverticulitis detected at CTC. (**a**) 2D axial CT image taken before carbon dioxide insufflation in a patient with a recent episode of diverticulitis showing air bubbles (arrows) around the sigmoid colon related to perforation and ongoing inflammation. Thus, the scheduled CTC was not performed and the patient was referred for therapeutic management. (**b**) 2D sagittal CTC image confirms the presence of air bubbles (arrows) around the sigmoid colon due to recent covered perforation

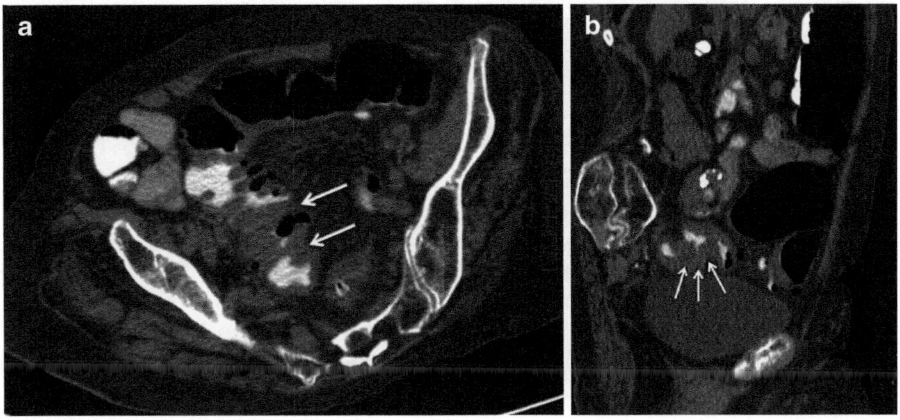

Fig. 14.13 CTC examination in a 66-year-old-woman with recurrent diverticulitis (DDSS 4). (**a**, **b**) Axial 2D image (**a**) and sagittal 2D CTC image (**b**) showing marked sigmoid wall thickening (arrows) and luminal narrowing associated with diverticula in the setting of sigmoid diverticular disease, classified as DDSS 4. The patient underwent elective surgery, and the pathology revealed diverticular disease with acute and chronic inflammation

14.2.2 Diverticular Disease Severity Score Based on CT Colonography

Wall thickening and lumen stenosis are the two CTC features that need to be investigated to describe the severity of the disease in follow-up, and, recently, a diverticular disease severity score (DDSS) based on CTC findings has been proposed [43]. The score is based on the varying degrees of these two CTC findings, i.e., wall thickening and lumen stenosis, and consists of four grades (DDSS 1–4). In the case of DDSS grade 4 (Fig. 14.13), where marked wall thickening is associated with severe luminal stenosis, surgical options should be considered. In practice, the simultaneous presence of severe stenosis and the inability to exclude CRC are both potential indications for surgery [48]. Moreover, this validated CTC-based DDSS score is a good predictor of chronic inflammation and fibrosis [49] and seems to have prognostic value in the follow-up of acute diverticulitis [50].

14.2.3 Differential Diagnosis Between Diverticular Disease and Colorectal Cancer

In patients with diverticular disease, it can be challenging to recognize a superimposed colorectal cancer (CRC), but these two entities are both relatively common in elderly patients and can therefore coexist. This differential diagnosis is particularly tricky in cases of marked wall thickening and severe luminal stenosis from diverticular disease. Some authors [36, 37] have described a number of CTC findings as being useful in differentiating these two disease entities. Of these various findings,

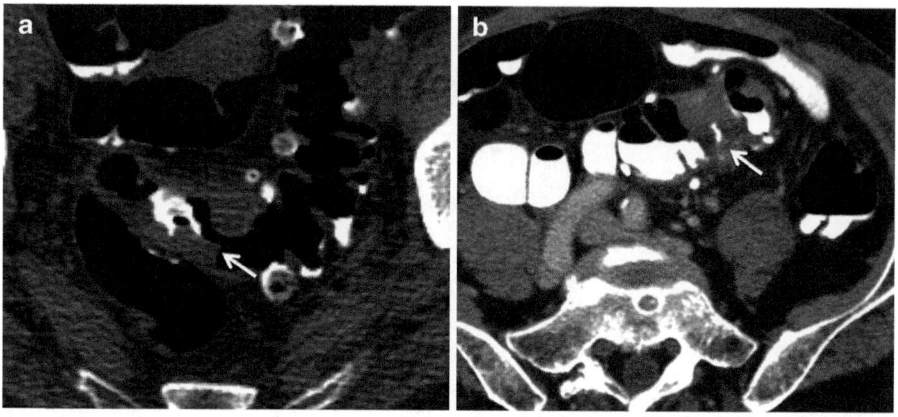

Fig. 14.14 Sigmoid diverticular disease versus cancer at CTC. (**a**) 2D axial CTC image in a 59-year-old-woman showing focal sigmoid wall thickening with severe luminal narrowing, shoulder formation (arrow), and diverticula adjacent to, but not within, the affected segment. The patient underwent a same-day colonoscopy with biopsies, and CRC diagnosis was confirmed. The pathology after surgery revealed adenocarcinoma (pT3N2b). (**b**) 2D axial CTC image showing circumferential segmental wall thickening and luminal narrowing of the sigmoid colon associated with multiple diverticula (arrow). The presence of diverticula is a key factor for excluding cancer. This was a diverticular stricture

the absence of diverticula in the affected segment and the presence of a shoulder phenomenon are the two most important findings for CRC (Fig. 14.14). Other CTC signs in favor of cancer include shorter length with straightening of the involved segment, the absence of mesenteric fascia thickening, the presence of distorted folds, and the presence of prominent local lymph nodes.

Lips et al. [37] described a prevalence of about 4–5% of their population where findings of advanced diverticular disease versus CRC are present. We believe that this prevalence could be substantially higher in some settings, including those patients recovering from a prior episode of acute diverticulitis with CTC. The above-mentioned criteria are useful for ruling out CRC, but sometimes the CTC findings will overlap. In these selected cases, referral to optical colonoscopy or flexible sigmoidoscopy may be necessary to allow for direct mucosal evaluation and biopsy. In other cases, the surgical option may be indicated regardless of the underlying cause.

14.2.4 Preoperative Surgical Information

There are a variety of treatment options for patients with chronic diverticular disease, leading to some controversy in the surgical guidelines [48]. In particular, new surgical guidelines [51–53] recommend a more conservative and case-by-case

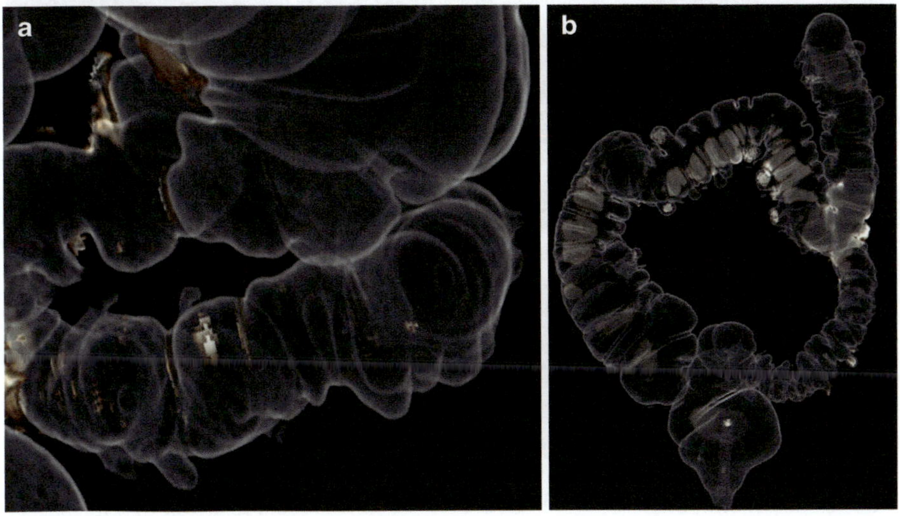

Fig. 14.15 Examples of a different distribution of diverticula in two patients who are candidates for elective surgery. (**a**) 3D computed tomography colonographic color map. The image shows diverticula limited to the sigmoid colon. (**b**) 3D computed tomography colonographic color map. The image shows diverticula spread in the whole colon

approach, taking into account multiple factors, including patient age, patient' s comorbidities (i.e., immune status), number of recurrent episodes of acute diverticulitis, the presence of complications, and patient preferences. Before elective surgery, surgeons could benefit from detailed anatomic information regarding the entire colon, and CTC, in our opinion, represents the test of choice for providing this. In this regard, CTC is clearly superior to both optical colonoscopy and the barium enema. In particular, CTC provides detailed information on colon anatomy, total number and distribution of diverticula (Fig. 14.15), and the degree of wall thickening and luminal stenosis. Surgical treatment is often considered when CTC detects unsuspected complications, such as abscess or fistula. CTC can also guide clinicians and surgeons when the appropriate therapeutic management is uncertain. For example, CTC diagnosis of unsuspected severe luminal stenosis could be a key factor in deciding on a surgical option. The surgical approach is generally laparoscopic, and surgeons could benefit from information about the vascular map derived from CTC (Fig. 14.16) [54, 55]. Of course, to obtain this level of detail requires a contrast-enhanced CTC protocol, adding an arterial contrast phase to the standard portal venous phase. In general, the initial position (e.g., prone) is obtained prior to the IV contrast, allowing for assessment of enhancement.

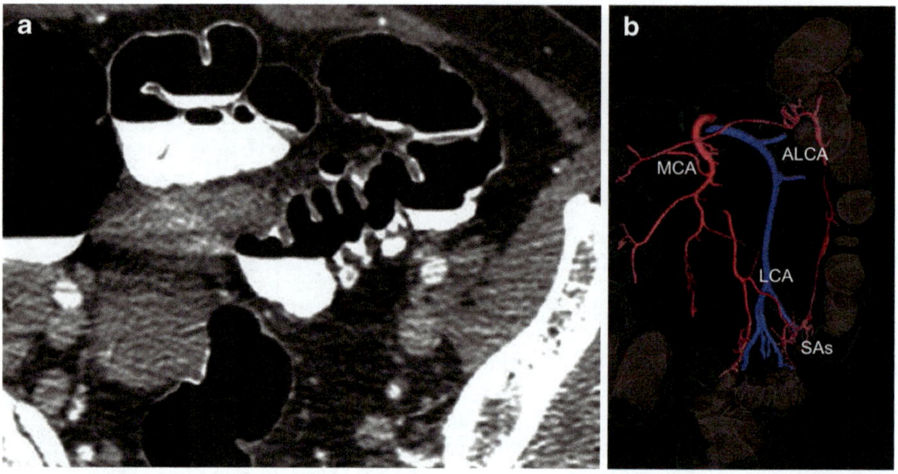

Fig. 14.16 Examples of a vascular 3D map provided by CT colonography. (**a**) 2D axial CTC image showing multiple diverticula limited to the sigmoid colon. (**b**) 3D-fused image demonstrating the sigmoid arteries (SAs) branching from the left colic artery (LCA) and the accessory left colic artery (ALCA) branching from the middle colic artery (MCA). LCA and SAs run anteriorly to the inferior mesenteric vein

References

1. Andeweg CS, Mulder IM, Felt-Bersma RJ, et al. Guidelines of diagnostics and treatment of acute left-sided colonic diverticulitis. Dig Surg. 2013;30:278–92.
2. Lameris W, van Randen A, Bipat S, et al. Graded compression ultrasonography and computed tomography in acute colonic diverticulitis: meta-analysis of test accuracy. Eur Radiol. 2008;18:2498–511.
3. Liljegren G, Chabok A, Wickbom M, et al. Acute colonic diverticulitis: a systematic review of diagnostic accuracy. Colorectal Dis. 2007;9:480–8.
4. Fozard JB, Armitage NC, Schofield JB, et al. ACPGBI position statement on elective resection for diverticulitis. Color Dis. 2011;13(suppl 3):1–11.
5. Nederlandse Vereniging voor Heelkunde. Richtlijn "Diagnostiek en behandeling acute diverticulitis van het colon" (Dutch Society of Surgery. Guideline "Diagnosis and Treatment of Acute Colonic Diverticulitis"). 2012. http://heelkunde.nl/uploads/mu/22/mu22HtlbEpr-SLLyAdT5nQ/NVvH-richtlijn-Acute-diverticulitis-van-het-colon-2012.pdf. Accessed June 2013.
6. Schreyer AG, Layer G. S2k guidelines for diverticular disease and diverticulitis: diagnosis, classification, and therapy for the radiologist. Fortschr Röntgenstr. 2015;187:676–84.
7. Schultz JK, Azhar N, Binda GA, et al. European Society of Coloproctology: guidelines for the management of diverticular disease of the colon. Color Dis. 2020;22(Suppl 2):5–28. https://doi.org/10.1111/codi.15140. Epub 2020 Jul 7
8. Oh KY, Gilfeather M, Kennedy A, et al. Limited abdominal MRI in the evaluation of acute right upper quadrant pain. Abdom Imaging. 2003;28:643–51.
9. Heverhagen JT, Sitter H, Zielke A, et al. Prospective evaluation of the value of magnetic resonance imaging in suspected acute sigmoid diverticulitis. Dis Colon Rectum. 2008;51:1810–5.
10. Halligan S, Wooldrage K, Dadswell E, Kralj-Hans I, von Wagner C, et al. Computed tomographic colonography versus barium enema for diagnosis of colorectal cancer or large polyps in symp-

tomatic patients (SIGGAR): a multicentre randomised trial. Lancet. 2013;381(9873):1185–93. https://doi.org/10.1016/S0140-6736(12)62124-2. Epub 2013 Feb 14
11. Neri E, Faggioni L, Cerri F, Turini F, Angeli S, et al. CT colonography versus double-contrast barium enema for screening of colorectal cancer: comparison of radiation burden. Abdom Imaging. 2010;35(5):596–601. https://doi.org/10.1007/s00261-009-9568-x. Epub 2009 Sep 24
12. Stevenson G. Colon imaging in radiology departments in 2008: goodbye to the routine double contrast barium enema. Can Assoc Radiol J. 2008;59(4):174–82.
13. Jensen DM, Machicado GA, Jutabha R, et al. Urgent colonoscopy for the diagnosis and treatment of severe diverticular haemorrhage. N Engl J Med. 2000;342:78–82.
14. Bloomfeld RS, Rockey DC, Shetzline MA. Endoscopic therapy of an acute diverticula hemorrhage. Am J Gastroenterol. 2001;96:2367–72.
15. Smoot RL, Gostout CJ, Rajan E, et al. Is early colonoscopy after admission for acute diverticular bleeding needed? Am J Gastroenterol. 2003;98:1996–9.
16. Hizaya K, Miura N, Matsumoto T, Iida M. Colonic diverticular bleeding: precise localization and successful management by a combination of CT angiography and interventional radiology. Abdom Imaging. 2009;34:777–9.
17. Loffroy R, Multidetector CT. Angiography for the detection of colonic diverticular bleeding: when, how, and why? Dig Dis Sci. 2013;58:1822–4.
18. Nagata N, Niikura R, Aoki T, Moriyasu S, Sakurai T, et al. Role of urgent contrast-enhanced multidetector computed tomography for acute lower gastrointestinal bleeding in patients undergoing early colonoscopy. J Gastroenterol. 2015;50:1162–72.
19. Barat M, Paisant A, Calame P, et al. Unenhanced CT for clinical triage of elderly patients presenting to the emergency department with acute abdominal pain. Diagn Interv Imaging. 2019;100:709–19.
20. Millet I, Sebbane M, Molinari N, et al. Systematic unenhanced CT for acute abdominal symptoms in th elderly patients improves both emergency deprtment diagnosis and prompt clinical management. Eur Radiol. 2017;27:868–77.
21. Expert panel on gastrointestinal imaging, Galgano SJ, MM MN, Peterson CM, et al. ACR appropriateness criteria left lower quadrant pain suspected diverticulitis. J Am Coll Radiol. 2019;16:S141–9.
22. Hinchey EJ, Schaal PG, Richards GK. Treatment of perforated diverticular disease of the colon. Adv Surg. 1978;12:85–109.
23. Klarenbeek BR, de Korte N, van der Peet DL, Cuesta MA. Review of current classifications for diverticular disease and a traslation into clinical practice. Int J Color Dis. 2012;27:207–14.
24. Tursi A, Brandimarte G, Di Mario F, Andreoli A, Annunziata ML, et al. Development and validation of an endoscopic classification of diverticular disease of the colon: the DICA classification. Dig Dis. 2015;33(1):68–76. https://doi.org/10.1159/000366039. Epub 2014 Dec 17
25. Sartelli A, Moore FA, Ansaloni L, Di Saverio S, Coccolini F, et al. A proposal for a CT driven classification of left colon acute diverticulitis. World J Emerg Surg. 2015;10:3.
26. Ambrosetti P. Value of CT for acute left-colonic diverticulitis: the Surgeon's view. Dig Dis. 2012;30:51–5.
27. Stoker J, van Randen A, Lameris W, Boermeester MA. Imaging patients with acute abdominal pain. Radiology. 2009;253:31–46.
28. van Randen A, Lameris W, Nio CY, et al. Inter-observer agreement for abdominal CT in unselected patients with acute abdominal pain. Eur Radiol. 2009;19:1394–407.
29. Chintapalli KN, Chopra S, Ghiatas AA, et al. Diverticulitis versus colon cancer: differentiation with helical CT findings. Radiology. 1999;210:429–35.
30. Shen SH, Chen JD, Tiu CM, et al. Differentiating colonic diverticulitis from colon cancer: the value of computed tomography in the emergency setting. J Chin Med Assoc. 2005;68:411–8.
31. Granlund J, Svensson T, Granath F, et al. Diverticular disease and the risk of colon cancer: a population based case-control study. Aliment Pharmacol Ther. 2011;34:675–81.
32. Huang WY, Lin CC, Jen YM, et al. Association between colonic diverticular disease and colorectal cancer: a nationwide population-based study. Clin Gastroenterol Hepatol. 2014;12:1288–94.

33. Flor N, Maconi G, Cornalba GP, Pickhardt PJ. The current role of radiologic and endoscopic imaging in diagnosis and foloow-up of colonic diverticular disease. AJR Am J Roentgenol. 2016;207:15–24.
34. Hjern F, Jonas E, Holmstrom B, Josephson T, Mellgren A, Johansson C. CT colonography versus colonoscopy in the follow-up of patients after diverticulitis. A prospective, comparative study. Clin Radiol. 2007;62:645–50.
35. De Cecco CN, Ciolina M, Annibale B, et al. Prevalence and distribution of colonic diverticula assessed with CT colonography. Eur Radiol. 2016;26(3):639–45. https://doi.org/10.1007/s00330-015-3866-1. Epub 2015 Jun 24
36. Gryspeerdt S, Lefere P. Chronic diverticulitis vs. colorectal cancer: findings on CT colonography. Abdom Imaging. 2012;37(6):1101–9. https://doi.org/10.1007/s00261-012-9858-6.
37. Lips LM, Cremers PT, Pickhardt PJ, Cremers SE, Janssen-Heijnen ML, de Witte MT, Simons PC. Sigmoid cancer versus chronic diverticular disease: differentiating features at CT colonography. Radiology. 2015;275(1):127–35. https://doi.org/10.1148/radiol.14132829. Epub 2014 Nov 26
38. Flor N, Rigamonti P, Di Leo G, et al. Technical quality of CT colonography in relation with diverticular disease. Eur J Radiol. 2012;81(3):e250–4.
39. Pichkardt PJ, Kim D. CT colonography. Pitfalls in interpretation. Radiol Clin N Am. 2013;51:69–88.
40. Sanford M, Pickhardt PJ. Diagnostic performance of primary 3-dimensional computed tomography colonography in the setting of colonic diverticular disease. Clin Gastroenterol Hepatol. 2006;4:1039–47.
41. Flor N, Sardanelli F, Pickhardt PJ. Diagnostic accuracy of CT colonography for the detection of polyps in the diverticular disease. Scand J Gastroenterol. 2014;49(3):383–4.
42. Theranian S, Klinge M, Saul M, et al. Prevalence of colorectal cancer and advanced adenoma in patients with acute diverticulitis: implications for follow-up colonoscopy. Clin Endosc. 2020;91:634–40.
43. Flor N, Rigamonti P, Pisani Ceretti A, et al. Diverticular disease severity score based on CT colonography. Eur Radiol. 2013;23(10):2723–9.
44. Buchach CM, Kim DH, Pickhardt PJ. Performing an additional decubitus series at CT colonography. Abdom Imaging. 2011;36(5):538–44. https://doi.org/10.1007/s00261-010-9666-9.
45. Pickhardt PJ, Bakke J, Kuo J, Robbins JB, Lubner MG, del Rio AM, Kim DH. Volumetric analysis of colonic distention according to patient position at CT colonography: diagnostic value of the right lateral decubitus series. AJR Am J Roentgenol. 2014;203:W623–8.
46. Shinners TJ, Pickhardt PJ, Taylor AJ, Jones DA, Olsen CH. Patient-controlled room air insufflation versus automated carbon dioxide delivery for CT colonography. AJR Am J Roentgenol. 2006;186:1491–6.
47. Taylor SA, Halligan S, Goh V, Morley S, Bassett P, Atkin W, Bartram CI. Optimizing colonic distention for multi-detector row CT colonography: effect of hyoscine butylbromide and rectal balloon catheter. Radiology. 2003;229(1):99–108.
48. Köhler L, Sauerland S, Neugebauer R, et al. Diagnosis and treatment of diverticular disease. Results of a consensus development conference. Surg Endosc. 1999;13(4):430–6.
49. Flor N, Pickhardt PJ, Maconi G, et al. CT colonography followed by elective surgery in patients with acute diverticulitis: a radiological-pathological correlation study. Abdom Radiol (NY). 2021;46:491–7.
50. Flor N, Maconi G, Sardanelli S, et al. Prognostic value of the diverticular disease severity score based on CT colonography: follow-up in patients recovering from acute diverticulitis. Acad Radiol. 2015;22:1503–9.
51. Hall J, Hardiman K, Lee S, et al. The american society of colon and rectal surgeons clinical practice guidelines for the treatment of left-sided colonic diverticulitis. Dis Colon Rectum. 2020;63:728–47.
52. Sartelli A, Weber DG, Kluger Y, et al. 2020 update of the WSES guidelines for the management of acute colonic diverticulitis in the emergency setting. World J Emer Surg. 2020;15:32.

53. Francis NK, Sylla P, Abou-Khalil M, et al. EAES and SAGES 2018 consensus conference on acute diverticulitis management: evidence-based recommendations for clinical practice. Surg Endosc. 2019;33:2726–41.
54. Matsuki M, Okuda J, Kanazawa S, Kanamoto T, Inada Y, Tatsugami F, et al. Virtual CT colectomy by three-dimensional imaging using multidetector-row CT for laparoscopic colorectal surgery. Abdom Imaging. 2005;30:698–707.
55. Flor N, Campari A, Ravelli A, Lombardi MA, Pisani Ceretti A, et al. Vascular map combined with CT Colonography for evaluating candidates for laparoscopic colorectal surgery. Korean J Radiol. 2015;16:821–6.

Endoscopy

15

Walter Elisei and Jaroslaw Regula

15.1 Introduction

Diverticular disease is characterized by the presence of sac-like protrusions (diverticula), which form when the colonic mucosa and submucosa herniate through defects in the muscular layer of the colon wall. Diverticula can be detected in both the left and right colon. Left-sided diverticula are pseudo-diverticula as herniation does not occur through all colonic layers, whereas diverticulosis occurring in the right colon is true diverticula, with herniation through all colonic layers [1]. For many years, it has been believed that diverticulosis exclusively affects the Western world and occurs due to a lack of fiber in the diet and increased pressure in the colonic wall [2, 3]. However, recent data have revealed an increase in the prevalence of colonic diverticulosis throughout the world [4]. In Western countries, the prevalence of diverticulosis increases with age. Fewer than 20% of individuals younger than 40 years of age are noted to have diverticulosis on colonoscopy compared to more than 60% of individuals older than 70 years. Of them, only a few develop complications such as acute diverticulitis or diverticular bleeding. In a recent prospective study, Ala I. Sharara et al. have shown that in a total of 826 consecutive patients who underwent colonoscopy for colorectal screening, incidental diverticulosis was noted in 224 of 823 patients (27.2%) (mean age 62.3 ± 8.2 years; M:F = 1.15). Diverticula were restricted to the left colon in 151 patients (67.4%),

W. Elisei (✉)
Division of Gastroenterology, A.O. San Camillo – Forlanini, Rome, Italy
e-mail: walter_elisei@hotmail.com

J. Regula
Department of Oncological Gastroenterology, Maria Sklodowska-Curie National Research Institute of Oncology and Department of Gastroenterology, Hepatology and Clinical Oncology, Centre of Postgraduate Medical Education, Warsaw, Poland
e-mail: jregula@coi.waw.pl

© The Author(s), under exclusive license to Springer Nature Switzerland AG 2022
A. Tursi et al. (eds.), *Colonic Diverticular Disease*,
https://doi.org/10.1007/978-3-030-93761-4_15

were right-sided in 13 (5.8%), and diffuse (right and left) in 51 (22.8%). Over a mean follow-up of 7.0 ± 1.7 years, DD developed in 6 out of 144 patients (4.2%; 4 acute cases of diverticulitis, 1 probable case of diverticular bleeding, and 1 acute case of diverticulitis and diverticular bleeding). Two patients were hospitalized, and none required surgery. The time to event was 5.1 ± 1.6 years, and the incidence rate was 5.9 per 1000 patient years. On multivariate analysis, it was determined that age, gender, obesity, exercise, fiber intake, alcohol use, constipation, or use of NSAIDs were not associated with DD [5]. Regarding the risk of diverticulitis occurrence, based on a study of the Veterans Affairs Greater Los Angeles Healthcare System, only about 4% of patients with diverticulosis develop acute diverticulitis, contradicting the common belief that diverticulosis has a high rate of progression [6].

In conclusion, diverticulosis of the colon is an incidental finding and does not affect the safety or accuracy of colonoscopy. However, the presence of severe sigmoid diverticulosis does increase the risk of perforation because of fixed angulation of the colon and potential confusion as to the location of the true lumen when multiple large diverticular orifices are encountered [7–9]. Up to now, colonoscopy represents the most important diagnostic and therapeutic tool in the hands of clinicians [10]. Here, we present and select interesting and rather atypical images of colonic diverticula (Figs. 15.1, 15.2, 15.3, and 15.4).

In summary, colonoscopy plays a key role in different clinical settings of diverticular disease (DD) (Table 15.1):

1. colonic diverticular bleeding;
2. differential diagnosis of colon disease (SCAD vs IBD);
3. assessment after an episode of acute diverticulitis (AD); and,
4. as a prognostic tool in patients with diverticular disease.

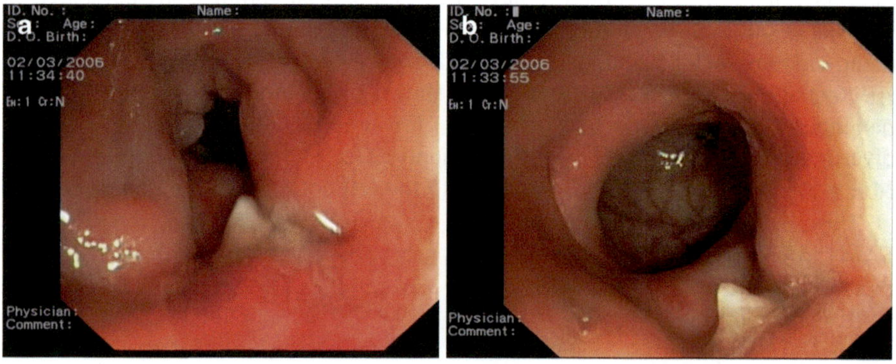

Fig. 15.1 Purulent diverticulitis. (**a**) Inflammatory changes of the sigmoid wall with pus coming out of the diverticulum; (**b**) thick pus forming "Mount Fuji" appearance

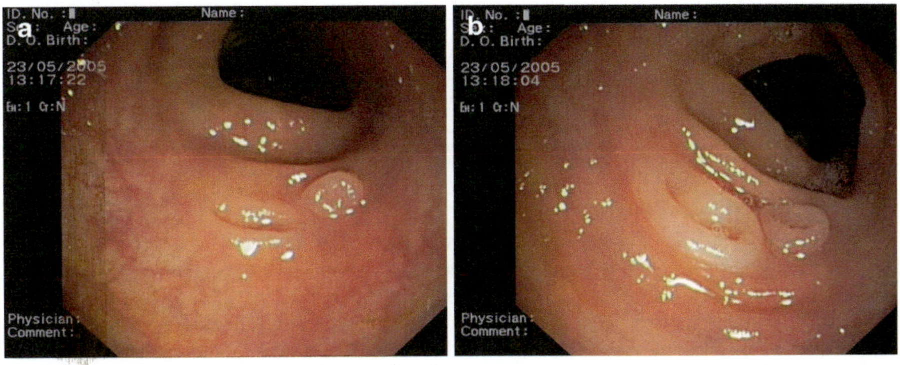

Fig. 15.2 Two sigmoid diverticula at different time points; peristalsis causes one of the diverticula inverts. (**a**) One of the diverticula that appear as a polyp; (**b**) one minute later, both diverticula look more typical

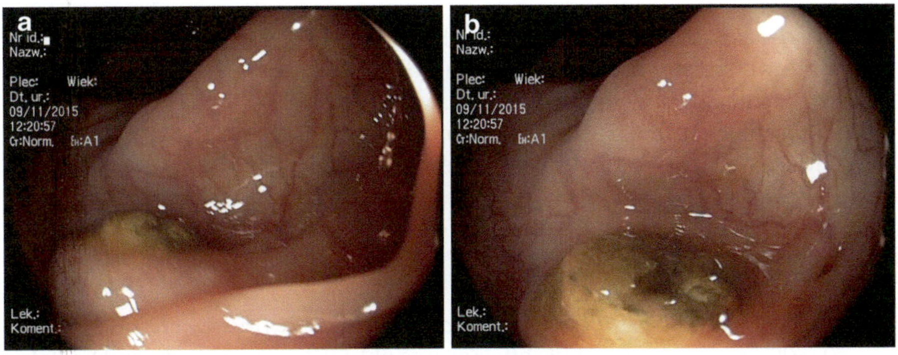

Fig. 15.3 Diverticula with impacted stool: (**a**) back view; (**b**) frontal view

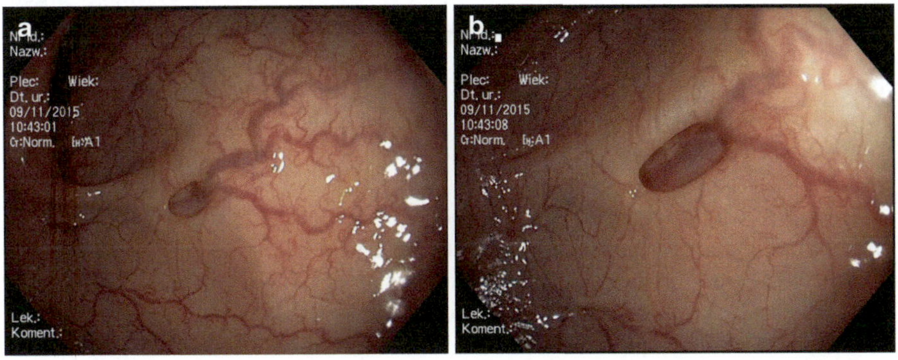

Fig. 15.4 Blood vessels that are at the bottom of the diverticula: (**a**) overview; (**b**) close view

Table 15.1 Indications of colonoscopy in diverticular disease

Clinical setting	Indication
Diverticulosis surveillance	No
Colonic diverticular bleeding	Yes[a]
Differential diagnosis of colon disease (SCAD vs IBD)	Yes
Following acute diverticulitis (AD)	Yes[b]
Symptomatic diverticular disease	Yes

[a] Electively when bleeding has stopped; as primary intervention in managing colonic diverticular bleeding; as primary imaging in patients with recurrent episodes of LGIB in which CT angiography was nondiagnostic

[b] In persistent symptomatic patients in order to exclude other disease (inflammatory bowel disease, colorectal cancer …); after resolution of acute diverticulitis if a high-quality examination of the colon has not been recently performed; after resolution of complicated acute diverticulitis

15.2 Colonoscopy in Colonic Diverticular Bleeding

Colonic diverticular bleeding is a complication of DD and is the most common cause of lower gastrointestinal bleeding (LGIB) affecting 3–15% of patients with colonic diverticulosis, with a mortality rate of 2–3%. Risk factors of diverticular bleeding include alcohol consumption, smoking, and usage of NSAIDs/antiplatelet drugs. Moreover, risk factors of diverticular rebleeding are age (>62 years), diverticulitis (recurrence), chronic renal failure, and peripheral vascular disorders.

In patients with suspected colonic diverticular bleeding, colonoscopy is generally indicated:

(a) *Electively when bleeding has stopped spontaneously (this condition occurs in 70–80% of cases):* to exclude other causes of LGIB (vascular ectasia, Dieulafoy lesions, colonic neoplasia, etc.).
(b) *As the primary intervention in managing colonic diverticular bleeding:* urgent colonoscopy, within 24 h, to find signs of diverticular bleeding (active bleeding, visible vessel, or adherent clot).
(c) *As the primary imaging in patients with recurrent episodes of LGIB in which CT angiography was nondiagnostic:* the rebleeding rate in colonic diverticular bleeding ranged from 20% to 38% [11–13].

To improve the diagnostic and therapeutic yield, attention must be paid to the timing of colonoscopy and bowel preparation. Urgent colonoscopy for acute LGIB is associated with a shorter length of hospital stay and lower hospitalization costs. Unprepped colonoscopy is not recommended for low cecal intubation rate (55–70%) and high risk of bowel perforation.

Endoscopic hemostasis is indicated only for a diverticulum with stigmata of recent hemorrhage (SRH), but the detection rates of SRH are relatively low. The goal of colonoscopy in colonic diverticular bleeding is to identify the site of bleeding and perform hemostasis. However, it should also be considered that the endoscopic hemostasis techniques are generally guided by access to the bleeding site.

Endoscopic therapy for the treatment of acute diverticular bleeding includes epinephrine injection, thermal coagulation, endoclip placement, endoscopic band ligation (EBL), endoscopic detachable snare ligation (EDSL), over-the-scope clip (OTSC), and hemostatic powder [14–16].

In two studies, epinephrine injection and electrocoagulation have been demonstrated to provide an immediate hemorrhagic control in 25–86% of patients with active bleeding, with an early rebleeding rate ranging from 25% to 40% [17, 18]. In some studies, hemoclips have been used for the treatment of acute diverticular bleeding, showing a 88–100% hemorrhage control without recurrent bleeding episodes or adverse events during hospitalization but with a late rebleeding from 17% to 24% [14–16]. Setoyama et al. [19] in comparative study regarding endoscopic hemostasis using EBL (after marking the site of bleeding with a clip, the diverticulum was pulled via suction into the cap of the endoscopic ligator, and the elastic O-ring was released) vs endoclips (when the hemorrhage source was located at the neck of the diverticulum, endoclips were placed directly onto the vessel if technically feasible, and, if not feasible, the diverticulum was closed in a zipper fashion) concluded that EBL should be considered superior to endoclips for the treatment of colonic diverticular bleeding and that the EBL procedure should be attempted as the initial therapy, especially for the right-side disease. Wedi E. et al., in a case series of six patients, with a high operative and rebleeding risk, for the treatment of diverticular bleeding, demonstrated that using the OTSC system is a safe and effective new option for patients in whom the bleeding diverticulum can be identified endoscopically [20].

Multiple modalities of thermal coagulation are available, including monopolar/bipolar hemostatic forceps, bipolar probes, and heater probes. Four reports published around 2000 showed data for bipolar probes used with or without epinephrine injection. Primary hemostasis was achieved in 80–100% of cases, with an average of 97%, and the early rebleeding rate was 0–50%. In 33 cases covered by 4 reports, the average rates of early rebleeding and need for surgery or TAE were 24% and 12%, respectively. No adverse events were reported in these studies or in other articles including case reports. These data suggest that bipolar probes might not provide the expected levels of efficacy for hemostasis [21]. In a case report, hemostatic powder was used after a failure of conventional strategy in massive diverticular bleeding. Hemostasis was rapidly achieved by a spray catheter application of 2 g of topical hemostatic powder inside the lumen of the diverticulum. No rebleeding occurred at follow-up of 30 days, even after readministration of dual antiplatelet therapy [22].

In conclusion, accumulating recent evidence has suggested that in the short term, outcomes of early rebleeding ligation therapy (EBL and EDSL) are superior to those of conventional endoscopic hemostasis (epinephrine injection, thermal coagulation with a bipolar probe, and endoscopic clipping). Conventional endoscopic hemostasis rarely causes perforation or diverticulitis, and ligation therapy induces diverticulitis in less than 1%. There are two case reports on delayed perforation in the sigmoid colon 4–5 days after EBL [21].

15.3 Colonoscopy in Differential Diagnosis of Colon Disease (SCAD Vs IBD)

Segmental colitis associated with diverticulosis (SCAD) is a chronic inflammatory process localized in the interdiverticular mucosa of the colonic area presenting diverticulosis and therefore mainly in the sigmoid colon. By definition, the diverticular ostia are spared from any inflammation. The rectum and the remaining segments of the colon (without diverticulosis) are also spared from inflammation [23].

The disease is relatively rare, with a prevalence of 0.25–1.4% in the general population and 1.15–11.4% amongst DD patients. The mean age at diagnosis is early to mid-60s, with a slightly higher male preponderance. The pathogenesis is multifactorial and includes genetic susceptibility, alteration in the bowel microbiome, local ischemia, mucosal prolapse, and more. The clinical presentation and the endoscopic and histological appearance vary in the four major subtypes. Type A is characterized endoscopically by red patches involving the colonic folds and diverticular sparing with neutrophil and lymphocyte infiltrates limited to the crypt epithelium. Types B and D are characterized by ulcerative colitis (UC)-like changes endoscopically and histologically, with erosions and hyperemic areas involving the colonic folds and severe inflammation involving the overall diverticula containing the mucosa. Histological changes in both subtypes involve crypt distortion and crypt abscesses. Type C is characterized by Crohn's disease-like changes, with isolated aphthous ulcers and transmural inflammatory changes [24, 25].

There are histological similarities between SCAD and IBD, but, by endoscopic examination, both entities can be easily differentiated from other forms of colitis. Differentiation may be helped with the following statements: (a) in SCAD, the inflammatory process involves the interdiverticular mucosa in the colonic area presenting diverticulosis and therefore is mainly located in the sigmoid colon; (b) in SCAD, the rectum and proximal colon are endoscopically and histologically normal; (c) in ulcerative colitis, the rectum is nearly always affected; and (d) Crohn's disease may affect the colon and other gastrointestinal parts [26].

15.4 Colonoscopy Following Acute Diverticulitis (AD)

Acute diverticulitis is the most important complication of diverticular disease. The diagnosis of acute colonic diverticulitis is based on the clinical presentation of left lower quadrant pain, fever, and leukocytosis, and on characteristic findings on computed tomography (CT) scan [27–29].

Regarding the role of endoscopy in acute diverticulitis or following an attack of acute diverticulitis, Galatin et al. in a systematic review and comparison of guidelines confirmed that there is a disagreement concerning indications for colonoscopy in acute diverticulitis [30]. However, there is an agreement that colonoscopy should be performed after acute diverticulitis is resolved in the majority of patients. Colonoscopy is usually avoided in patients with suspected acute diverticulitis because air inflation and instrumental manipulation are considered as a high risk of bowel perforation. Expert opinion is in favor of performing these tests when the acute process has resolved, usually after approximately 6 weeks to avoid the potential risk of converting a sealed perforation into a free perforation and to rule out the presence of other diseases, such as cancer and inflammatory bowel disease.

However, when imaging studies are equivocal, colonoscopy may be required to correctly differentiate acute diverticulitis from a segmental colonic abnormality caused by Crohn's disease, bacterial infection, ischemia, cancer, or Clostridium difficile colitis occurring in association with diverticulosis In this situation, gentle colonoscopy with minimal air insufflation can be safely carried out. If a diagnosis of acute diverticulitis is confirmed, many experts would terminate the procedure at that point.

In a randomized prospective study, Lahat A et al. demonstrated the feasibility and safety of early colonoscopy during hospitalization in patients with acute diverticulitis and no pericolic air on CT. It was as safe as late colonoscopy, which is the current practice, and showed better compliance (93.3% of the hospitalized patients underwent colonoscopy, compared with only 75.6% of the ambulatory group; $p = 0.03$) [31]. Obviously, if a patient has something in their evaluation that would dictate any need for a colonoscopy (i.e., diagnostic dilemma, concerning radiographic finding, due for elective routine screening), colonoscopy should be performed.

Earlier studies searching for associations between diverticular disease and colorectal cancer have described a clear overall association, suggesting that long-term inflammation can lead to cancer. However, the issue is still debated. In 2008, Morini et al. [32], by describing associations between diverticulosis and colorectal cancer, showed that some studies were positive, some negative, and some inconclusive. Those studies were usually retrospective, case–control, cohort, or cross-sectional, and the number of patients included was mostly around 1000. That analysis also showed associations between diverticulosis and colorectal adenomas. The mechanisms of the link (if it existed) between two diseases was usually speculated. Most frequently, the authors listed the presence of longstanding chronic inflammation, including segmental colitis associated with diverticula, alterations in the extracellular matrix in the involved colon segments promoting carcinogenesis, and deregulated cell proliferation measured by increased numbers of aberrant crypt foci. Most recently, it has also been suggested that probable microbiome changes observed in diverticular disease may also be responsible for promoting carcinogenesis. However, all those hypotheses lacked strong evidence.

The most recent studies have been mainly characterized by much larger cohorts of studied patients. Two of those require a detailed description as they lead to the final and logical conclusions concerning the association between diverticular disease and colorectal cancer. The first important study was conducted in Sweden by Granlund et al. [33]. This was a huge nation-wide case–control study involving 41,037 patients with colorectal cancer identified by the Swedish Cancer Registry. Each case was matched with 2 controls without cancer (82,074 patients). Cases and controls were then searched for the episode of hospitalizations with the diagnosis of diverticular disease. Odds ratios for receiving the diagnosis of colon cancer were calculated after hospital discharge for diverticular disease. Furthermore, cancer mortality was calculated for those cases with and without diverticular disease. Results are important and meaningful. The odds ratio for receiving the diagnosis of colon cancer was extremely high at 31.49 (95% CI 19.00–52.21) within 6 months following hospitalization for diverticular disease. The risk of diagnosis of colon cancer was, however, not increased at all from the time of 12 months after hospitalization. Among patients with colon cancer, the mortality was not different between patients with and without diverticular disease. Moreover, the authors strongly recommended that patients with diverticular disease should have a high-quality diagnostic workup within the first 12 months after the initial episode of diverticular disease.

The second large study was performed in Taiwan [34]. The authors first retrieved a cohort of 41,359 patients with diverticular disease from the National Health Research Institute database. Of those patients, 28,909 had diverticulitis and 12,450 had diverticulosis. These patients were matched with 4 controls comprising 165,436 individuals without diverticular disease. In the initial analysis, the risk of colorectal cancer was significantly increased (adjusted HR = 4.54, 95% CI 4.19–4.91). However, in the proper analysis performed after excluding the first 12 months of follow-up, the adjusted hazard ratio was not increased at all (HR = 0.98, 95% CI 0.85–1.13). The risk was also not increased for both subcohorts with diverticulosis and diverticulitis. The authors drew similar conclusions as in the Swedish study: diverticular disease does not increase the risk of colorectal cancer. The risk is only increased within the first year after diagnosis of diverticular disease, which rather suggests the misclassification and misdiagnosis of diverticular disease.

Finally, Brar et al. [35] subdivided their study population into complicated and uncomplicated diverticulitis. This subgroup analysis only considered patients with pericolic or pelvic abscess at the time of presentation for the complicated diverticulitis group because those presenting with obstruction or fistula were managed surgically. In their analysis, they found that 9 patients (5.4%) in the uncomplicated group had advanced adenoma, whereas, in those patients presenting with abscess, 14 patients (18.9%) had advanced adenoma. Four patients (5.4%) presenting with complicated diverticulitis were found to have invasive malignancy, whereas there were none identified in the uncomplicated diverticulitis group. The investigators also looked at age as a risk factor for advanced neoplasia. On multivariate analysis, both age (OR = 1.04, 95% CI 1.01–1.08) and the presence of intra-abdominal abscess (OR = 4.15, 95% CI 1.68–10.3) were determined to be independent risk factors. Looking at patients with complicated diverticulitis, Lau et al. [36] found that the odds of malignancy with the presence of abscess is 6.7-fold (95% CI 2.4–18.7), 4-fold (95% CI 1.1–14.9) with local perforation, and 18-fold (95% CI 5.1–63.7) in patients with concomitant fistula as compared to uncomplicated diverticulitis. Therefore, in patients above the age of 50 or those presenting with complicated diverticulitis, colonoscopy should be considered (Figs. 15.5 and 15.6).

In conclusion, colonoscopy following acute diverticulitis is useful in the following conditions:

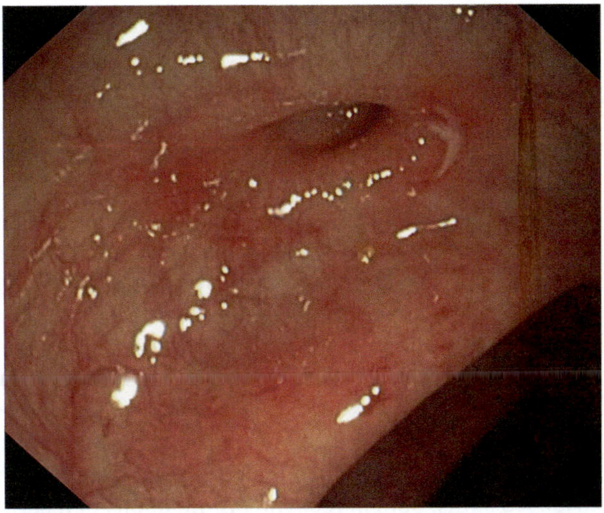

Fig. 15.5 Diverticulitis with erosion

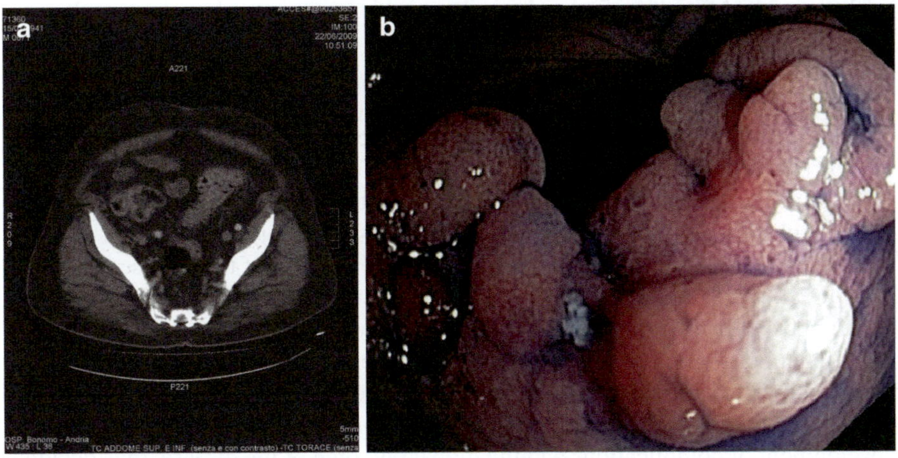

Fig. 15.6 (**a**) An 80-year-old man was admitted to a hospital due to acute complicated diverticulitis and treated with support treatment and intravenous antibiotics. (**b**) Due to persistence of anemia and mild abdominal pain, he underwent colonoscopy 3 weeks later, with detection of colon cancer in the sigmoid colon

(a) in persistent symptomatic patients to exclude other diseases (IBD, colorectal cancer);
(b) after resolution of acute diverticulitis if a high-quality examination of the colon has not been recently performed [37]; and,
(c) after resolution of complicated acute diverticulitis [38] to rule out colorectal cancer.

15.5 Colonoscopy as a Predictive Tool for Diverticular Disease Outcomes

Different images can be found during colonoscopy in patients with diverticula: non-inflamed diverticula, segmental colitis associated with diverticulosis (SCAD), diverticulitis with or without complications, and bleeding diverticula. In addition, colonoscopy may reveal indirect signs of previous acute diverticulitis, such as rigidity of the colonic wall and substenosis or stenosis of the intestinal lumen. Colonoscopy is also essential for establishing the diagnosis of SCAD, which is a chronic colitis occurring only in the left colon, in the presence of diverticula. Rather than a complication of diverticular disease, SCAD is currently believed to be an independent clinical disease falling in the subset of inflammatory bowel disease. The endoscopic findings of SCAD are erythema, erosions, granularity, and fragility of the mucosa, and the involvement of the colonic mucosa can be diffuse or, more often, "patched." [39]. Colonoscopy, in patients with diverticulosis, requires advanced skills, both in recognizing situations of a particular risk (acute diverticulitis with or without perforation signs) and in special situations such as massive diverticulosis with difficult-to-find colonic lumen, the presence of narrow angles and rigid, fixed lumen, or to passing stenosis. The use of endoscopes with different calibers and stiffness (such as pediatric endoscopes or enteroscopes) can be useful in some cases, providing further help to endoscopists. Sometimes we suggest the use of a transparent cap, especially in training endoscopists. Moreover, the current use of CO_2 instead of air may decrease the patient's discomfort. Recently, an international study group on diverticular disease has introduced and validated the DICA (Diverticular Inflammation and Complications Assessment) classification to establish, with an objective and reproducible score, the severity of the disease associated with diverticula. The DICA score purely consists of endoscopic parameters such as the number of diverticula (in the right and left colon), the presence of inflammatory signs (edema/hyperemia, erosions, SCAD), the presence of complications of stigmata, such as stiffness or luminal stenosis, and the presence of complications, such as bleeding and pus [40]. The main aim of the DICA score is to predict the future development of complications and the global outcome of the disease, thus deciding whether medical therapy is needed. In summary, the role of endoscopy in diverticular disease is paramount for staging the severity of the disease, its complications, and for the selection of an appropriate medical or surgical treatment.

References

1. Tursi A, Papagrigoriadis S. Review article: the current and evolving treatment of colonic diverticular disease. Aliment Pharmacol Ther. 2009;30:532–46.
2. Floch M, Bina I. The natural history of diverticulitis – fact and theory. J Clin Gastroenterol. 2004;38(Suppl.1):S2–7.
3. Aldoori WH, Giovannucci EL, Rimm EB, Wing AL, Trichopoulos DV, Willett WC. A prospective study of diet and the risk of symptomatic diverticular disease in men. Am J Clin Nutr. 1994;60:757–64.

4. Tursi A. Diverticulosis today: unfashionable and still under-researched. Ther Adv Gastroenterol. 2016;9:213–28.
5. Sharara AI, Ziade N, Shayto RH, Rustom LBO, Chehab H, Rimmani HH, Hanna K, Chalhoub JM, Sarkis FS, Rahal MA, Soweid A, Mourad FH, Barada K, Harb AH. The natural history of incidental colonic diverticulosis on screening colonoscopy. Can J Gastroenterol Hepatol. 2018;2018:3690202. https://doi.org/10.1155/2018/3690202.
6. Shahedi K, Fuller G, Bolus R, Cohen E, Michelle V, Shah R, Agarwal N, Kaneshiro M, Atia M, Sheen V, Kurzbard N, van Oijen MGH, Yen L, Hodgkins P, Erder MH, Spiegel B. Long-term risk of acute diverticulitis among patients with incidental diverticulosis found during colonoscopy. Clin Gastroenterol Hepatol. 2013;11(12):1609–13. https://doi.org/10.1016/j.cgh.2013.06.020. Epub 2013 Jul 12
7. Kavin H, Sinicrope F, Esker A. Management of perforation of the colon at colonoscopy. Am J Gastroenterol. 1992;87:161.
8. Kozarek RA, Earnest DL, Silverstein ME, et al. Air-pressureinduced colon injury during diagnostic colonoscopy. Gastroenterology. 1980;78(1):7–14.
9. Brayco CM, Kozarek RA, Sanowski RA, et al. Diverticular rupture during colonoscopy. Fact or fancy? Dig Dis Sci. 1984;29:427.
10. Peery AF, Barrett PR, Park D, et al. A high-fiber diet does not protect against asymptomatic diverticulosis. Gastroenterology. 2012;142:266–72.
11. Suzuki K, Uchiyama S, Imajyo K, Tomeno W, Sakai E, Yamada E, Tanida E, Akiyama T, Watanabe S, et al. Risk factors for colonic diverticular hemorrhage: Japanese multicenter study. Digestion. 2012;85:261–5.
12. Nagata N, Niikura R, Aoki T, Shimbo T, Kishida Y, Sekine K, Tanaka S, Watanabe K, Sakurai T, et al. Colonic diverticular hemorrhage associated with the use of nonsteroidal anti-inflammatory drugs, low-dose aspirin, antiplatelet drugs, and dual therapy. J Gastroenterol Hepatol. 2014;19:1786–93.
13. Longstreth GF. Epidemiology and outcome of patients hospitalized with acute lower gastrointestinal hemorrhage: a population-based study. Am J Gastroenterol. 1997;92:419–24.
14. Yen EF, Uri Ladabaum V, Muthusamy R, Cello JP, McQuaid KR, Shah JN. Colonoscopic treatment of acute diverticular hemorrhage using endoclips. Dig Dis Sci. 2008;53(9):2480–5.
15. Kaltenbach T, Watson R, Shah J, Friedland S, Sato T, Shergill A, McQuaid K, Soetikno R. Colonoscopy with clipping is useful in the diagnosis and treatment of diverticular bleeding. Clin Gastroenterol Hepatol. 2012;10(2):131–7.
16. Wong Kee Song LM. Baron TH. Endoscopic management of acute lower gastrointestinal bleeding Am J Gastroenterol. 2008;103(8):1881–7.
17. Chaudhry V, Hyser MJ, Gracias VH, Gau FC. Colonoscopy: the initial test for acute lower gastrointestinal bleeding. Am Surg. 1998;64(8):723–8.
18. Green BT, Rockey DC, Portwood G, Tarnasky PR, Guarisco S, Branch MS, Leung J, Jowell P. Urgent colonoscopy for evaluation and management of acute lower gastrointestinal hemorrhage: a randomized controlled trial. Am J Gastroenterol. 2005;100(11):2395–402. https://doi.org/10.1111/j.1572-0241.2005.00306.x.
19. Setoyama T, Ishii N, Fujitaina Y. Endoscopic band ligation (EBL) is superior to endoscopic clipping for the treatment of colonic diverticular hemorrhage. Surg Endosc. 2011;25:3574–8. https://doi.org/10.1007/s00464-011-1760-8.
20. Wedi E, von Renteln D, Jung C, Tchoumak I, Roth V, Gonzales S, Leroy J, Hochberger J. Treatment of acute colonic diverticular bleeding in high risk patients, using an over-the-scope clip: a case series. Endoscopy. 2016;48:E383–5.
21. Kaise M, Nagata N, Ishii N, Omori J, Goto O, Iwakiri K. Epidemiology of colonic diverticula and recent advances in the management of colonic diverticular bleeding. Dig Endosc. 2020;32(2):240–50.
22. Grassia R, Iiritano E, Vjero K, Cereatti F, Capone P, Buffoli F. Severe acute diverticular bleeding: successful treatment with hemostatic powder. Gastrointest Endosc. 2017;86(1):239–40.
23. Koutroubakis IE, et al. The spectrum of segmental colitis associated with diverticulosis. Int J Color Dis. 2005;20(1):28–32.

24. Schembri J, Bonello J, Christodoulou DK, Katsanos KH, Ellul P. Segmental colitis associated with diverticulosis: is it the coexistence of colonic diverticulosis and inflammatory bowel disease? Ann Gastroenterol. 2017;30:257–61.
25. Tursi A, Elisei W, Giorgetti GM, et al. Segmental colitis associated with diverticulosis: a 5-year follow-up. Int J Color Dis. 2012;27:179–85. https://doi.org/10.1007/s00384-011-1296-3.
26. Tursi A, et al. Histopathology of segmental colitis associated with diverticulosis resembles inflammatory bowel diseases. J Clin Gastroenterol. 2015;49(4):350–1.
27. Hulnick DH, Megibow AJ, Baithazar EJ, et al. Computed tomography in the evaluation of diverticulitis. Radiology. 1984;152:491–5.
28. Kaiser AM, Jiang JK, Lake JP, et al. The management of complicated diverticulitis and the role of computed tomography. Am J Gastroenterol. 2005;100:910–7.
29. Hachigian MP, Honickman S, Eisenstat TE, et al. Computed tomography in the initial management of acute left sided diverticulitis. Dis Colon Rectum. 1992;35:1123–9.
30. Galatin et al. Int J Color Dis 2008; 33: 261–272.
31. Lahat A, et al. Feasibility and risk of early colonoscopy in acute diverticulitis: a prospective controlled study. Endoscopy. 2007;39:521–4.
32. Morini S, Zullo A, Hassan C, et al. Diverticulosis and colorectal cancer. Between lights and shadows. J Clin Gastroenterol. 2008;42:763–70.
33. Granlund J, Svensson T, Granath F, et al. Diverticular disease and the risk of colon cancer—a population-based case-controlstudy. Aliment Pharmacol Ther. 2011;34:675–81.
34. Huang W-Y, Lin C-C, Jen Y-M, et al. Association between colonic diverticular disease and colorectal cancer: a nationwide population-based study. Clin Gastroenterol Hepatol. 2014;12:1288–94.
35. Brar MS, Roxin G, Yaffe PB, Stanger J, MacLean AR, Buie WD. Colonoscopy following nonoperative management of uncomplicated diverticulitis may not be warranted. Dis Colon Rectum. 2013;56:1259–64.
36. Lau KC, Spilsbury K, Farooque Y, Kariyawasam SB, Owen RG, Wallace MH, Makin GB. Is colonoscopy still mandatory after a CT diagnosis of left-sided diverticulitis: can colorectal cancer be confidently excluded? Dis Colon Rectum. 2011;54:1265–70.
37. Stollman N, et al. American Gastroenterological Association Institute guideline on the management of acute diverticulitis. Gastroenterology. 2015;149(7):1944–9.
38. Agarwal AK, Karanjawala BE, Maykel JA, Johnson EK, Steele SR. Routine colonic endoscopic evaluation following resolution of acute diverticulitis: is it necessary? World J Gastroenterol. 2014;20(35):12509–16. https://doi.org/10.3748/wjg.v20.i35.12509.
39. Tursi A. The role of colonoscopy in managing diverticular disease of the colon. J Gastrointestin Liver Dis. 2015;24(no1):85–93.
40. Tursi A, Brandimarte G, Di Mario F, et al. Development and validation of an endoscopic classification of diverticular disease of the colon: the DICA classification. Dig Dis. 2015;33:68–76.

Diverticular Inflammation and Complication Assessment (DICA) Classification

16

Antonio Tursi, Giovanni Brandimarte, and Francesco Di Mario

16.1 Introduction

Diverticulosis of the colon is an acquired deformity of the colonic wall, which shows an increasing prevalence worldwide [1]. It is estimated that it affects more than 75% of people older than 70 years [2] and that no more than 20% of those people may have occurrence of symptoms, the so-called diverticular disease (DD) [2].

There are several approaches to classify DD. Imaging-based classifications are the most used classifications in this setting, in particular, the classification based on abdominal computerized tomography (CT) (e.g., modified Hinchey, Buckey, or Ambrosetti classification) [3–5]. There are also some clinical classifications that look at the clinical appearance of the disease (e.g., the classification of the Scientific Committee of the European Association for Endoscopic Surgery, the Sheth

Conflict of interest statement: none declared.
Source of funding: none.

A. Tursi (✉)
Territorial Gastroenterology Service, Local Sanitary Agency Barletta-Andria-Trani, Barletta, Italy

Department of Medical and Surgical Sciences, Post-graduate School of Digestive Diseases, Catholic University, Rome, Italy
e-mail: antotursi@tiscali.it

G. Brandimarte
Division of Internal Medicine and Gastroenterology, "Cristo Re" Hospital, Rome, Italy
e-mail: giovannibrandimarte56@gmail.com

F. Di Mario
Gastroenterology Unit, "Ospedale Maggiore" University Hospital, University of Parma, Parma, Italy
e-mail: francesco.dimario@unipr.it

© The Author(s), under exclusive license to Springer Nature Switzerland AG 2022
A. Tursi et al. (eds.), *Colonic Diverticular Disease*,
https://doi.org/10.1007/978-3-030-93761-4_16

classification, and the Hansen–Stock classification) [6–8]. However, most of them are focused on the severity of diverticulitis rather than on the overall spectrum of DD and are thus not widely used in clinical practice.

Surprisingly, an endoscopic classification of the disease was lacking until 2015, despite several findings suggesting a need for it:

(a) diverticulosis of the colon is the most frequent anatomical alteration detected at colonoscopy [9];
(b) the number of colonoscopies performed for colorectal cancer screening or for any other colonic diseases is increasing worldwide. For example, in the USA, 19 million colonoscopies are performed each year [10];
(c) Due to this large number of exams, it is quite frequent to find not only diverticulosis but also signs of endoscopic inflammation without any clinical suspicion of acute diverticulitis. In fact, endoscopic signs of diverticular inflammation may be recognized in about 1% of patients undergoing colonoscopy, in the absence of any clinical sign of suspected acute diverticulitis [11, 12];
(d) the extension of diverticulosis through the colon is a risk factor for diverticulitis recurrence [13];
(e) the detection of persisting endoscopic inflammation following an attack of acute diverticulitis is a risk factor for recurrence of the disease [14].

Considering all of these findings, it is hypothesized that patients differ from each other. For example, it was hypothesized that a patient having only scattered diverticula in the sigmoid colon may differ from a patient having diffuse diverticulosis and rigidity of the colon or having diverticular inflammation, but we did not know whether these differences have a prognostic significance. Moreover, the meaning of the terms currently used for describing diverticulosis, from 'scattered diverticulosis' and 'diffuse diverticulosis' to 'diverticular inflammation', are not an objective and reproducible endoscopic description.

For these reasons, in 2015, we published the first endoscopic classification of diverticulosis/DD, assessing its reproducibility and clinical validity [15]. The development of this endoscopic classification, called "Diverticular Inflammation and Complication Assessment" (DICA), was divided into three parts: construction of the classification by selecting the most relevant endoscopic variables; development of the classification by assessing the reproducibility level of the endoscopic score by an interobserver variation study; and validation of the classification, in which the final items were reassessed to establish a new concordance of the classification and to finally validate it.

The main steps in the implementation process were as follows: (1) the promoters of the DICA classification (Antonio Tursi, Giovanni Brandimarte, and Francesco Di Mario) selected a panel of experts in gastrointestinal endoscopy; (2) visualization of the videos and assessment of the endoscopic variables under examination were performed during a plenary session lasting 2 days by the members of the expert group (interobserver agreement); and (3) a new visualization of the videos and assessment of the modified endoscopic variables under examination were performed 3 months later by the same experts using internet access (intraobserver agreement).

16.2 Construction of the Classification

To select the endoscopic items, the promoters (Antonio Tursi, Giovanni Brandimarte, and Francesco Di Mario) reviewed 300 videos displaying their gastroenterological structures and showing colonic diverticulosis/DD. After visualization, they selected four main items on which to build the classification: (1) diverticulosis extension; (2) number of diverticula in each colonic district; (3) the presence of inflammation; and (4) the presence of complications. At the beginning of the developmental process, each endoscopic item was developed as follows:

1. Diverticulosis extent: Sigmoid colon, descending colon, transverse colon, ascending colon, and cecum.
2. Number of diverticula in each region: Grade I: ≤5, grade II: 5–10, grade III: 10–20, and grade IV: >20.
3. Presence of inflammation: Four different types of inflammation were identified: (a) edema: congestion of the diverticular opening, with loss of the submucosal vascular pattern; (b) hyperemia: hyperemia of the diverticular opening, with loss of the submucosal vascular pattern; and (c) erosions: small fibrinous ulcerations. In case of contemporaneous detection of different severities of inflammation at colonoscopy in the same region (e.g., some diverticula with hyperemia and others with erosions), the most severe grade of inflammation was reported.
4. Presence of complications: Five different complications were identified: (a) rigidity of the colon: slight distension of the diverticular region at inflation; (b) passing stenosis: whether a standard colonoscope could be passed through the narrowed lumen; (c) incomplete colonic exploration (due to not passing stenosis or an elevated risk of perforation): when the standard colonoscope could not be passed through the narrowed lumen or when the presence of some anatomical characteristics (e.g., several diverticula with rigidity at the spleen flexure) increased the risk of perforation, it was advised to suspend the examination; (d) segmental colitis associated with diverticulosis (SCAD): inflammation of the interdiverticular mucosa that does not involve the diverticular opening [16]; and (e) bleeding.

After the identification of the endoscopic items and their gradation, the next step was the construction of a numerical classification in which the power of each variable was related to its importance. For example, sigmoid diverticulosis was graded with 2 points because in the Western world diverticulosis occurred more frequently in the left than in the right colon. At the same time, the detection of inflammation, as well as that of the complication, was graded according to the progressive severity of inflammatory findings. At the end of this construction, four different numerical DICA were identified: DICA 0: when the sum of the points was up to 4; DICA 1: when the sum of the points was from 5 to 7; DICA 2: when the sum of the points was from 8 to 12; and DICA 3: when the sum of the points was over 13.

16.3 Development of the Classification

A total of 32 expert endoscopists, from university hospitals, first-level secondary and tertiary hospitals, and territorial endoscopic centers, who knew the DICA classification, were involved in the construction of the DICA. In all, 30 videos of diverticulosis/DD were assessed at this time, and the overall Fleiss' kappa for inter-rater reliability was 0.686 (95% CI 0.596–0.701). Fleiss' kappa was 0.755 for grade 0 (95% CI 0.689–0.783), 0.557 for grade 1 (95% CI 0.501–0.578), 0.521 for grade 2 (95% CI 0.498–0.583), and 0.895 for grade 3 (95% CI 0.863–0.910).

However, a four-step DICA score was considered too complex by these experts, and items and subitems assessed were considered too much or too complex. For example, the experts found it highly difficult to differentiate between a low and medium number of diverticula or between severe and mild stenosis. After plenary discussion, the definitive DICA classification therefore comprised the following items and subitems and related scores (Table 16.1):

1. Diverticulosis extent: left colon (2 points), right colon (1 point);
2. Number of diverticula (in each region): grade I: ≤15 (0 point) (Fig. 16.1), grade II: >15 (1 point) (Fig. 16.2);

Table 16.1 Items and subitems in constructing DICA classification

Diverticulosis extension: • Left Colon (2 points); • Right Colon (1 point)	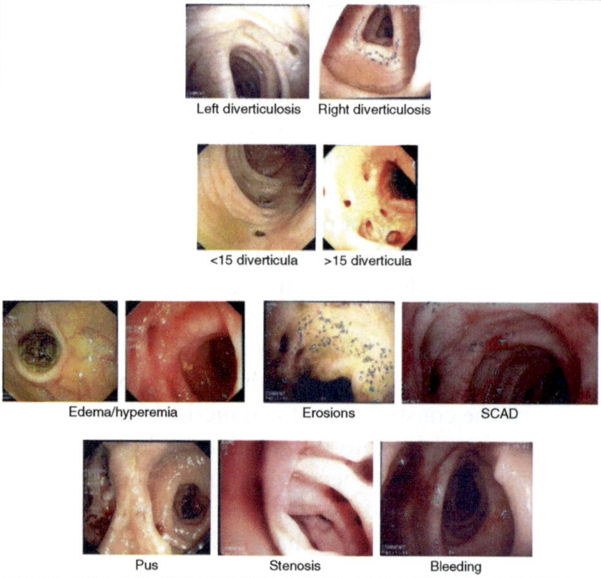
Number of diverticula per district: • Less than 15 (0 points); • More than 15 (1 point)	
Presence and type of inflammatory findings: • Edema/Hyperemia (1 point); • Erosions (2 points); • SCAD (3 points)	
Presence of endoscopic complications: • Rigidity (4 points); • Pus (4 points); • Stenosis (4 points); • Diverticular bleeding (4 points)	

DICA score	Numeric values
DICA1	1–3 points
DICA 2	4–7 points
DICA 3	>7 points

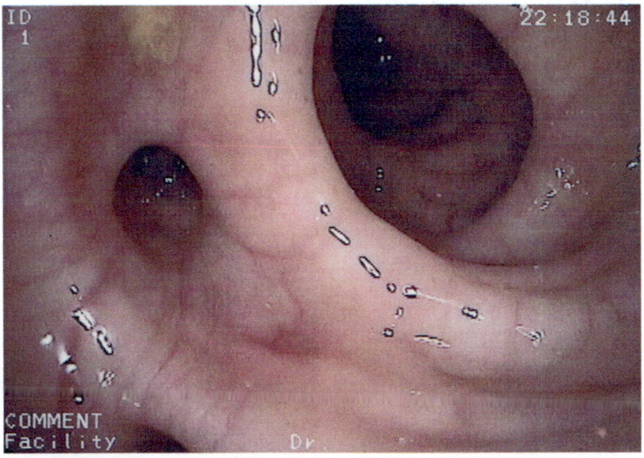

Fig. 16.1 Less than 15 diverticula

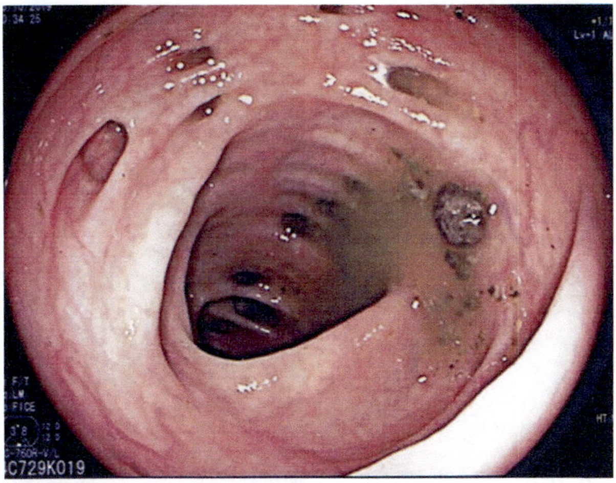

Fig. 16.2 More than 15 diverticula

3. Presence of inflammation: edema/hyperemia (1 point) (Fig. 16.3), erosions (2 points) (Fig. 16.4), SCAD (3 points) (Fig. 16.5). If different types of inflammation are detected at colonoscopy in the same region (e.g., some diverticula with hyperemia and others with erosions), the most severe grade of inflammation was reported;
4. Presence of complications (all of them scored with 4 points): (a) rigidity of the colon: slight distension of the diverticular region at inflation, and also comprising mild stenoses in which the standard colonoscope could be passed through the narrowed lumen (Fig. 16.6); (b) stenosis: not passing stenosis or narrowed lumen, with an elevated risk of perforation due to the presence of some anatomical characteristics (e.g., several diverticula at the splenic flexure) (Fig. 16.7); (c) pus: purulent material coming from the diverticular opening (Fig. 16.8); and (d) bleeding (Fig. 16.9).

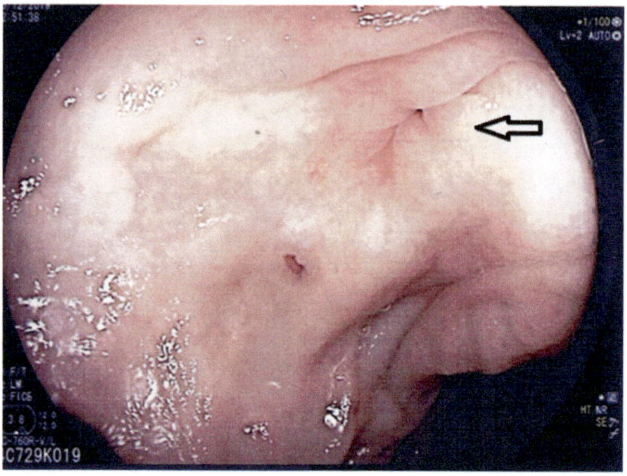

Fig. 16.3 Diverticular edema (arrow)

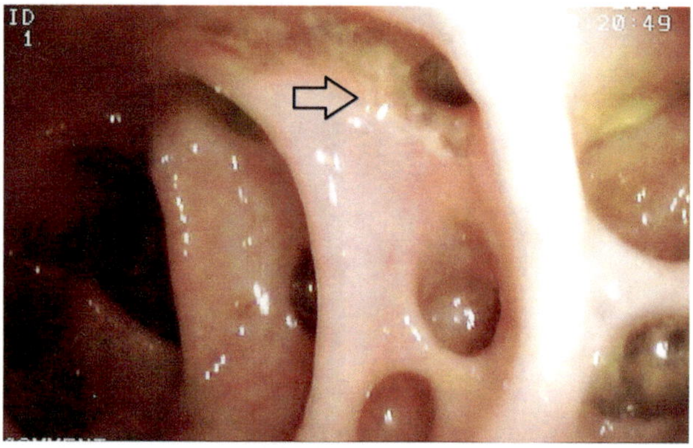

Fig. 16.4 Erosion of the diverticular opening (arrow)

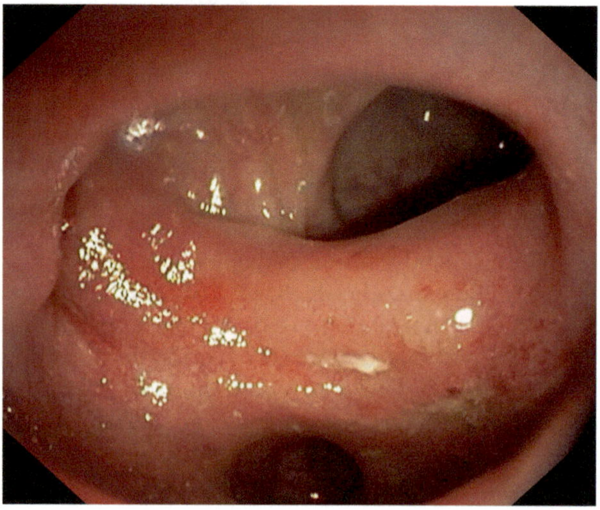

Fig. 16.5 Segmental colitis associated with diverticulosis

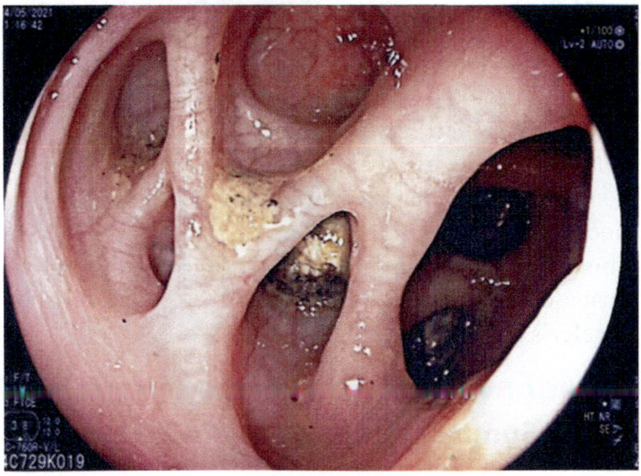

Fig. 16.6 Rigidity of the colonic lumen in the diverticular district

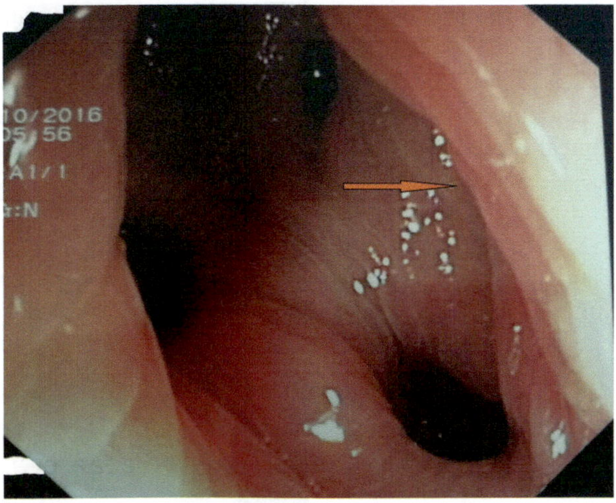

Fig. 16.7 Diverticular stenosis (arrow)

The definitive DICA score was therefore constructed as follows: DICA 1: when the sum of the points was up to 3—this was a simple diverticulosis, probably without the risk of complications; DICA 2: when the sum of the points was from 4 to 7—this was a mild DD, probably with a lower risk of complications; and DICA 3: when the sum of the points was over 7—this was a severe DD, probably with higher risk of complications.

At this step, 70 consecutive videos of patients who underwent colonoscopy, due to abdominal symptoms (abdominal pain, bleeding, constipation, diarrhea) and in whom a first diagnosis of diverticulosis/DD was made, were recorded. Among them, 30 videos were selected according to the quality of the images (complete endoscopic exploration of the colon, adequate colonic cleansing, and adequate visualization of the diverticula with or without inflammation and/or complications). Videos were visualized during a plenary session as six blocks of five videos each,

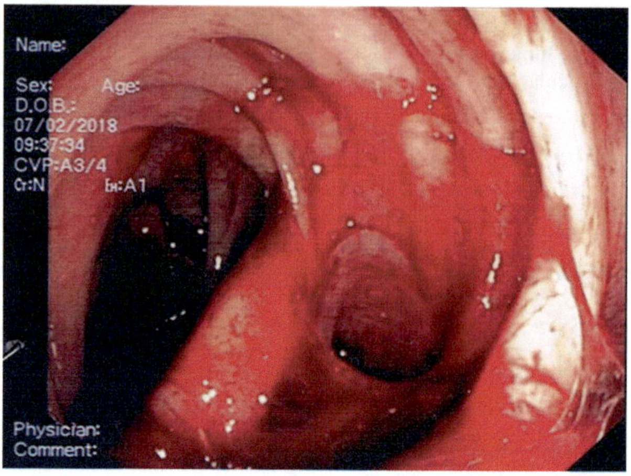

Fig. 16.8 Diverticular bleeding

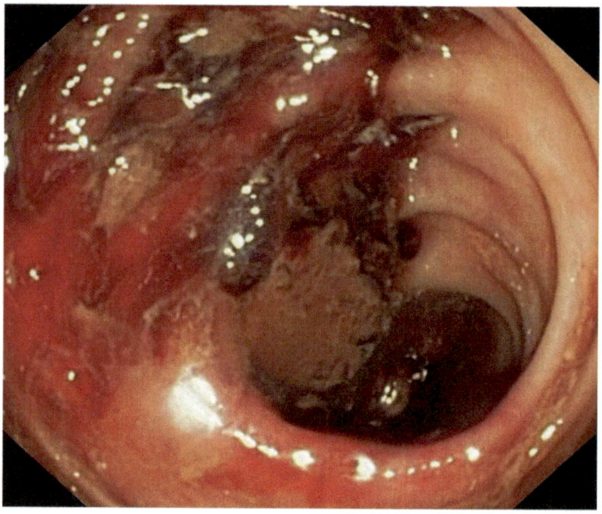

Fig. 16.9 Bleeding and purulent material coming from the diverticula

with each block followed by a discussion of the results. Moreover, five videos were repeated with a new numeration to have an intraobserver agreement assessment. After visualization, all items were reassessed under plenary discussion. After modifying the items and the complexity of the classification, Fleiss' kappa in using the DICA increased to 0.847 (95% CI 0.812–0.893). Fleiss' kappa was 0.878 for grade 1 (95% CI 0.832–0.895), 0.765 for grade 2 (95% CI 0.735–0.786), and 0.891 for grade 3 (95% CI 0.845–0.7923). With respect to the intraobserver agreement, kappa was 0.91 (95% CI 0.886–0.947).

The videos were visualized again 6 months later by internet access. Each expert accessed the videos by a case-sensitive password and reassessed them according to the final DICA classification. The videos had a different distribution from the first visualization to have a more sensitive interobserver agreement. Moreover, five videos were repeated again with a new numeration to have an intraobserver agreement assessment. Each expert was blinded to the clinical and laboratory characteristics of the patient under examination, as well as to the answers provided by the other experts. Again, a high agreement rate was recorded for each DICA score.

16.4 Validation of the Classification

DICA score validation was carried out by estimating the correlation between the calculated index and the inflammatory indices: erythrocyte sedimentation rate (ESR) and C-reactive protein (CRP) expression. ESR and CRP were selected because they correlated with the severity of DD [12]. The correlation between the calculated index and the symptoms experienced by patients at the time of colonoscopy was also assessed. In this manner, four main symptoms were assessed: abdominal pain, bleeding, constipation, and diarrhea. In particular, abdominal pain was considered the main symptom characterizing DD [17], and it was assessed using a 4-point verbal scale (none, mild, moderate, or severe), assigning numerical values of 0–3. Mild pain was defined as an occasional disturbance that did not limit normal activities, moderate pain as pain that interfered with normal-day life activities, and severe pain as pain that rendered the patient unable to perform normal activities.

DICA score severity correlated with both the ESR ($p = 0.0001$) and CRP values ($p = 0.0001$). A significant correlation was found between the pain score and the DICA score ($p = 0.0001$), whereas no differences were found between distribution of the associated symptoms in the three DICA scores.

16.5 Validation of the Classification in Real Life

The next step in developing this classification was to validate it in real life. This was performed by two studies.

Since this classification was created and developed in Italy, the first study was conducted in an Italian national setting [18]. The promoters (Antonio Tursi, Giovanni Brandimarte, and Francesco Di Mario) selected a panel of 66 endoscopists from university hospitals, first-level secondary and tertiary hospitals, and territorial endoscopic centers, to assess the reproducibility of the DICA classification in a clinical setting. All the endoscopists involved knew the DICA classification, but not all of them used it in their practice: 31 endoscopists did use the DICA classification in their practice from at least 3 months prior to the plenary session, and thus were named “experts”; 35 endoscopists did not use the DICA classification in their practice, and thus were named “not experts”.

Visualization of the videos and assessment of the endoscopic variables under examination were performed during a plenary session lasting 2 days by the members of the group. Each participant assessed the videos using their own tablet, had 10 min to evaluate and rate each video, and the response was anonymously collected via electronic data collection. At the end of the second day, a discussion of the results was conducted. The promoters of the study took part in the discussion but did not interfere with the decisions of the group.

Overall, 1320 visualizations were performed. The overall agreement levels among the total group of raters were as follows: DICA 1, 70.2%; DICA 2, 70.5%; and DICA 3, 81.3%. The free-marginal κ varied as follows: DICA 1 = 0.553, DICA 2 = 0.558, and DICA 3 = 0.719. The overall agreement levels among the expert group of raters were as follows: DICA 1, 78.8%; DICA 2, 80.2%; and DICA 3, 88.5%. The free-marginal κ varied as follows: DICA 1 = 0.682, DICA 2 = 0.712, and DICA 3 = 0.828 (Table 16.2). Significantly, no differences were found between the experts and the not experts in using the DICA classification.

The second study was conducted in an International setting during the third International Symposium on Diverticular Disease, held in Madrid (Spain) in April 2019 [19]. A total of 96 doctors from Europe (Bulgaria, Croatia, Germany, Hungary, Italy, Romania, Poland, Portugal, Slovakia, Spain, The Netherlands, and Russia), Africa (Tunisia), America (Brazil, Mexico, United States, and Venezuela), and Australia were involved (63 of them (82.9%) were endoscopists). The DICA classification was known by 62 (81.6%) doctors and used routinely by 37 (48.7%) doctors.

Overall, 960 visualizations were performed. The overall agreement level for the DICA classification was 91.8% with a free-marginal kappa of 88% (95% CI 80–95). The overall agreement levels were: DICA 1, 85.2%; DICA 2, 96.5%; and DICA 3, 99.5%. The free-marginal κ was: DICA 1 = 0.753, DICA 2 = 0.958, and DICA 3 = 0.919. The agreement about the main endoscopic items was 83.4% (k 67%) for diverticular extension, 62.6% (k 65%) for the number of diverticula in each district, 86.8% (k 82%) for the presence of inflammation, and 98.5 (98%) for the presence

Table 16.2 Agreement about DICA scores and items in the Italian real life setting

	DICA 1		DICA 2		DICA 3	
Raters	Overall agreement	Free marginal K	Overall agreement	Free marginal K	Overall agreement	Free marginal K
All	0.702	0.553	0.705	0.558	0.813	0.719
Experts	0.788	0.682	0.802	0.712	0.885	0.828
Not experts	0.612	0.420	0.590	0.410	0.628	0.440

	All		Expert		Not expert	
Items	Overall agreement	Free marginal K	Overall agreement	Free marginal K	Overall agreement	Free marginal K
Diverticulosis extent	0.767	0.650	0.787	0.680	0.744	0.620
Number of diverticula	0.758	0.520	0.769	0.539	0.741	0.480
Presence of inflammation	0.579	0.440	0.609	0.479	0.571	0.430
Presence of complications	0.780	0.730	0.797	0.747	0.778	0.720

Table 16.3 Agreement about DICA scores and items in the International real life setting

	DICA 1		DICA 2		DICA 3	
Raters	Overall agreement (%)	Free marginal K	Overall agreement (%)	Free marginal K	Overall agreement (%)	Free marginal K
All	85.2	0.753	96.5	0.958	99.5	0.919
Users	91	0.880	90	0.812	100	1
Not users	88	0.820	89	0.800	99	0.900

	All		Expert		Not expert	
Items	Overall agreement (%)	Free marginal K	Overall agreement (%)	Free marginal K	Overall agreement (%)	Free marginal K
Diverticulosis extent	83.4	0.670	98.3	0.820	88.3	0.620
Number of diverticula	82.6	0.650	89	0.690	81.3	0.600
Presence of inflammation	86.8	0.820	91	0.910	83.5	0.810
Presence of complications	98.5	0.980	99	0.990	97	0.920

Free marginal multirater kappa (κ) coefficient:
=0: pure chance
<0.4: poor agreement
0.41 to 0.60: moderate agreement
>0.80: very good agreement

of complications (Table 16.3). Significantly, no differences were found between doctors using and not using the DICA classification in terms of the agreement.

16.6 Predictive Value of the Classification: A Retrospective Study

This classification has also shown a significant role in predicting the outcomes of the disease according to the severity of the DICA score. This role was first demonstrated in a retrospective study [20].

A multicenter, international, retrospective cohort study, involving 21 centers from Italy, Brazil, Norway, and Venezuela, enrolled 1651 patients (793 M, 858 F, mean age 66.6 ± 11.1 years): 939 (56.9%) patients were classified as DICA 1, 501 (30.3%) as DICA 2, and 211 (12.8%) as DICA 3. The aim of the study was to assess the role of the DICA classification in predicting the risk of acute diverticulitis occurrence/recurrence and the risk of surgery according to the DICA score severity. During a median follow-up of 24 (9–38) months, acute diverticulitis occurred/recurred in 263 (15.9%) patients, whereas surgery due to DD complications was necessary in 57 (21.7%) cases.

Both the univariate ($\chi^2 = 405.029$; $p < 0.0001$) and the multivariate analyses (hazard ratio = 4.319, 95% CI 3.639–5.126, $p < 0.0001$) found that the DICA score was the only factor significantly associated with the occurrence/recurrence of diverticulitis and surgery during the follow-up.

This study also analyzed whether the current scheduled treatment advised for DD patients, ranging from rifaximin to mesalazine or probiotics, may be able to influence the outcome of the disease according to the severity of the DICA score. The study found that only in DICA 2 patients, scheduled therapies were effective in the prevention of AD occurrence/recurrence with a hazard ratio of 0.598 (95% CI 0.391–0.914, $p = 0.006$); among them, only mesalazine-based therapies were significantly able to reduce the risk of AD occurrence/recurrence and the need for surgery with hazard ratios of 0.2103 (95% CI 0.122–0.364) and 0.459 (95% CI 0.258–0.818), respectively.

16.7 Predictive Value of the Classification: Prospective Studies

The next step was to assess the predictive value of this classification in a prospective study.

A multicenter, international, prospective cohort study, involving 43 centers from Italy, Brazil, The United Kingdom, Lithuania, Poland, Romania, and Venezuela, enrolled 2215 patients: 1377 (62.15%) patients were classified as DICA 1, 599 (27.04%) as DICA 2, and 239 (10.80%) as DICA 3.

The patients were followed-up for 3 years, and the results at the second year of follow-up are currently available [21]. At 2 years of follow-up, acute diverticulitis occurred in 123 (5.5%) patients: 32 (2.3%) patients in the DICA 1 group, 53 (8.9%) patients in the DICA 2 group, and 32 (16.4%) patients in the DICA 3 group ($p = 0.0001$) (Fig. 16.10); surgery occurred in 35 (1.6%) patients: 2 (0.1%) patients in the DICA 1 group, 15 (2.5%) patients in the DICA 2 group, and 18 (7.6%) patients in the DICA 3 group ($p = 0.0001$) (Fig. 16.11). Again, the DICA classification shows a significant role in predicting the outcome of diverticulosis/DD.

Another recent real-life study has tried to identify some factors associated with the severity of the endoscopic appearance of diverticulosis/DD according to the DICA classification [21], by analyzing a cohort of 11,086 patients, 5635 with diverticulitis and 5451 without diverticulosis. Blood hypertension, diabetes, and angiotensin receptor blocker use occurred more frequently in the study group, whereas the prevalence of colorectal cancer (CRC) was significantly lower. Age > 70 years, BMI > 30, and blood hypertension were factors independently related to the presence of diverticulosis, whereas diabetes and CRC were significantly associated with the absence of diverticulosis. Female sex, age, smoking, appendectomy, proton pump inhibitors, and acetylsalicylic acid use were directly related to the severity of diverticular disease, whereas CRC and colonic polyp occurrence were inversely related to the severity of diverticular disease, significantly. Female sex, age > 70 years, and smoking were significantly related to the severity of diverticular disease. CRC and colonic polyps were significantly less in DICA 3 patients. Moreover, DICA 3 patients were more often symptomatic, at higher risk of hospital

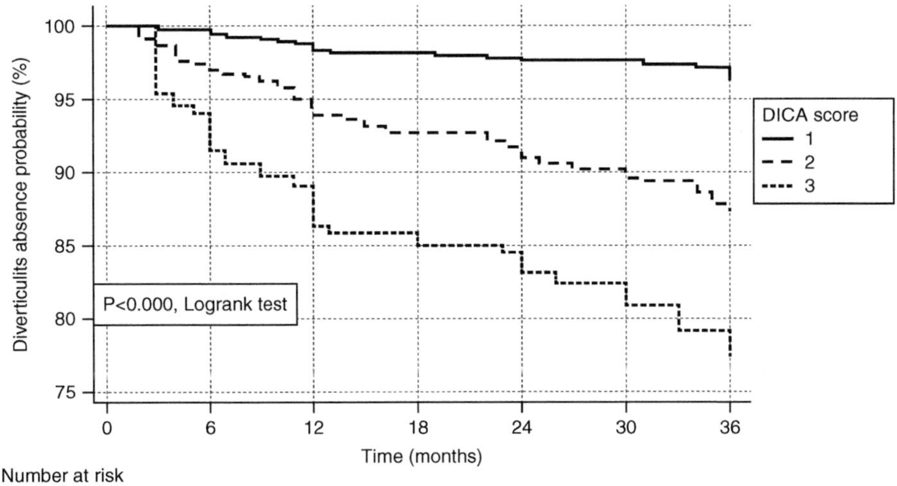

Number at risk

	0	6	12	18	24	30	36
Group: 1	1363	1344	1303	1300	702	452	0
Group: 2	590	566	531	523	352	250	0
Group: 3	236	211	192	188	112	92	0

Fig. 16.10 Acute diverticulitis occurrence/recurrence according to the DICA score after 2 years of follow-up

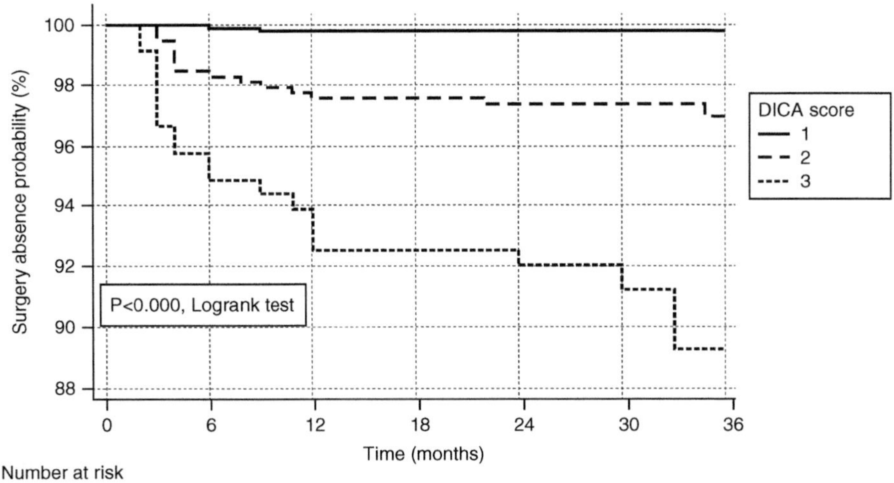

Number at risk

	0	6	12	18	24	30	36
Group: 1	1374	1353	1312	1309	712	452	0
Group: 2	594	569	534	526	355	249	0
Group: 3	236	211	192	188	112	92	0

Fig. 16.11 Surgery occurrence due to diverticular complications according to the DICA score after 2 years of follow-up

admission ($p < 0.0001$), had longer hospital stay (9 days, range 6–15, $p = 0.012$), and higher mean costs (1964 €, range 1173–3467, $p = 0.017$).

16.8 Conclusions

The DICA classification has been shown to have an important role as a predictive tool for the outcome of the disease in terms of acute diverticulitis occurrence/recurrence and surgery due to complications of the disease. Its importance is demonstrated by evidence that suggests that it is becoming the standard endoscopic classification in the field of diverticular disease [22–29].

Further studies are required to investigate whether some scheduled treatments can positively influence the outcome of the disease according to the DICA score.

References

1. Tursi A. Diverticulosis today: unfashionable and still under-researched. Ther Adv Gastroenterol. 2016;9:213–28.
2. Tursi A, Scarpignato C, Strate LL, Lanas A, Kruis W, Lahat A, Danese S. Colonic diverticular disease. Nat Rev Dis Primers. 2020;6:20.
3. Lohrmann C, Ghanem N, Pache G, Makowiec F, Kotter E, Langer M. CT in acute perforated sigmoid diverticulitis. Eur J Radiol. 2005;56:78–83.
4. Wasvary H, Turfah F, Kadro O, Beauregard W. Same hospitalization resection for acute diverticulitis. Am Surg. 1999;65:632–5.
5. Ambrosetti P, Becker C, Terrier F. Colonic diverticulitis: impact of imaging on surgical management – a prospective study of 542 patients. Eur Radiol. 2002;12:1145–9.
6. Köhler L, Sauerland S, Neugebauer E. Diagnosis and treatment of diverticular disease: results of a consensus development conference. The scientific Committee of the European Association for endoscopic surgery. Surg Endosc. 1999;13:430–6.
7. Sheth AA, Longo W, Floch MH. Diverticular disease and diverticulitis. Am J Gastroenterol. 2008;103:1550–6.
8. Hansen O, Graupe F, Stock W. Prognostic factors in perforating diverticulitis of the large intestine (in German). Chirurg. 1998;69:443–9.
9. Everhart JE, Ruhl CE. Burden of digestive diseases in the United States part II: lower gastrointestinal diseases. Gastroenterology. 2009;136:741–54.
10. Peery AF, Crockett SD, Murphy CC, et al. Burden and cost of gastrointestinal, liver, and pancreatic diseases in the United States: update 2018. Gastroenterology. 2019;156:254–72.
11. Ghorai S, Ulbright TM, Rex DK. Endoscopic findings of diverticular inflammation in colonoscopy patients without clinical acute diverticulitis: prevalence and endoscopic spectrum. Am J Gastroenterol. 2003;98:802–6.
12. Tursi A, Elisei W, Giorgetti GM, Aiello F, Brandimarte G. Inflammatory manifestations at colonoscopy in patients with colonic diverticular disease. Aliment Pharmacol Ther. 2011;33:358–65.
13. Hall JF, Roberts PL, Ricciardi R, et al. Long-term follow-up after an initial episode of diverticulitis: what are the predictors of recurrence? Dis Colon Rectum. 2011;54:283–8.
14. Tursi A, Elisei W, Giorgetti GM, et al. Detection of endoscopic and histological inflammation after an attack of colonic diverticulitis is associated with higher diverticulitis recurrence. J Gastrointestin Liver Dis. 2013;22:13–9.

15. Tursi A, Brandimarte G, Di Mario F, et al. Development and validation of an endoscopic classification of diverticular disease of the colon: the DICA classification. Dig Dis. 2015;33:68–76.
16. Tursi A. Segmental colitis associated with diverticulosis: complication of diverticular disease or autonomous entity? Dig Dis Sci. 2011;56:27–34.
17. Tursi A, Brandimarte G, Di Mario F, et al. International Consensus on Diverticulosis and Diverticular Disease. Statements from the 3rd International Symposium on Diverticular Disease. J Gastrointestin Liver Dis. 2019;28(suppl. 4):57–66.
18. Tursi A, Brandimarte G, Di Mario F, et al. DICA Italian group. The "DICA" endoscopic classification for diverticular disease of the colon shows a significant interobserver agreement among community endoscopists. J Gastrointestin Liver Dis. 2019;28:23–7.
19. Tursi A, Brandimarte G, Di Mario F, et al. The DICA endoscopic classification for diverticular disease of the colon shows a significant interobserver agreement among community endoscopists: an International Study. J Gastrointestin Liver Dis. 2019;28(suppl. 4):39–44.
20. Tursi A, Brandimarte G, Di Mario F, et al. Predictive value of the Diverticular Inflammation and Complication Assessment (DICA) endoscopic classification on the outcome of diverticular disease of the colon: an international study. United European Gastroenterol J. 2016;4:604–13.
21. Tursi A, Violi A, Cambie' G, et al. Risk factors for endoscopic severity of diverticular disease of the colon and its outcome: a real-life case-control study. Eur J Gastroenterol Hepatol. 2020;32:1123–9.
22. Yamada E, Kuriyama H, Uchida E, et al. Association between endoscopic findings related to colonic diverticula and bowel habits: a multicenter study in Japan. J Gastroenterol Hepatol. 2017;32:1938–42.
23. Gavrić A, Drobne D, Štabuc B. Akutni divertikulitis – novosti [in slovenian]. Gastroenterolog. 2017;1:39–42.
24. García-Zermeño KR, Valdovinos-Díaz MA, Raña-Garibay R, Abreu y Abreu AT, Remes-Troche JM. Rifaximina-alfa en el tratamiento de la enfermedad diverticular. Evidencia y conceptos actuales [in español]. Med Int Méx. 2019;35:912–26.
25. Sabelnikova EA, Bordin DS. Classification of DICA as an effective tool for prognosis and choice of therapy for diverticular disease [in russian]. Effect Pharmacother. 2019;29:66–71.
26. Lahat A, Necula D, Yavzori M, et al. Prolonged recurrent abdominal pain is associated with ongoing underlying mucosal inflammation in patients who had an episode of acute complicated diverticulitis. J Clin Gastroenterol. 2019;53:e178–85.
27. Rutter MD, Evans R, Hoare Z, et al. WASh multicentre randomised controlled trial: water-assisted sigmoidoscopy in English NHS bowel scope screening. Gut. 2021;70:845–52.
28. Lukosiene JI, Reichert MC, Lammert F, et al. Environmental and dietary risk factors for colonic diverticulosis and diverticulitis. J Gastrointestin Liver Dis. 2021;30:66–72.
29. Brandimarte G, Tursi A, Di Mario F, et al. Predictive value of the "DICA" endoscopic classification on the outcome of diverticular disease of the colon: a 1-year analysis from the international, multicenter, prospective study. Falk Symposium 217 "West meets East: Functional meets Organic in Gastrointestinal Disease". Singapore, 29–30 November 2019;abstract book: 26–7.

Part V

Medical Treatment of Symptomatic Uncomplicated Diverticular Disease

High-Fiber Diet

17

Gian Marco Giorgetti, Annarita Eramo, Valeria Clemente, Guilherme Piovezani Ramos, and Odery Ramos

17.1 Introduction

Colonic diverticula are common in Western countries, affecting up to 60% of subjects over 70 years of age [1]. In about 80% of patients, colonic diverticula remain asymptomatic, whereas approximately 20% of them may develop abdominal symptoms (symptomatic uncomplicated diverticular disease, SUDD). SUDD is defined by the presence of nonspecific episodes of abdominal pain from a diverticular source, without evidence of an inflammatory process and alteration in bowel habits.

The geographic variability of diverticular disease and its correlation with a Western diet have long suggested diet as a fundamental factor in the pathogenesis of the disorder. Autopsy series from 1920 to 1940 identified diverticulosis present in 2–10% of individuals. More recent autopsy studies have shown that the presence of diverticulosis has increased up to 20–50%. This sharp rise in the incidence of diverticulosis is largely attributed to dietary changes, mainly the dietary decline of intake of fibers from cereal grains. In 1971, Burkitt and Painter first proposed the initial hypothesis of fiber deficiency as the etiology of diverticular disease. They recorded transit times and stool weights of more than 1200 individuals in the UK and rural Uganda [2]. The UK

G. M. Giorgetti (✉) · A. Eramo · V. Clemente
Division of Nutritional and Digestive Endoscopy, "S. Eugenio" Hospital, Rome, Italy
e-mail: gianmarcogiorgetti@hotmail.com; annarita.eramo@aslroma2.it; valeria.clemente@aslroma2.it

G. P. Ramos
Division of Gastroenterology and Hepatology, Mayo Clinic, Rochester, MN, USA
e-mail: ramos.gui@mayo.edu

O. Ramos
Division of Gastroenterology, Department of Internal Medicine, Hospital del Clinical, Universidade federal do Paranà, Curitiba, Brazil
e-mail: oderyramos@gmail.com

© The Author(s), under exclusive license to Springer Nature Switzerland AG 2022

A. Tursi et al. (eds.), *Colonic Diverticular Disease*,
https://doi.org/10.1007/978-3-030-93761-4_17

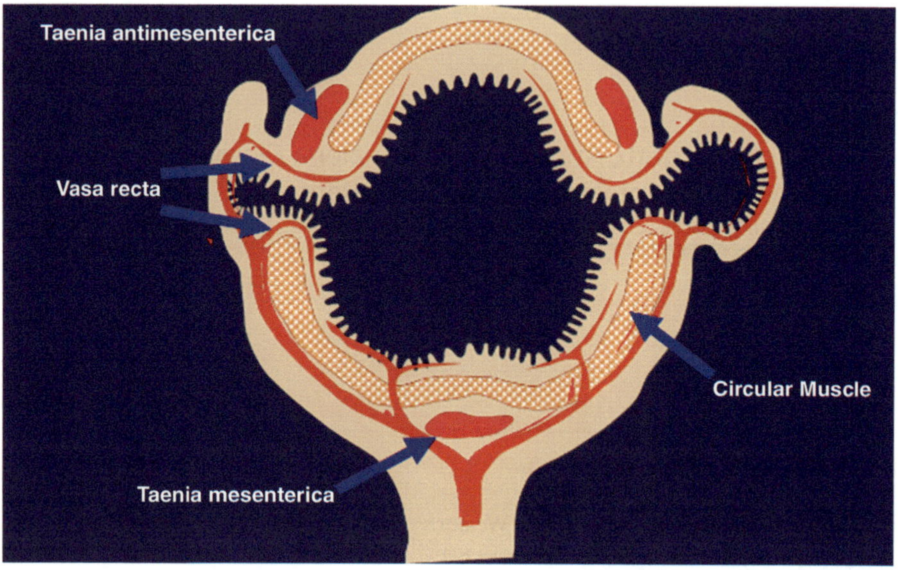

Fig. 17.1 Pathogenesis of diverticula

patients, consuming a low-fiber diet, had transit times of about 80 h and mean stool weights of 110 g/day. In contrast, rural Ugandans, consuming extremely high-fiber diets, had transit times of 34 h and mean stool weights of more than 450 g/day. The longer transit times and smaller stool volumes were believed to increase intraluminal pressure, predisposing to diverticular herniation. The hypothesis is that decreased dietary fiber intake results in decreased intestinal contents and smaller size of the lumen. This in turn results in the transmission of muscular contraction pressure to the wall of the colon, rather than to the contents of the lumen. The result of increased pressure on the wall is the formation of diverticula at the weakest point on the wall, namely, the sites of penetration by blood vessels, called the vasa recta [3] (Fig. 17.1).

The main goals for managing SUDD include both the reduction of abdominal symptoms and the prevention of acute diverticulitis. A standard therapeutic approach still remains to be defined. Fibers have been suggested in the treatment of SUDD patients, for increasing fecal mass, regularizing bowel movements, and favoring health-promoting species of the intestinal microbiota (Fig. 17.2).

17.2 Characteristics of Dietary Fibers

Dietary fibers are defined as the edible parts of plants or analogous carbohydrates, which are resistant to digestion and absorption in the human small intestine, with complete or partial fermentation in the colon. Fiber intake may be achieved by consuming fruits, vegetables, and cereal grains (dietary fibers), and/or by diet supplementation with specific commercial preparations containing fibers (supplemental

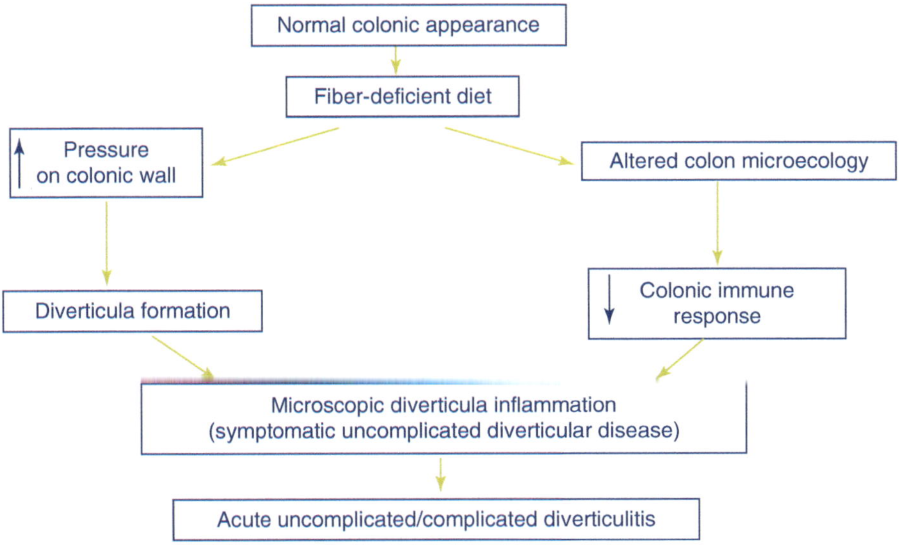

Fig. 17.2 New understanding about the pathogenesis of diverticular disease

fibers) [4, 5]. Fruit fiber is a relatively small component of the total fiber consumed in populations following a Western dietary pattern [4].

Total fiber is the sum of dietary fibers and functional fibers. As all fibers are not hydrolyzed by human digestive enzymes, their constituent sugars are not absorbed in the small intestine. Fibers entering the large intestine may be fermented by the gut microbiota or may be resistant to fermentation, passing through the digestive tract relatively unchanged. Dietary fibers are heterogeneous, regarding their origin, chemical composition, and physicochemical properties with additional subcategorization based on the degree of polymerization (e.g., chain length). With regard to their origin, plant-based fibers can be separated into fibers derived from cereals and grains, fruits, vegetables, nuts, and legumes. The physicochemical characteristics of fibers include fermentability, solubility, and viscosity, and these properties influence not only fermentation but also the therapeutic effects of consumption. Fibers that are highly fermentable while also possessing high solubility and viscosity include β-glucan, inulin, and pectins. These fibers are naturally found in whole grains, such as oats and barley, and in fruits, such as apples (pectin).

Soluble fibers are fermented to a large extent more proximally in the gastrointestinal tract (e.g., the ileam and the ascending colon) by a wide variety of anaerobic bacteria, such as bifidobacteria and Bacteroides, which result in an increase in bacterial biomass, an increase in fecal mass, a change in intracolonic pH, and production of short-chain fatty acids (SFCAs) and various gases as metabolic end products [6]. SCFAs resulting from this colonic fermentation of fibers will have systemic effects following absorption into the portal circulation. These include metabolic effects such as postprandial hypoglucemia and hypolipidemia [7]. Moreover, SCFAs exhibit anti-inflammatory properties, particularly related to modulation of specific microbiome signatures, which may also play a role in the pathogenesis of DD.

Amongst the soluble fibers, pectin is a major fruit prebiotic that has been extensively studied and shown to promote a healthy, anti-inflammatory colonic microbiota ecosystem with greater microflora diversity than inulin. Collectively, this soluble fiber supports a higher anti-inflammatory microbial profile by: (1) increasing the Bacteroidetes/Firmicutes ratio and increasing the abundance of Bifidobacterium and Clostridium cluster XIV, resulting in enhanced colonic mucosal barrier integrity and function, increased mucosal immunity, increased butyrate production, and a decrease in enteric pathogens; (2) promoting Eubacterium eligens, which upregulates pectinolytic enzymes; and (3) supporting certain Faecalibacterium prausnitzii strains while utilizing the fermentation of pectin to exert anti-inflammatory effects [8].

Insoluble fibers, such as cellulose, are generally poorly fermented by gut microbes, but their presence in the diet serves almost exclusively as bulking agents, which result in shorter transit time and increased fecal mass. They are partially fermented in the distal colon, where the transit time is slower and bacterial densities are higher. Psyllium is also a nonfermentable fiber; however, its high solubility and viscosity results in unique therapeutic effects, including improved glycemic control and reduced blood cholesterol levels [6].

The adequate daily intake of fiber is 14 g of total fiber per 1000 kcal, or 25 g for adult women and 38 g for adult men. These numbers come mostly from studies related to fiber use and its benefits on protection against coronary heart disease. The mean intake of dietary fiber in the United States is 17 g/day with only 5% of the population meeting the adequate intake, whereas, in Europe, the intake may vary from 16 to 29 g/day. Grain-based foods (not including desserts) are the major sources of dietary fiber, with grain mixtures (e.g., pasta meals, pizza, and noodle soups) being the highest source of dietary fiber at 17.8%, followed by fruits at 14.9%, and vegetables at 13.7%. Owing to low consumption, higher-fiber foods, such as dry beans, peas, other legumes, nuts, and seeds, contribute to only 6.3% of dietary fiber intake [9].

A growing number of human studies on specific fruit sources show varying levels of prebiotic effects depending on the fruit source and daily amount consumed. Generally, a minimum of two whole fruit servings daily, especially those containing ≥2.5 g fiber/serving (e.g., Kiwi, prunes), is required to stimulate significant colonic prebiotic activity (higher SCFA production, increased levels of Bifidobacteria, reduced levels of pathogenic bacteria, and protection against persistent bacterial diarrhea in children and adults) compared to ≤1 whole fruit serving/day, which is common in Western diets [8].

17.3 Dietary Fibers and Diverticular Disease

Diverticular disease has historically been considered a disease of both diet and lifestyle. In the past, the high prevalence of diverticular disease was attributed to insufficient fiber intake. Recent studies, however, have indicated that after controlling for

Table 17.1 Main studies on dietary fibers in diverticular disease

Author, year	Study type	Dietary fibers/supplemental
Brodribb A.J.M., 1977	Double-blind trial	Dietary fibers
Aldoori WH 1994	Prospective	Dietary fibers
Aldoori WH 1998	Prospective	Dietary fibers
Latella G., 2003	Open RCT	Supplemental
Cuomo R, 2014	Consensus conference	Dietary fibers
Carabotti M, 2017	Review	Dietary fibers
Carabotti M, 2018	Review	Dietary fibers
Eberhardt F, 2019	Review	Dietary fibers
Tursi A, 2020	Review	Dietary fibers/supplemental

other risk factors, dietary fiber intake is not associated with the prevalence of diverticulosis detected at colonoscopy. On the other hand, a number of population-based studies have shown that fiber intake is inversely associated with the risk of diverticulitis. For instance, in a prospective study of 51,529 US male health professionals followed up for more than 4 years, a significant inverse association was recorded between dietary fiber intake and risk of development of clinically evident diverticular disease [10]. Individuals consuming 30 g of fiber per day have been shown to have a 41% reduction in risk compared to persons with a low fiber intake. Insoluble fibers from fruits and vegetables were noted to be more protective than cereal fibers [11]. These results provide further support for the recommendation that patients with asymptomatic diverticular disease might benefit from increasing their fruit and vegetable fiber intake, a stance endorsed by the American Dietetic Association [12]. The main characteristics of the included studies are summarized in Table 17.1. However, it is not clear whether a specific type or source of fiber is more beneficial in reducing the risk of diverticulitis. During acute phases, it may be advisable to limit the sources of insoluble fibers, which could cause further damage to inflammatory processes at the local level, while maintaining a minimum supply of fibers in its soluble forms (pectins, gums, fruity, and some hemicellulose), especially contained in some types of fruit.

Although dietary and supplementary fibers have been proposed for symptomatic relief in SUDD patients, the therapeutic benefit is not yet fully understood. In SUDD patients, fibers might act through: (a) conferring benefits by increasing fecal mass and promoting the regularity of bowel movements and (b) acting as prebiotics in the colon by favoring health-promoting species of the intestinal microbiota, especially bifidobacteria and lactobacilli. Indeed, the gut microbiota shifts rapidly in response to dietary changes, particularly with fiber intake. However, evidence for a therapeutic benefit of a high-fiber diet in the treatment of DD is conflicting [4]. A systematic review evaluating multiple studies over a period of 40 years tried to assess the impact of a high-fiber diet on the treatment of more than 736 SUDD patients, mostly female in their seventh decade of life. Major limitations were involved in this analysis, including a wide variety of amounts considered as "high" fiber intake, which ranged from 20 to 96 g/day, and different outcomes and follow-up times, in addition to lack of reports of type of fiber consumed (soluble vs. insoluble). As an example of one of the clinical trials assessed, Brodribb et al. performed a randomized double-blind trial of a high-fiber diet in 18 patients with symptomatic diverticular disease [13]. Despite a considerable placebo effect being noted at 1 month, at 3 months, a significant reduction in bowel symptoms was seen in patients on the high-fiber diet. These findings suggest that patients should gradually increase their dietary fiber consumption over weeks and also be aware that their symptoms might initially worsen before they improve, which could take months. In a subsequent study, no improvement in symptom end points was reported despite a decline in transit times and increases in stool weight and frequency [13]. Despite these conflicting data, some amelioration of symptoms in patients with uncomplicated disease can be reasonably expected with a high-fiber diet.

In addition to assessing the role of a high-fiber diet, another major consideration is the addition of supplementary fiber sources and their impact on diverticular disease. A systematic review assessing this theme evaluated articles published over the past 37 years and identified 10 studies with more than 1707 patients, with a majority of them females over 60 years of age [4]. Study designs varied, but were in majority randomized controlled trials assessing different types of supplementations including glucomannan, ispaghula, bran, Plantago ovata, and methylcellulose. With regard to fiber solubility, soluble fibers were used in five studies, both insoluble and soluble fibers were used in two studies, and in three studies, insoluble fibers were used. Notably, the fiber intake of the diet was not reported and many studies included added interventions to fiber supplementation, including the addition of the selective antibiotic rifaximin. For instance, three studies assessed the efficacy of glucomannan (2 or 4 g/day) when compared to glucomannan together with cyclic rifaximin, measured by the improvement of abdominal symptoms in SUDD patients. In all three studies, a significant reduction of abdominal symptoms in the treatment arm with just glucomannan was achieved. In two of these three studies, the glucomannan treatment arm had a similar occurrence of diverticulitis as the antibiotic arm, whereas in the study by Latella et al., the incidence of episodes of diverticulitis in the group treated with rifaximin was lower than that in the group treated with glucomannan alone [14].

A more recent systematic review has aimed to update the evidences on the efficacy of fiber treatment, both dietary and supplemental, in terms of reduction in symptoms and prevention of acute diverticulitis (AD) in SUDD patients. In all, 19 studies were included, 9 with dietary fibers and 10 with supplemental fibers. The authors concluded that, mostly based on low-quality evidence study designs, both dietary and supplemental fibers could be beneficial in the treatment of SUDD. Nonetheless, owing to methodological limitations and the heterogeneity of therapeutic regimens employed a summary of the outcome measures is not permitted. On the basis of these data, fiber supplements are suggested in Danish and Polish guidelines, whereas Italian guidelines argue that fiber supplementation alone produces controversial results in terms of symptom relief [15].

One particular observation is related to the use of antibiotics concomitant with fibers. Antimicrobial drugs have been shown to reduce H_2 production and gas-related symptoms and to increase mean stool weight in subjects taking fibers, most likely for a reduced fiber degradation. All the above findings provide rationale for antibiotic use in diverticular disease. Both the reduction in gas production and the increase in fecal mass can reduce intraluminal pressure and therefore improve, thus leading to a decrease in the enlargement of diverticula and in the generation of new diverticula. Fibers in combination with the selective antibiotic rifaximin have been shown to be associated with a greater prevalence of symptom-free disease when compared to fibers alone. The combination of rifaximin with fibers has also been shown to be more effective than fibers alone in preventing acute diverticulitis [16].

One additional concern with the use of fibers in patients with diverticular disease is as follows. Historically, physicians have advised individuals with diverticular disease to avoid nuts, seeds, popcorn, corn, and other high-residue foods [17, 18]. This recommendation stems from the theory that luminal trauma is a causal mechanism for both diverticulitis [19]. Nuts, seeds, popcorn, and corn are presumed to be particularly likely to abrade the mucosa or to lodge within small diverticula [20]. However, the biological mechanisms responsible for diverticular complications remain poorly understood. Aside from luminal trauma, the potential inciting factors include elevated colonic pressures, compromised colon wall integrity, and altered bacterial flora [21, 22]. In contrast to this paradigm, utilizing a questionnaire-based protocol, the Health Professionals Follow-Up Study has demonstrated an inverse association between nut and popcorn consumption and the risk of diverticulitis. In this large, prospective study of men without a known diverticular disease, nut, corn, and popcorn consumption did not increase the risk of diverticulosis or diverticular complications [23]. Based on these data and the aforementioned benefits of fibers obtained from these food resources, the recommendation to avoid these foods to prevent diverticular complications should be reconsidered.

17.4 Conclusions

In conclusion, the role of diet in preventing diverticular disease has long been debated in the treatment of diverticular disease, with fibers in the center of recommendations. Even though high-quality evidence is still lacking, a high-fiber diet seems to decrease the likelihood of SUDD in asymptomatic patients and may provide symptom relief in patients with active disease. Recent studies have proposed that its use in combination with selective antibiotics may also yield further symptom control in patients with active SUDD, given modulation of the gut microbiome processing the ingested fibers. Nonetheless, the type, amount, and form of administration are still widely variable, thus making outcome assessment and specific recommendation guidance unclear. Further studies are needed to determine the best regimen of both high-fiber diets and supplementation in patients with DD, in addition to further comprehend the prebiotic effect of specific fiber regimens in modulating the gut microbiome and, consequently, intestinal inflammation in patients with SUDD.

References

1. Parra-Blanco A. Colonic diverticular disease: pathophysiology and clinical picture. Digestion. 2006;73(Suppl. 1):47–57.
2. Burkitt DP, Walker AR, Painter NS. Effect of dietary fiber on stools and the transit-times, and its role in the causation of disease. Lancet. 1972;2:1408–12.
3. Ünlu C, Daniels L, Vrouenraets BC, Boermeester MA. A systematic review of high-fibre dietary therapy in diverticular disease. Int J Color Dis. 2012;27:419–27.
4. Carabotti M, Annibale B, Severi C, Lahner E. Role of fiber in symptomatic uncomplicated diverticular disease: a systematic review. Nutrients. 2017;9(161):1–14. Published online 2017 Febr 20. https://doi.org/10.3390/nu9020161.
5. Tursi A, Scarpignato C, Strate LL, Lanas A, Kruis W, Lahat A, et al. Colonic diverticular disease. Nat Rev Dis Primers. 2020;6(1):20. https://doi.org/10.1038/s41572-020-0153-5.
6. Holscher HD. Dietary fiber and prebiotics and the gastrointestinal microbiota. Gut Microbes. 2017;8(2):172–84.
7. Roberfroid M. Dietary fiber, inulin, and oligofructose: a review comparing their physiological effects. Crit Rev Food Sci Nutr. 1993;33(2):103–48.
8. Dreher ML. Whole fruits and fruit fiber emerging health effects. Nutrients. 2018;10(12):1–54. Published online 2018 Nov 28. https://doi.org/10.3390/nu10121833.
9. Dahl WJ, Stewart ML. Position of the academy of nutrition and dietetics: health implications of dietary fiber. J Acad Nutr Diet. 2015;115(11):1861–70.
10. Aldoori WH, Giovannucci EL, Rimm EB, Wing AL, Trichopoulos DV, Willett WC. A prospective study of diet and the risk of symptomatic diverticular disease in men. Am J Clin Nutr. 1994;60:757–64.
11. Aldoori WH, Giovannucci EL, Rockett HR, Sampson L, Rimm EB, Willett WC. A prospective study of dietary fiber types and symptomatic diverticular disease in men. J Nutr. 1998;128:714–9.
12. Marlett J, McBurney M, Slavin J. Position of the American dietetic association: health implications of dietary fiber. J Am Diet Assoc. 2002;102:993–1000.
13. Brodribb AJ. Treatment of symptomatic diverticular disease with a high-fiber diet. Lancet. 1977;1:664–6.
14. Latella G, Pimpo MT, Sottili S, Zippi M, Viscido A, Chiaramonte M, et al. Rifaximin improves symptoms of acquired uncomplicated diverticular disease of the colon. Int J Color Dis. 2003;18:55–62.
15. Carabotti M, Annibale B. Treatment of diverticular disease: an update on latest evidence and clinical implications. Drugs Context. 2018;7:212526. https://doi.org/10.7573/dic.212526.
16. Cuomo R, Barbara G, Pace F, Annese V, Bassotti G, Binda GA, et al. Italian consensus conference for colonic diverticulosis and diverticular disease. United European Gastroenterol J. 2014;2(5):413–42.
17. Eberhardt F, Crichton M, Dahl C, Nucera R, Jenkins J, Marx W. Role of dietary fibre in older adults with asymptomatic (AS) or symptomatic uncomplicated diverticular disease (SUDD): Systematic review and meta-analysis. Maturitas. 2019;130:57–67.
18. Horner JL. Natural history of diverticulosis of the colon. Am J Dig Dis. 1958;3(5):343–50.
19. Jacobs DO. Clinical practice. Diverticulitis N Engl J Med. 2007;357(20):2057–66.
20. Bogardus ST Jr. What do we know about diverticular disease? A brief overview. J Clin Gastroenterol. 2006;40(7 Suppl 3):S108–11.
21. Floch MH, Bina I. The natural history of diverticulitis: fact and theory. J Clin Gastroenterol. 2004;38(5 Suppl):S2–7.
22. Korzenik JR. Case closed? Diverticulitis: epidemiology and fiber. J Clin Gastroenterol. 2006;40(7 Suppl 3):S112–6.
23. Strate LL, Liu YL, Syngal S, Aldoori WH, Giovannucci EL. Nut, corn, and popcorn consumption and the incidence of diverticular disease. JAMA. 2008;300(8):907–14.

Non-Absorbable Antibiotics 18

Carmelo Scarpignato and Neil Stollman

18.1 Introduction

The spectrum of colonic diverticular disease is wide and ranges from asymptomatic diverticula to symptomatic uncomplicated diverticular disease (SUDD), uncomplicated diverticulitis, and, eventually, complicated diverticulitis. As a consequence, the therapeutic approach in each clinical scenario will depend on the severity of the disease [1].

Asymptomatic diverticulosis does not require any pharmacological treatment. However, a healthy lifestyle (regular physical exercise, maintaining ideal body weight, abstention from smoking) and intake of a high-fiber diet are recommended to reduce its progression to SUDD, acute diverticulitis, and its complications [2]. Most people with diverticulosis will not progress to symptomatic disease; the proportion of subjects with diverticulosis that eventually develop SUDD or acute diverticulitis is unknown.

C. Scarpignato (✉)
Department of Health Sciences, United Campus of Malta, Msida, Malta

Faculty of Medicine, Chinese University of Hong Kong, Shatin, Hong Kong, China
e-mail: carmelo.scarpignato@gmail.com

N. Stollman
Division of Gastroenterology, Alta Bates Summit Medical Center, East Bay Center for Digestive Health, Oakland, CA, USA

School of Medicine, University of California San Francisco (UCSF), San Francisco, CA, USA
e-mail: neil@stollman.com

© The Author(s), under exclusive license to Springer Nature Switzerland AG 2022
A. Tursi et al. (eds.), *Colonic Diverticular Disease*,
https://doi.org/10.1007/978-3-030-93761-4_18

18.2 Pharmacological Treatment of SUDD

In patients with SUDD, pharmacological treatment should be aimed at reducing both the intensity and the frequency of symptoms as well as preventing complications [1, 3, 4]. Most symptoms in SUDD are mild-to-moderate but they impair the patients' quality of life, which can potentially be improved by medical treatment [5]. Typical symptoms of SUDD include pain (often, but not always, in the lower or left lower quadrant of the abdomen), bloating, and changes in bowel habits. Such symptoms are also observed in patients with irritable bowel syndrome (IBS), and distinguishing between these two clinical entities can be challenging [3, 6].

Diverticular disease has historically been considered a disease of diet and lifestyle, and a high-fiber diet has been and still is suggested for these patients. As pointed out by a recent systematic review [7], despite some evidence that a high-fiber diet or dietary fiber supplements may reduce symptoms in patients with SUDD, the quality of evidence is extremely low, due to substantial methodological limitations of the studies, the heterogeneity of the regimens employed, and the lack of specifically designed studies.

In addition to fibers, the therapeutic armamentarium in diverticular disease has been relying on antibiotics and, more recently, on the poorly absorbable antibiotic, rifaximin [8, 9], the locally delivered anti-inflammatory drug, mesalazine [10, 11], and probiotics [12, 13], alone or in combination. This chapter will focus specifically on poorly absorbed antibiotics in SUDD.

18.3 Rationale for Antibiotic Use in SUDD

The rationale for the use of antibiotics in diverticular disease is based on the conception that diverticula (pouches of the colonic wall) – in predisposed individuals – favor fecal entrapment, bacterial overgrowth, and potential breakdown of the epithelial lining, involved in bacterial translocation, mucosal inflammation, symptoms, and potential complications [14].

It is now well established that intestinal microecology plays a key role in determining symptoms in patients with diverticular disease [1, 3]. Small intestinal bacterial overgrowth (SIBO, defined as a bacterial concentration $\geq 10^3$ CFU/ml in small bowel aspirates [15]), which represents the most widely characterized form of dysbiosis, is frequently found in patients with diverticular disease [16, 17], and its role seems to be crucial in symptom development [18]. In addition to the absolute number of organisms, a *variety of microbiota play a critical role* in the manifestation of signs and symptoms of overgrowth [19]. For example, a predominance of bacteria that metabolize bile salts to unconjugated or insoluble compounds may lead to fat malabsorption or bile acid diarrhea. In contrast, microorganisms that preferentially metabolize carbohydrates to short-chain fatty acids and gas may cause bloating, but not diarrhea, since the metabolic products are usually absorbed. Gram-negative coliforms, such as the *Klebsiella* species, may produce toxins that damage the mucosa, interfering with the absorptive function and causing fluid secretion, thereby mimicking tropical sprue. As a consequence, some investigators have assumed the diagnosis of SIBO, provided that the bacterial species, isolated in the jejunal aspirate, are those that normally colonize the large bowel (e.g., *Enterobacteriaceae*, *Pseudomonas* spp., *Bacteroides* spp.) or that the same species are absent from saliva and gastric juice [20–22]. Indeed, small intestinal permeability (a hallmark of SIBO [23]) is increased in subjects whose small bowel is populated by colonic-type bacteria but not in those with salivary-type flora [24].

Bacteria activate the immune system through specific receptors known as Toll-like receptors (TLRs) [25]. Bacterial lipopeptides and lipopolysaccharides are recognized by TLR-2 and TLR-4, which are involved in the generation of innate and adaptive immunity [25]. As a matter of fact, Cianci et al. [26] showed that, compared to controls, TLR-2 and TLR-4 expression on immune cell subpopulations and on the colonic mucosa is altered in patients with SUDD. By studying the distribution of gut-homing lymphocytes in peripheral blood, the same investigators found that – compared to controls – both CD4+ and CD8+/CD103+ were significantly higher in patients, while no difference was evident between lymphocytes in the diverticular sigmoid mucosa [27].

Bacteria-induced immune activation can drive low-grade mucosal inflammation, which sensitizes both intrinsic primary efferent neurons and extrinsic primary afferent neurons, generating neural and smooth muscle dysfunction. These disturbances can in turn lead to symptom development and persistence [18] (Fig. 18.1). Indeed, bacterial metabolism is the major source of intestinal gas such as H_2, CO_2, and CH_4 via carbohydrate fermentation [28]. Excessive production of bowel gas can play a role in triggering abdominal symptoms such as bloating, pain, and discomfort [29]. Antimicrobial drugs have been shown to reduce colonic H_2 production [30, 31] and gas-related symptoms [32, 33], with significant symptom improvement correlating with reduction in H_2 breath excretion [34].

Antimicrobial therapy causes an increase in the mean stool weight in subjects on constant fiber intake, most likely because of a reduced fiber degradation consequent to the decline in bacterial population [35]. Both the reduction in gas production and the increase of fecal mass reduce the intraluminal pressure, thus improving symptoms and decreasing the enlargement and stretching of the diverticula as well as—potentially—the generation of new diverticula [36].

Although the involvement of the gut microbiota in the pathophysiology of diverticular disease has long been hypothesized, only recently has a clear evidence base become available. An early study found a shift in bacterial phyla abundance in SUDD, with a decrease in Bacteroidetes and an increase in Firmicutes [37]. Interestingly,

Fig. 18.1 Potential role of intestinal bacterial overgrowth in symptom development in patients with diverticular disease (derived from Colecchia et al. [18])

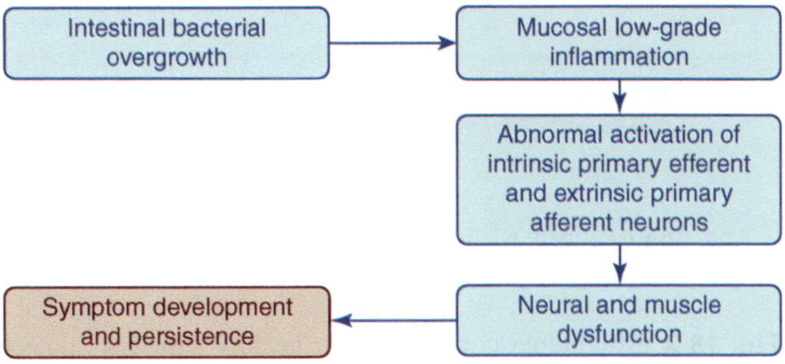

these changes are similar to those observed in patients with IBS [38]. In addition, in line with the potential role of microbial pathogens in diverticular disease complications, a study showed a global increase in all fecal phyla, as well as an increase in Proteobacteria in patients with acute diverticulitis [39].

A recent descriptive, cross-sectional pilot study has assessed the tissue low-grade inflammation, the microbiota and the metabolome in patients with diverticular disease [40]. The results showed that compared with controls, patients with diverticula (regardless of symptoms) had a >70% increase in colonic macrophages (Fig. 18.2). Their fecal microbiota were depleted of Clostridium cluster IV, a class comprising several groups with potential anti-inflammatory properties. In addition, compared to asymptomatic patients, patients with SUDD showed a depletion in Clostridium cluster IX, Fusobacterium, and Lactobacillaceae, all bacterial groups with potential anti-inflammatory properties or producers of short-chain fatty acids (Fig. 18.3). Interestingly, the depletion of microbiota members with anti-inflammatory activity

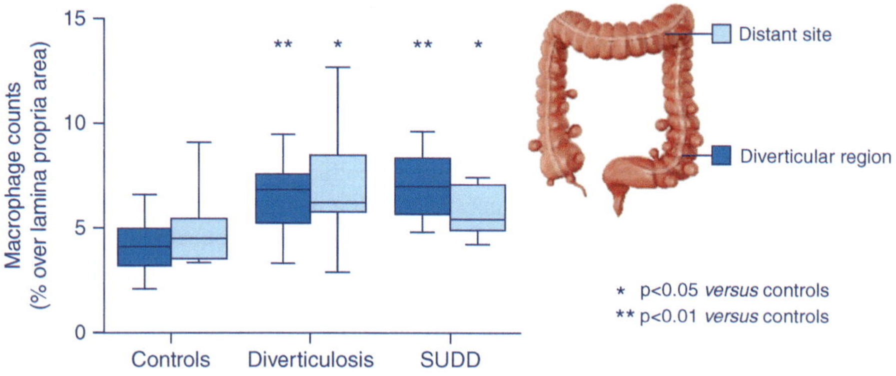

Fig. 18.2 Low-grade inflammation in diverticular disease (redrawn from Barbara et al. [40])

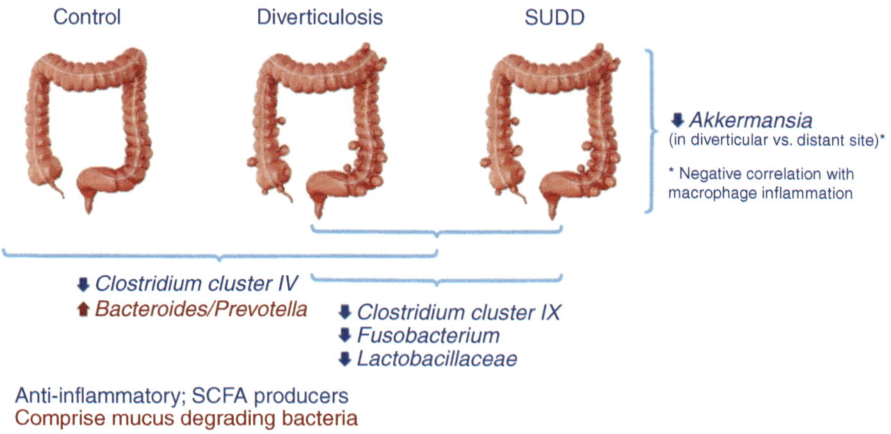

Fig. 18.3 Microbiota composition in healthy subjects, subjects with diverticulosis or patients with SUDD (drawn from data in Barbara et al. [40])

was associated with mucosal macrophage infiltration. This study also showed a decrease in the mucus-degrading bacteria Akkermansia in the colonic tract affected by the diverticula, compared with distant unaffected sites [40]. A report by Tursi and colleagues [41] assessed the fecal microbiota from 15 patients with SUDD, with asymptomatic diverticulosis, and 16 healthy controls. Their results showed that the overall bacterial abundance of dominant bacterial groups, including Bacteroides/Prevotella, *Clostridium coccoides*, *Bifidobacterium*, *Lactobacillus*, and *Escherichia coli*, was not different among the three groups. Interestingly, the amount of *Akkermansia muciniphila* species was significantly higher in patients bearing diverticula than in controls. Methodological and population differences exist between these two studies [40, 41], which may explain the differences in findings.

It is worth emphasizing that many of these studies have significant drawbacks and limitations, including reduced sample size, poorly defined inclusion criteria, disparate patient populations, and variable methodology, leading to often inconsistent (and sometimes conflicting) results [42]. As a consequence, the available studies evaluating both fecal and mucosa-associated microbiota in diverticular disease do not allow drawing *definite* conclusions on the precise alterations (if any) of intestinal microecology associated with the disease. However, the evidence to date does suggest that asymptomatic diverticulosis is not associated with significant changes in the gut microbiome, but significant changes do occur in the microbiota composition when diverticulosis evolves into SUDD or acute diverticulitis (in particular, depletion of taxa with purported anti-inflammatory activity) [3, 42]. These data are consistent with the idea that the microbiota could be involved in the progression of diverticulosis to SUDD and diverticulitis but not in the pathogenesis of diverticulosis per se.

In addition to cataloguing the microorganisms themselves, there is ongoing work evaluating the metabolome in diverticular disease. Six molecules (namely, 3-hydroxykynurenine, ethanolamine, 3-methylglutarate, 3-aminoisobutyrate, and the unassigned molecules X-5.43 and X-2.83) have been identified in urinary metabolite analysis, which are capable of distinguishing between patients with diverticular disease and healthy controls, with accuracy greater than 95%. These metabolites may be considered as biomarkers of the disease and could be useful diagnostic tools in the near future [40]. Another study [41], using nuclear magnetic resonance-based metabolomics data, showed significant discrimination between healthy controls and diverticulosis, as well as between diverticulosis and SUDD. Nonetheless, the profile of metabolites identified in the two studies [40, 41] was not the same; in the last investigation, two molecules (hippurate and methanol) differed between healthy controls and asymptomatic diverticulosis, whereas two others (3,5-dihydroxybenzoate and compound U16) showed a trend toward a significant difference [41]. Clearly, more research in a larger sample size of patients is needed to define specific metabolites to be considered as suitable biomarkers for the diagnosis of diverticular disease.

Taken together, the above results indicate the presence of dysbiosis in patients with diverticular disease and suggest an imbalance in favor of bacteria with proinflammatory and pathogenetic potential, particularly in patients with SUDD and at sites with the most abundant presence of diverticula. Although further large-scale studies, specifically aimed at identifying consistent microbiota and metabolome signatures with reliable diagnostic values, are needed, these findings represent a rationale for microbiota-directed therapies in the treatment of diverticular disease.

18.4 Antibiotics for SUDD: Which Ones?

Although it is clear that several non-antimicrobial drug classes are able to affect the gut microbiota [43, 44], with 24% of them displaying anticommensal activity at concentrations lower than those achieved in the small and large bowel [43], diet, prebiotics, probiotics, and antibiotics are the most widely used and effective nutritional and pharmacological means for modifying intestinal microecology [19].

It is well known that systemic antimicrobials have many detrimental effects on the gut microbiota [45]. Both molecular- and cultivation-based approaches have revealed ecological disturbances in the microbiota after antibiotic administration, in particular, for specific members of the bacterial community that are susceptible or alternatively resistant to the antibiotic in question. A consistently observed consequence of antibiotic treatment has been a temporary decrease in microbial diversity and a long-term persistence of antibiotic-resistant genes [46]. In addition, systemic drugs have all adverse events [47] and drug-to-drug interactions [47]. In this context, development of *poorly absorbed antibiotics* with a favorable impact on the gut microbiota has been a useful addition to our therapeutic armamentarium. These antimicrobial drugs are not systemically available, and this will minimize both antimicrobial resistance and adverse events. Indeed, they have been proved to be safe in all patient populations studied, including young children.

18.5 Are There Pathophysiological Features Other than the Gut Microbiota that Can Benefit from Poorly Absorbed Antibiotics?

Additional pathophysiological pathways involved in the symptom development of SUDD are visceral hypersensitivity [48], extended to the rectum [49], an abnormal neuromuscular function [50], and an altered anticipatory response to thermal pain [51]. All these features are, at least partially, mediated by the ongoing low-grade inflammation and upregulation of neuropeptides and are common in patients with IBS, whose symptoms overlap with those of SUDD [3, 52]. Indeed, a large proportion of patients with SUDD fulfill the Rome III criteria for IBS [53]. In addition to the demographic and clinical characteristics (SUDD patients are older, more frequently males, with severe, long-lasting, and localized, mainly in the left lower quadrant, abdominal pain) [3], fecal calprotectin may also help in differentiating these two clinical conditions. Indeed, despite the presence of low-grade intestinal inflammation (mostly driven by mast cells in IBS [54] and by macrophages in SUDD [40]) in both patient populations, this inflammatory marker was found to be increased in SUDD but not in IBS patients, with its concentration significantly

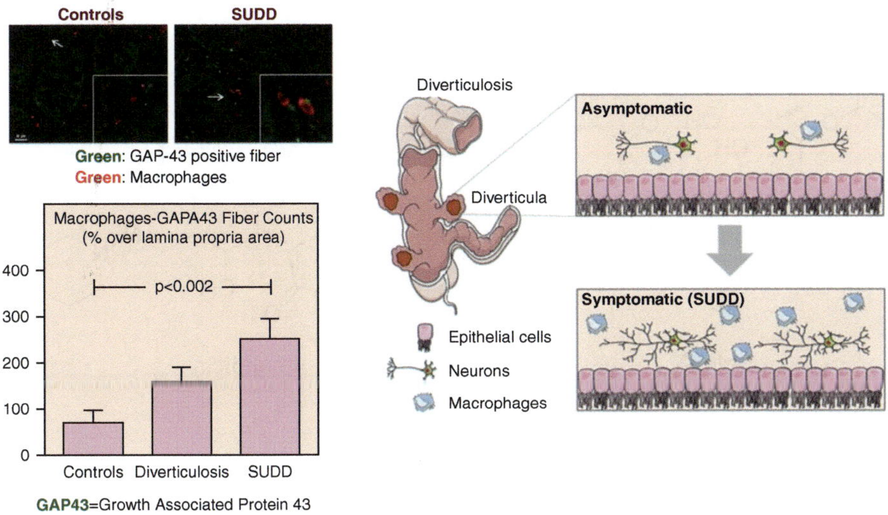

Fig. 18.4 Extensive Axonal Sprouting and Increased Macrophage Infiltration in Colonic Tissue of Patients with SUDD (redrawn from Barbaro et al. [56] and De Simone et al. [57])

correlated with the severity of abdominal pain [55]. Similarly, Barbara's laboratory [56] has recently shown that the colonic mucosa of patients with SUDD is characterized by nerve fiber outgrowth and that a higher number of macrophages are located in close proximity to these fibers (Fig. 18.4). These findings strongly suggest the role of inflammation in symptom generation [57].

Studies in animal models have also demonstrated a relationship between the presence of mucosal inflammation and altered sensory motor function [58]. In several instances, neuromuscular dysfunction was shown to persist after mucosal inflammation has subsided, likely maintained by locally produced mediators. It is therefore plausible that the low-grade mucosal inflammation, driven by bacteria-induced immune activation, could represent an additional target for rifamycins, the leading class of antibiotics employed in SUDD that are endowed with an intrinsic anti-inflammatory activity [59–61].

18.5.1 Rifaximin: Experimental and Clinical Pharmacology

Rifaximin (4-deoxy-4′-methylpyrido[1′,2′-1,2]imidazo[5,4-c]rifamycin SV) is a synthetic rifamycin derivative (Fig. 18.5) designed to achieve low gastrointestinal (GI) absorption while retaining good antibacterial activity [62]. Like all the members of the rifamycin family, it exerts its antibiotic effect through inhibition of bacterial ribonucleic acid (RNA) synthesis by binding to the β-subunit of bacterial deoxyribonucleic acid-dependent RNA polymerase [63]. Both experimental and clinical pharmacology show that this compound has a broad spectrum of antibacterial action covering Gram-positive and Gram-negative organisms, both aerobes and

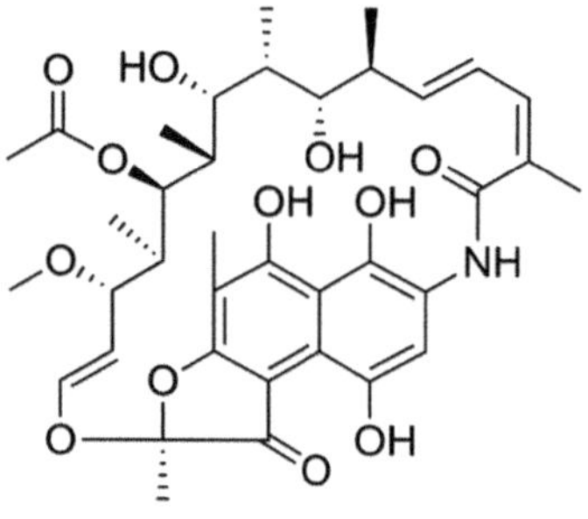

Rifamycin SV

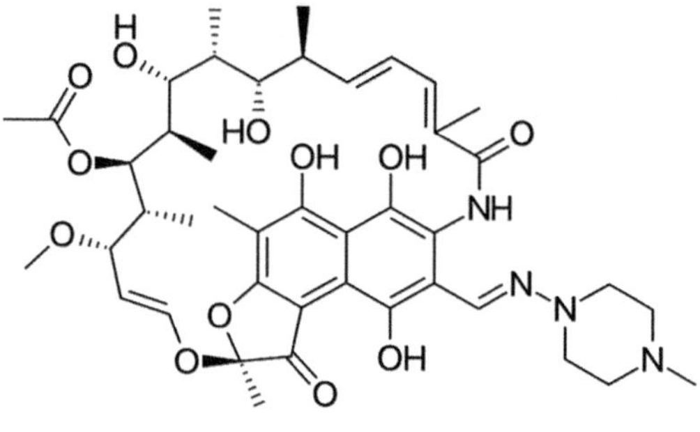

Rifampicin

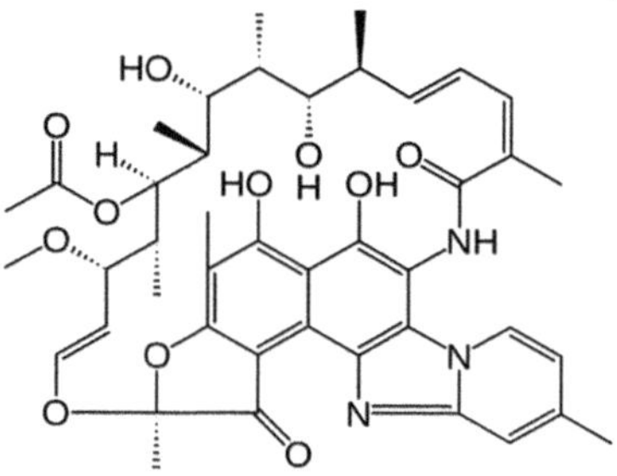

Rifaximin

Fig. 18.5 Chemical structure of rifaximin and its parent compounds, rifamycin SV and rifampicin

anaerobes [62]. Being virtually nonabsorbed, its bioavailability within the GI tract is rather high with intraluminal and fecal drug concentrations that largely exceed the minimum inhibitory concentration values observed in vitro against a wide range of pathogenic organisms [64]. Therefore, the GI tract represents the primary therapeutic target and GI infections were the original indication. The appreciation of the role of gut dysbiosis and SIBO in several organic and functional GI diseases [21] has increasingly broadened the clinical use of rifaximin, which is now extended to hepatic encephalopathy, small intestine bacterial overgrowth, inflammatory bowel disease, and colonic diverticular disease.

Amongst the antimicrobial treatments employed to eradicate SIBO [33], rifaximin seems to be the most suitable antibiotic, as it is highly effective and safe. A systematic review and meta-analysis [65] of 32 studies (involving 1331 patients) found an ITT overall eradication rate of 70.8% (95% CI 61.4–78.2; $I^2 = 89.4\%$). The overall rate of adverse events was only 4.6% (95% CI 2.3–7.5; $I^2 = 63.6\%$). In the subset of studies ($n = 10$) allowing the analysis, improvement or resolution of symptoms in patients with eradicated SIBO was found to be 67.7% (95% CI 44.7–86.9; $I^2 = 91.3\%$). Meta-regression identified three covariates (drug dose, study design, and co-therapy) independently associated with an increased eradication rate (Fig. 18.6).

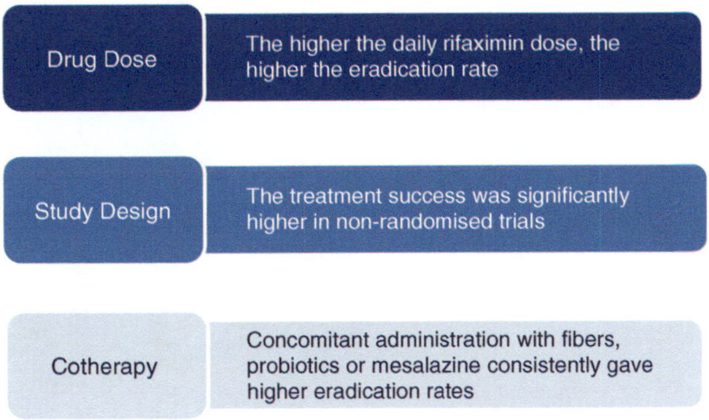

Fig. 18.6 Meta-analysis of rifaximin studies in SIBO eradication. Covariates independently associated with an increased eradication rate (drawn from thata in Gatta and Scarpignato [65])

Although rifaximin has antibiotic properties, it seems to have a minimal negative impact on the overall gut microbiota. In addition, the drug has shown *eubiotic* effects since it stimulates the growth of beneficial bacterial species, including Lactobacilli and Bifidobacteria [66, 67]. A recent investigation [68] in patients with intestinal inflammatory conditions (including diverticular disease) has found that the clinical improvement following rifaximin treatment was associated with an increase in the abundance of *Faecalibacterium prausnitizii*, an important butyrate-producing bacterium endowed with anti-inflammatory properties [69]. These results were independent of the underlying disease and were not accompanied by a significant alteration of the *overall* gut microbial ecology.

Rifaximin has also demonstrated anti-inflammatory properties [70]. In particular, it suppressed intestinal and systemic inflammation by preserving the epithelial function (and limiting bacterial translocation) and/or by a *direct* anti-inflammatory activity, as it is able to inhibit cytokine and chemokine synthesis from LPS-activated THP-1 monocytes and macrophages in vitro [61]. In intestinal epithelial cells, rifaximin caused a robust attenuation of the generation of inflammatory mediators caused by LPS (via abrogating its binding with NF-κB) and increased the generation of TGF-β. In addition, exposure of human colon biopsies from inflammatory bowel disease patients to rifaximin reduced mRNA levels of IL-8, Rantes (Regulated on Activation, Normal T-cell Expressed and Secreted), MIP-3α, and TNF induced by LPS [71]. Silencing the human nuclear pregnane-X receptor (PXR) decreased the anti-inflammatory activity of rifaximin, suggesting a mechanism involving this receptor. Indeed, the drug was found to be a gut-specific ligand for the PXR [72], a master gene, critical for maintenance of intestinal integrity.[73, 74]

A recent experimental study [75] has confirmed the anti-inflammatory activity of rifaximin in a model of diclofenac-induced intestinal inflammation, where the drug decreased myeloperoxidase (MPO) and cytokine tissue concentrations as well as the fecal excretion of calprotectin. In-depth investigations also showed that—in a human monocyte cell line (THP-1), a well-established model to study monocyte/macrophage functions—this antibiotic is able to modulate the activity of the inflammasome NLRP3 (nucleotide-binding oligomerization domain, leucine-rich repeat,

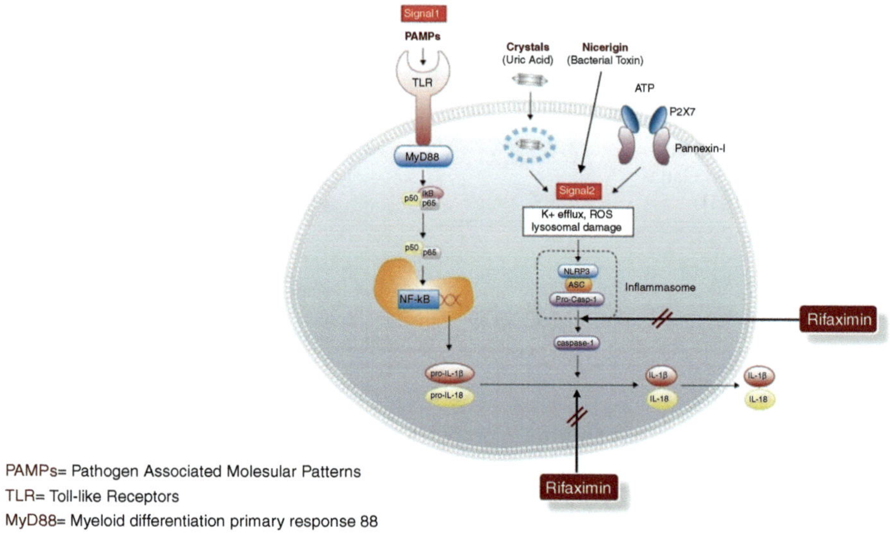

Fig. 18.7 Anti-inflammatory Activity of Rifaximin: Modulation of the Inflammasome Functions and Signaling Pathways (from Tursi et al. [70])

and pyrin domain-containing protein 3) by preventing the caspase-1-dependent activation and release of IL-1**β** [75]. This observation provides compelling evidence for an intrinsic anti-inflammatory activity of rifaximin (Fig. 18.7).

18.6 Rifamycin SV: MMX Formulation

The broad-spectrum, semisynthetic rifamycin SV was derived from rifamycin B and introduced into clinical practice as an intravenous regimen for the treatment of tuberculosis in 1962, replaced later on by rifampicin, an orally active compound [76].

An oral modified-release formulation of rifamycin SV (which is poorly absorbed), using the patented multimatrix (MMX) technology [77], has been recently developed to deliver high concentrations of the antibiotic into the colon, with a homogeneous distribution along all colonic segments, particularly the most distal one [78].

In the MMX formulation, rifamycin SV is dispersed in the lipophilic matrix that is surrounded by a hydrophilic matrix. The lipophilic matrix protects the active ingredient from dissolution in the intestinal aqueous fluids before it reaches the cecum. In addition, the gastro-resistant polymer film surrounding the core does not disintegrate at a pH lower than 7. The film gradually transforms into a viscous gel mass at the distal ileum and the rectosigmoid. Rifamycin SV then disaggregates and is released in proximity to the mucosa during its movement toward the rectum [77, 78].

While rifamycin SV shares the spectrum of antibacterial activity [76] and its anti-inflammatory activities [61, 79] with the other members of the family, the pharmacokinetics of the MMX formulation is different. Indeed, its poor bioavailability has been further reduced by the MMX technology. In healthy volunteers, the estimated mean absolute bioavailability of a single dose (two 200 mg tablets) of rifamycin SV-MMX was 0.04% under fasting conditions [80]. Quantifiable (>2.00 ng/mL) rifamycin SV plasma concentrations were reported infrequently and were randomly distributed following single and multiple (400 mg twice daily for 3 days) doses of rifamycin SV-MMX. Indeed, plasma concentrations never exceeded 10 ng/mL following multiple doses. Urinary excretion of rifamycin SV was negligible, whereas the total elimination of the unchanged rifamycin SV with feces represented 87% of the administered oral dose [80].

Rifamycin SV-MMX is currently approved in the USA and some European countries for the treatment of travelers' diarrhea caused by noninvasive strains of *Escherichia coli* in adults, but it is not recommended for use in patients with diarrhea complicated by fever and/or bloody stools or due to pathogens other than noninvasive strains of *E. coli* [78]. Rifamycin SV-MMX was well tolerated in this patient population, with the overall incidence of adverse effects overlapping that of placebo [78].

Since the MMX formulation releases rifamycin SV mainly into the distal colon, the region most commonly affected by diverticula, its use in SUDD may be worthwhile. While a preliminary study [81] showed some benefit in the treatment of acute uncomplicated diverticulitis, no data are available for rifamycin SV-MMX so far in patients with SUDD, in whom a randomized clinical trial is planned.

18.7 Rifaximin Efficacy in SUDD

Numerous trials with rifaximin in patients with SUDD have been reported in Italy and several European and South American countries since the first trial in 1992 [82]. Their results will be reviewed here.

18.7.1 Rifaximin in Combination with Dietary Fibers

In a double-blind, placebo-controlled, randomized clinical trial (RCT) [83], as well as in open studies (for review, see [8]) and their meta-analyses [9, 84], the combination of rifaximin and (soluble or insoluble) fibers was more effective in reducing symptoms in patients with SUDD than fibers alone (Fig. 18.8). As the number needed to treat (NNT) was found to be three [9], the treatment is clearly cost-effective.

The combination of rifaximin (administered for 7–10 days, every month) and soluble fibers such as konjac glucomannan (a plant extract capable of absorbing up to 200 times its weight in water [85]) was highly effective in treating SUDD, a finding confirmed in real-life studies from both gastroenterology and general practice [86–88]. In a real-life study [87], after 3 months of cyclic rifaximin, the severity of symptoms markedly decreased and as many as 75% of patients were free from abdominal pain. In a subgroup of patients, in whom the symptom pattern suggested

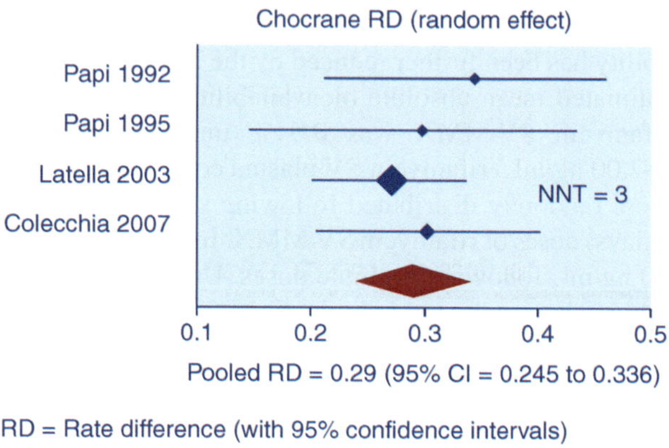

Fig. 18.8 Efficacy of rifaximin for symptom relief in SUDD: meta analysis of RCTs (from Bianchi et al. [47])

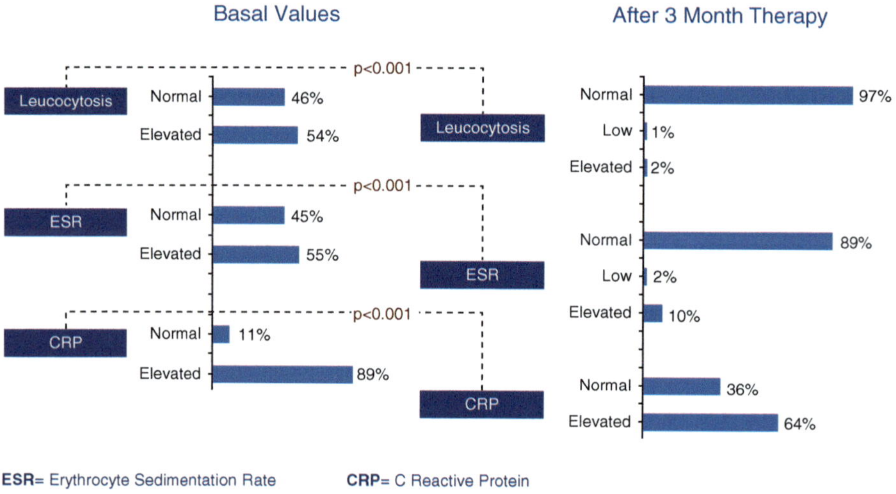

Fig. 18.9 Effect of cyclic rifaximin on inflammatory parameters in patients with SUDD: A Polish real-life study (from Moniuszko & Rydzewska [87])

the presence of diverticulitis, inflammatory indexes were measured and found to significantly decrease after treatment (Fig. 18.9).

Besides soluble fibers, diet supplementation with bran (at least 20 g daily) has also been tried. In both studies [16, 89], administration of rifaximin improved the benefits of dietary fiber, likely by preventing its bacterial degradation. However, like in IBS [90, 91], both the efficacy and tolerability of soluble fibers seem superior to those of insoluble fibers.

The durability of response has been demonstrated as well, including up to 8 years in one retrospective study [92]. However, the underlying pathophysiology of diverticulosis remains, and SUDD seems be a chronic relapsing disorder, similar to SIBO [93]. A cyclical (typically 7–10 days a month) treatment with rifaximin has been found effective. In patients who responded to the initial treatment, this therapy was able to maintain remission and prevent recurrences [94].

Both the GRIMAD (Italian Group for the Study of Diverticular Disease) consensus [95] and the SICCR (Italian Society of Colon and Rectal Surgery) [96] guidelines point out the benefit of *long-term cyclic administration* of rifaximin (in combination with soluble or insoluble fibers) in providing symptom relief for patients with SUDD, a recommendation shared by the Mexican [97], Danish [98], Polish [99], and Romanian [100] (but not German [101]) guidelines.

18.7.2 Rifaximin Alone

Although rifaximin has historically been administered in combination with dietary fiber supplements, one recent trial [102] has found that rifaximin *alone* (800 mg/day, 10 days a month) was more effective than dietary fibers in improving symptoms and quality of life in patients with SUDD.

18.7.3 Rifaximin in Combination with Prebiotics

In addition to fibers, the benefits of rifaximin–prebiotic treatment have also been recently reported in an investigation [103] evaluating the effectiveness of combined therapy with rifaximin and arabinogalactan–lactoferrin in symptom relief in patients with SUDD. After 6 months of combined treatment, there was a statistically significant reduction in the total severity score and improvement in each symptom score. Stool frequency normalized in all patients, regardless of the pretreatment bowel habits (diarrhea, constipation, or alternating bowel). As many as 31.7% had complete symptom resolution.

18.7.4 Rifaximin in Combination with Probiotics

Compared with antibiotic treatment, probiotics are less invasive and provide a more physiological approach to the treatment of microbial dysbiosis in patients with diverticular disease. Despite these potential benefits, the available evidence for the efficacy of probiotics in treating SUDD is limited [13]. Their use as *adjunct treatment* is however an attractive option. For instance, in a double-blind, placebo-controlled RCT [104], the combination of *Lactobacillus casei* DG and mesalazine (administered 10 days a month for 12 months) was able to maintain remission in almost 100% of patients with SUDD. However, administration of a probiotic (i.e., a *live* microorganism that, when administered in adequate amounts, confers a health benefit on the host [105]) together with an antibiotic could be counterproductive, unless bacteria are resistant to the antibiotic in question. This is the case of *Bifidobacterium longum* W11 [106], which displays a nontransmissible antibiotic resistance, due to a nucleotide polymorphism mutation in the rpoB gene, making it resistant to antibiotics of the rifamycin group, including rifaximin [107]. Administration of this probiotic with rifaximin to patients with SUDD resulted in better symptom improvement (particularly stool consistency) compared to that seen with the antibiotic alone [108]. The report was a retrospective one, with the intrinsic bias related to these types of studies. As a consequence, a well-designed, prospective trial is needed to confirm these preliminary results and to establish whether *B. longum* W11 can represent a useful adjuvant to rifaximin in the treatment of SUDD. Other single-strain or multistrain probiotics could be used *following* rifaximin treatment [109] to further improve the gut microbiota [110] and to prevent colonization with resistant bacteria [111], if any [112]. Although widely adopted in clinical practice, this biologically plausible and potentially useful approach has not yet been subjected to the scrutiny of a long-term clinical trial and should therefore not be considered as evidence-based.

18.7.5 Rifaximin in Combination with Mesalazine

Mesalazine is endowed with well-known anti-inflammatory activity [113] and also beneficial effects on the gut microbiota [114], which can synergize with those of rifaximin. In this connection, an open trial [115] explored the effectiveness of this combined treatment. All patients were administered 800 mg/day of rifaximin plus 2.4 g/day of mesalazine for 10 days, followed by 1.6 g/day of mesalazine for 8 weeks. At the end of the treatment, 78% of patients were completely asymptomatic.

18.7.6 Rifaximin for Primary Prevention of Acute Diverticulitis

Progression from SUDD to diverticulitis is uncommon because the disease course is often benign. In a prospective, long-term study [116], 97% of patients with SUDD had mild or no symptoms after a median follow-up of 66 months and only 2.5% of patients developed acute diverticulitis. Prevention (both primary and secondary) of acute diverticulitis is challenging. Although studies on medical therapies to reduce the occurrence and recurrence of diverticulitis are available, most of them are of poor quality and management is often empirical rather than evidence-based.

Two meta-analyses [9, 84] found that rifaximin in combination with fibers is more effective than fibers alone in preventing acute diverticulitis, a trend that is also observed in daily clinical practice [92]. However, the cost-effectiveness of rifaximin in this indication was quite low (NNT 59) [9].

18.7.7 Rifaximin for Secondary Prevention of Acute Diverticulitis

After an episode of acute diverticulitis, patients might present with recurrent or smoldering diverticulitis, stricture, and fistula and often develop chronic gastro-intestinal and non-gastrointestinal symptoms [117]. For example, one study found that, after a follow-up of 1 year, 40% of patients with CT-confirmed acute diverticulitis complained of mild-to-moderate abdominal pain and/or changes in bowel habits [118]. In a retrospective analysis of patients over an average follow-up period of 6.3 years, patients with acute diverticulitis had a 4.7-fold increased risk of being subsequently diagnosed with IBS [119]. The infection-associated gut dysbiosis and the resulting chronic low-grade mucosal inflammation might underlie this post-diverticulitis IBS (more appropriately termed as 'post-diverticulitis syndrome'), which has a pathophysiology similar to that of postinfection IBS [120]. The overall risk of acute diverticulitis recurrence is ~36% at 5 years [121]. Recurrence usually occurs <12 months after the initial episode, and the risk of complications is extremely low [122]. Several strategies have been applied to prevent recurrence of diverticulitis.

In a proof-of-concept study [123], the combination of cyclic rifaximin treatment and fiber supplements reduced the risk of diverticulitis recurrence in patients in remission (HR 2.64, 95% CI 1.08–6.46), a trend later confirmed in an observational study [124] (Table 18.1). Due to the intrinsic limitations of both studies, the current evidence favoring rifaximin use is low. An international, multicenter RCT [125] with a new rifaximin formulation (extended intestinal release) for secondary prevention of acute diverticulitis was initiated, but—due to the extremely slow recruitment rate—the study was suspended. However, an interim analysis is being conducted and the results are awaited.

A combination of mesalazine and rifaximin (both administered 7 days per month for 12 months) has also been tried in this clinical setting and seems to be more effective than rifaximin alone in the resolution of symptoms and prevention of diverticulitis (recurrence rate of 2.7 versus 13.0%, respectively, at the end of follow-up, Fig. 18.10) [126]. Furthermore, normalization of the inflammatory indices was

Table 18.1 Rifaximin for Secondary Prevention of Diverticulitis: Comparison of an Observational Study and a RCT (from data in Festa et al. [122] and Lanas et al. [121])

Studies	Year	N	Anticipated absolute effect		Difference (95% CIs)	HR (vs Mesalazine) or RR (vs Placebo)
			Without rifaximin	With rifaximin		
Festa et al.	2017	124	19%	5%	−14 (−14 to +3)	0.27
Lanas et al.	2013	167	19%	10%	−9 (−17 to −5)	0.54

Fig. 18.10 Prevention of recurrent diverticulitis: efficacy of rifaximin alone or rifaximin plus mesalazine (redrawn from Tursi et al. [124])

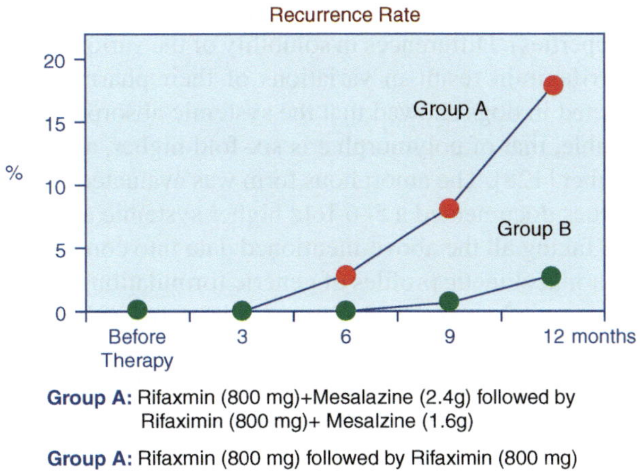

faster with the combined treatment. Although rifaximin use can be considered promising, the AGA guidelines do not consider the available evidence to be sufficient to recommend its use for the secondary prevention of diverticulitis [127].

18.7.8 Which Rifaximin?

All the studies in patients with SUDD have been performed using branded rifaximin formulations. The active ingredient contained in all rifaximin-based, brand name, medicinal products has been always characterized as a *crystalline* powder. Indeed, the European Pharmacopoeia, under the section **Characteristics**, specifically states "appearance: red-orange hygroscopic powder…". The same monograph states that rifaximin is endowed with crystalline polymorphism. Currently, five polymorphic forms of rifaximin, designated as **α**, **β**, **γ**, **δ**, and **ε**, have been identified. They are all rifaximin hydrates, characterized by different water content [128]. A noncrystalline form, designated as amorphous rifaximin, can also be generated through modifications of the synthetic and/or purification processes.

Amorphous or crystalline forms, despite containing the same active ingredient, may display extremely different chemical, physical, and mechanical properties (for instance, solubility and bioavailability, hygroscopicity, chemical stability, hardness, etc.), with remarkable impact on their respective utilization, manipulation, and absorption. In addition, possible interconversions among different polymorphs can seriously impact the maintenance of the prespecified characteristics of a given product (for instance, therapeutic efficacy in the case of drugs) [129, 130]. In particular, by virtue of variations of some parameters (such as, for instance, pressure and relative humidity), a metastable form can be converted into a more thermodynamically stable form or an anhydrous crystalline form can be converted into a hydrated crystalline form by adsorption of aqueous vapor from the environment. In some instances, the conversion of a crystalline form into another form can result in dramatic variations of the original properties [129, 130].

The different chemical–physical properties of polymorphs (stability, chemical reactivity, dissolution rate, and solubility) can considerably modify the bioavailability of every molecule (thus, affecting its pharmacokinetic and pharmacodynamic properties). Differences in solubility of the various crystalline and amorphous forms of rifaximin result in variations of their pharmacokinetics. Indeed, a study conducted in dogs showed that the systemic absorption of polymorphs **α** and **β** is negligible, that of polymorph **ε** is six-fold higher, and that of polymorph **γ** is 400-fold higher [128]. The amorphous form was evaluated in healthy volunteers, and its AUC values documented a 5–6-fold higher systemic absorption than rifaximin-**α** [131].

Taking all the above-mentioned data into consideration, it is conceivable that the pharmacokinetic profiles of generic formulations, which cannot contain rifaximin-**α** because of patent infringement, differ from those of the branded formulations. Indeed, patents covering the synthesis and pharmaceutical utilization of rifaximin polymorphs will expire in 2023. Generic formulations might thus contain the amorphous form, a different crystalline form, or a mixture of different polymorphs. In the latter setting, systemic absorption would be fully unpredictable. In a study

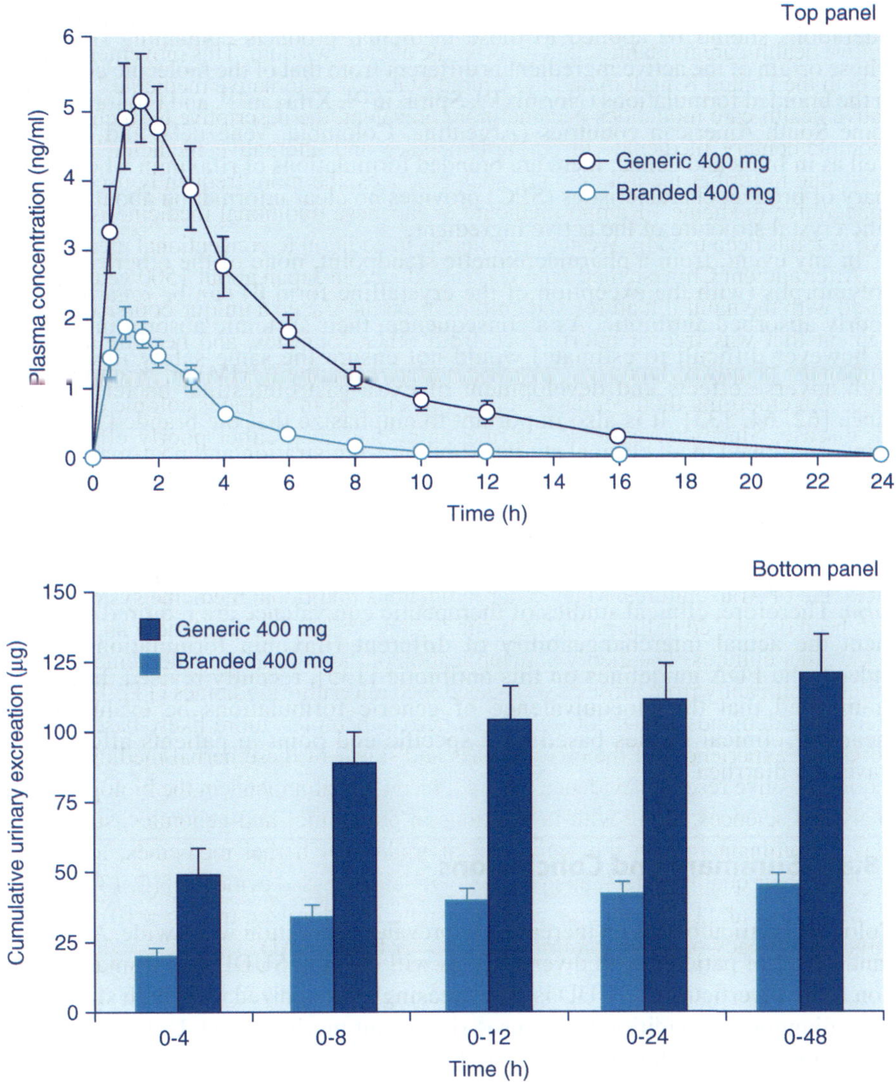

Fig. 18.11 Mean rifaximin plasma concentration-time (top panel) and cumulative urinary excretion (bottom panel) profiles followi ng administration of 400-mg single-dose generic or branded (polymorph-a) rifaximin to healthy volunteers. Each point or column represents the mean+SEM (vertical lines) obtained from 24 subjects (redrawn from Blandizzi et al. [130])

comparing a generic and the branded formulation [132], most pharmacokinetic parameters were significantly higher after administration of generic rifaximin than those after rifaximin-α. In particular, the differences for C_{max}, AUC, and cumulative urinary excretion between the generic formulation and the branded product ranged from 165% to 345% [132] (Fig. 18.11). As a consequence, generic rifaximin does not possess the features of a poorly absorbed antibiotic.

As the polymorph content is related to the manufacturing process, the same considerations should be applied to those medicinal products containing rifaximin, whose origin of the active ingredient is different from that of the molecule contained in the branded formulations (Normix™, Spiraxin™, Xifaxan™, and Flonorm™). In some South American countries (Argentina, Colombia, Venezuela, and Peru) as well as in India and China, there are branded formulations of rifaximin whose summary of product characteristics (SPC) provides no clear information about the specific crystal structure of the active ingredient.

In any event, from a pharmacokinetic standpoint, none of the other rifaximin polymorphs (with the exception of the crystalline form **β**) can be regarded as a poorly absorbed antibiotic. As a consequence, their systemic absorption (which is however difficult to estimate) would not ensure the same safety in terms of both adverse effects and development of extra-gastrointestinal bacterial resistance [62, 64, 133]. It is also important to emphasize that the branded formulations, employed in all clinical studies (both pre-registration and post-marketing), contained a crystalline active ingredient with dissolution and pharmacokinetic profiles overlapping those of polymorph-**α** known to be contained in the currently marketed formulation. For these reasons, *the results obtained with the crystalline form* **α** *cannot be extended to the other polymorphs or the amorphous form.* Therefore, clinical studies of therapeutic equivalence are required to document the actual interchangeability of different rifaximin formulations [134]. Indeed, the FDA guidelines on this antibiotic [135], recently revised, have recommended that the bioequivalence of generic formulations be evaluated by means of clinical studies based on a specific end point in patients affected by traveler's diarrhea.

18.8 Summary and Conclusions

Colonic diverticulosis is an increasingly prevalent condition worldwide. A significant subset of patients with diverticulosis will develop SUDD and a smaller portion acute diverticulitis. SUDD is an increasingly recognized (although still likely underdiagnosed) condition that causes significant morbidity [1]. Unfortunately, it is also undertreated, but we have been heartened by recent interest in pharmacological approaches targeting the gut microbiome with poorly absorbed antibiotics, mesalazine, and/or probiotics. Although there is a reasonable body of data supporting these approaches in SUDD, there remains much work to be done to more precisely define the agents, regimens, and patients most appropriate for this treatment. In particular, it should be established in which patients rifaximin is the most suitable approach and in which mesalazine could be preferable. Moreover, those patients, who can benefit most from the combined approach, should be identified in well-designed RCTs.

References

1. Tursi A, Scarpignato C, Strate LL, Lanas A, Kruis W, Lahat A, et al. Colonic diverticular disease. Nat Rev Dis Primers. 2020;6(1):20. https://doi.org/10.1038/s41572-020-0153-5.
2. Crowe FL, Appleby PN, Allen NE, Key TJ. Diet and risk of diverticular disease in Oxford cohort of European Prospective Investigation into Cancer and Nutrition (EPIC): prospective study of British vegetarians and non-vegetarians. BMJ. 2011;343(jul19 4):d4131. https://doi.org/10.1136/bmj.d4131.
3. Scarpignato C, Barbara G, Lanas A, Strate LL. Management of colonic diverticular disease in the third millennium: highlights from a symposium held during the united European gastroenterology week 2017. Ther Adv Gastroenterol. 2018;11:1756284818771305. https://doi.org/10.1177/1756284818771305.
4. Strate LL, Modi R, Cohen E, Spiegel BM. Diverticular disease as a chronic illness: evolving epidemiologic and clinical insights. Am J Gastroenterol. 2012;107(10):1486–93. https://doi.org/10.1038/ajg.2012.194.
5. Comparato G, Fanigliulo L, Aragona G, Cavestro GM, Cavallaro LG, Leandro G, et al. Quality of life in uncomplicated symptomatic diverticular disease: is it another good reason for treatment? Dig Dis. 2007;25(3):252–9. https://doi.org/10.1159/000103896.
6. Spiller RC, Humes DJ, Campbell E, Hastings M, Neal KR, Dukes GE, et al. The patient health questionnaire 12 somatic symptom scale as a predictor of symptom severity and consulting behaviour in patients with irritable bowel syndrome and symptomatic diverticular disease. Aliment Pharmacol Ther. 2010;32(6):811–20. https://doi.org/10.1111/j.1365-2036.2010.04402.x.
7. Carabotti M, Annibale B, Severi C, Lahner E. Role of fiber in symptomatic uncomplicated diverticular disease: a systematic review. Nutrients. 2017;9(2):161. https://doi.org/10.3390/nu9020161.
8. Latella G, Scarpignato C. Rifaximin in the management of colonic diverticular disease. Expert Rev Gastroenterol Hepatol. 2009;3(6):585–98. https://doi.org/10.1586/egh.09.63.
9. Bianchi M, Festa V, Moretti A, Ciaco A, Mangone M, Tornatore V, et al. Meta-analysis: long-term therapy with rifaximin in the management of uncomplicated diverticular disease. Aliment Pharmacol Ther. 2011;33(8):902–10. https://doi.org/10.1111/j.1365-2036.2011.04606.x.
10. Picchio M, Elisei W, Tursi A. Mesalazine to treat symptomatic uncomplicated diverticular disease and to prevent acute diverticulitis occurrence. A systematic review with meta-analysis of randomized, placebo-controlled trials. J Gastrointestin Liver Dis. 2018;27(3):291–7. https://doi.org/10.15403/jgld.2014.1121.273.pic.
11. Picchio M, Elisei W, Brandimarte G, Di Mario F, Malfertheiner P, Scarpignato C, et al. Mesalazine for the treatment of symptomatic uncomplicated diverticular disease of the colon and for primary prevention of diverticulitis: a systematic review of randomized clinical trials. J Clin Gastroenterol. 2016;50(Suppl 1):S64–9. https://doi.org/10.1097/MCG.0000000000000669.
12. Lahner E, Bellisario C, Hassan C, Zullo A, Esposito G, Annibale B. Probiotics in the treatment of diverticular disease. A systematic review. J Gastrointestin Liver Dis. 2016;25(1):79–86. https://doi.org/10.15403/jgld.2014.1121.251.srw.
13. Scarpignato C, Bertelé A, Tursi A. Probiotics for the treatment of symptomatic uncomplicated diverticular disease: rationale and current evidence. J Clin Gastroenterol. 2016;50(Suppl 1):S70–3. https://doi.org/10.1097/MCG.0000000000000641.
14. Humes DJ, Spiller RC. Review article: the pathogenesis and management of acute colonic diverticulitis. Aliment Pharmacol Ther. 2014;39(4):359–70. https://doi.org/10.1111/apt.12596.
15. Quigley EMM, Murray JA, Pimentel M. AGA clinical practice update on small intestinal bacterial overgrowth: expert review. Gastroenterology. 2020;159(4):1526–32. https://doi.org/10.1053/j.gastro.2020.06.090.

16. D'Inca R, Pomerri F, Vettorato MG, Dal Pont E, Di Leo V, Ferronato A, et al. Interaction between rifaximin and dietary fibre in patients with diverticular disease. Aliment Pharmacol Ther. 2007;25(7):771–9. https://doi.org/10.1111/j.1365-2036.2007.03266.x.
17. Tursi A, Brandimarte G, Giorgetti GM, Elisei W. Assessment of small intestinal bacterial overgrowth in uncomplicated acute diverticulitis of the colon. World J Gastroenterol. 2005;11(18):2773–6. https://doi.org/10.3748/wjg.v11.i18.2773.
18. Colecchia A, Sandri L, Capodicasa S, Vestito A, Mazzella G, Staniscia T, et al. Diverticular disease of the colon: new perspectives in symptom development and treatment. World J Gastroenterol. 2003;9(7):1385–9.
19. Simrén M, Barbara G, Flint HJ, Spiegel BM, Spiller RC, Vanner S, et al. Intestinal microbiota in functional bowel disorders: a Rome foundation report. Gut. 2013;62(1):159–76. https://doi.org/10.1136/gutjnl-2012-302167.
20. Quigley EM, Abu-Shanab A. Small intestinal bacterial overgrowth. Infect Dis Clin N Am. 2010;24(4):943–59. https://doi.org/10.1016/j.idc.2010.07.007.
21. Scarpignato C, Gatta L. Commentary: towards an effective and safe treatment of small intestine bacterial overgrowth. Aliment Pharmacol Ther. 2013;38(11–12):1409–10. https://doi.org/10.1111/apt.12531.
22. Adike A, DiBaise JK. Small intestinal bacterial overgrowth: nutritional implications, diagnosis, and management. Gastroenterol Clin N Am. 2018;47(1):193–208. https://doi.org/10.1016/j.gtc.2017.09.008.
23. Lauritano EC, Valenza V, Sparano L, Scarpellini E, Gabrielli M, Cazzato A, et al. Small intestinal bacterial overgrowth and intestinal permeability. Scand J Gastroenterol. 2010;45(9):1131–2. https://doi.org/10.3109/00365521.2010.485325.
24. Riordan SM, McIver CJ, Thomas DH, Duncombe VM, Bolin TD, Thomas MC. Luminal bacteria and small-intestinal permeability. Scand J Gastroenterol. 1997;32(6):556–63. https://doi.org/10.3109/00365529709025099.
25. Abreu MT. Toll-like receptor signalling in the intestinal epithelium: how bacterial recognition shapes intestinal function. Nat Rev Immunol. 2010;10(2):131–44. https://doi.org/10.1038/nri2707.
26. Cianci R, Frosali S, Pagliari D, Cesaro P, Petruzziello L, Casciano F, et al. Uncomplicated diverticular disease: innate and adaptive immunity in human gut mucosa before and after rifaximin. J Immunol Res. 2014;2014:696812. https://doi.org/10.1155/2014/696812.
27. Cianci R, Iacopini F, Petruzziello L, Cammarota G, Pandolfi F, Costamagna G. Involvement of central immunity in uncomplicated diverticular disease. Scand J Gastroenterol. 2009;44(1):108–15. https://doi.org/10.1080/00365520802321204.
28. Levitt MD, Bond JH Jr. Volume, composition, and source of intestinal gas. Gastroenterology. 1970;59(6):921–9.
29. Azpiroz F. Intestinal gas. In: Feldman M, Friedman LS, Brandt LJ, editors. Sleisenger and Fordtran's gastrointestinal and liver disease. 11th ed. Philadelphia, PA: Saunders; 2020. p. 244–51.
30. Bjørneklett A, Midtvedt T. Influence of three antimicrobial agents--penicillin, metronidazole, and doxycyclin--on the intestinal microflora of healthy humans. Scand J Gastroenterol. 1981;16(4):473–80. https://doi.org/10.3109/00365528109182001.
31. Rao SS, Edwards CA, Austen CJ, Bruce C, Read NW. Impaired colonic fermentation of carbohydrate after ampicillin. Gastroenterology. 1988;94(4):928–32. https://doi.org/10.1016/0016-5085(88)90549-5.
32. Di Stefano M, Strocchi A, Malservisi S, Veneto G, Ferrieri A, Corazza GR. Non-absorbable antibiotics for managing intestinal gas production and gas-related symptoms. Aliment Pharmacol Ther. 2000;14(8):1001–8. https://doi.org/10.1046/j.1365-2036.2000.00808.x.
33. Corazza GR, Di Stefano M, Scarpignato C. Treatment of functional bowel disorders: is there room for antibiotics? Digestion. 2006;73(Suppl 1):38–46. https://doi.org/10.1159/000089778.
34. Sharara AI, Aoun E, Abdul-Baki H, Mounzer R, Sidani S, Elhajj I. A randomized double-blind placebo-controlled trial of rifaximin in patients with abdominal bloating and flatulence. Am J Gastroenterol. 2006;101(2):326–33. https://doi.org/10.1111/j.1572-0241.2006.00458.x.

35. Kurpad AV, Shetty PS. Effects of antimicrobial therapy on faecal bulking. Gut. 1986;27(1): 55–8. https://doi.org/10.1136/gut.27.1.55.
36. Stollman NH, Raskin JB. Diagnosis and management of diverticular disease of the colon in adults. Ad hoc practice parameters Committee of the American College of Gastroenterology. Am J Gastroenterol. 1999;94(11):3110–21. https://doi.org/10.1111/j.1572-0241.1999.01501.x.
37. Lopetuso LR, Petito V, Graziani C, Schiavoni E, Paroni Sterbini F, Poscia A, et al. Gut microbiota in health, diverticular disease, irritable bowel syndrome, and inflammatory bowel diseases: time for microbial marker of gastrointestinal disorders. Dig Dis. 2018;36(1):56–65. https://doi.org/10.1159/000477205.
38. Rajilic-Stojanovic M, Biagi E, Heilig HG, Kajander K, Kekkonen RA, Tims S, et al. Global and deep molecular analysis of microbiota signatures in fecal samples from patients with irritable bowel syndrome. Gastroenterology. 2011;141(5):1792–801. https://doi.org/10.1053/j.gastro.2011.07.043.
39. Daniels L, Budding AE, de Korte N, Eck A, Bogaards JA, Stockmann HB, et al. Fecal microbiome analysis as a diagnostic test for diverticulitis. Eur J Clin Microbiol Infect Dis. 2014;33(11):1927–36. https://doi.org/10.1007/s10096-014-2162-3.
40. Barbara G, Scaioli E, Barbaro MR, Biagi E, Laghi L, Cremon C, et al. Gut microbiota, metabolome and immune signatures in patients with uncomplicated diverticular disease. Gut. 2017;66(7):1252–61. https://doi.org/10.1136/gutjnl-2016-312377.
41. Tursi A, Mastromarino P, Capobianco D, Elisei W, Miccheli A, Capuani G, et al. Assessment of fecal microbiota and fecal metabolome in symptomatic uncomplicated diverticular disease of the colon. J Clin Gastroenterol. 2016;50(Suppl 1):S9–S12. https://doi.org/10.1097/MCG.0000000000000626.
42. Ticinesi A, Nouvenne A, Corrente V, Tana C, Di Mario F, Meschi T. Diverticular disease: a gut microbiota perspective. J Gastrointestin Liver Dis. 2019;28(3):327–37. https://doi.org/10.15403/jgld-277.
43. Maier L, Pruteanu M, Kuhn M, Zeller G, Telzerow A, Anderson EE, et al. Extensive impact of non-antibiotic drugs on human gut bacteria. Nature. 2018;555(7698):623–8. https://doi.org/10.1038/nature25979.
44. Zhernakova A, Kurilshikov A, Bonder MJ, Tigchelaar EF, Schirmer M, Vatanen T, et al. Population-based metagenomics analysis reveals markers for gut microbiome composition and diversity. Science. 2016;352(6285):565–9. https://doi.org/10.1126/science.aad3369.
45. Sullivan A, Edlund C, Nord CE. Effect of antimicrobial agents on the ecological balance of human microflora. Lancet Infect Dis. 2001;1(2):101–14. https://doi.org/10.1016/S1473-3099(01)00066-4.
46. Jernberg C, Lofmark S, Edlund C, Jansson JK. Long-term impacts of antibiotic exposure on the human intestinal microbiota. Microbiology. 2010;156(Pt 11):3216–23. https://doi.org/10.1099/mic.0.040618-0.
47. Richardson WL, Hammert WC. Adverse effects of common oral antibiotics. J Hand Surg Am. 2014;39(5):989–91. https://doi.org/10.1016/j.jhsa.2014.01.021.
48. Humes DJ, Simpson J, Smith J, Sutton P, Zaitoun A, Bush D, et al. Visceral hypersensitivity in symptomatic diverticular disease and the role of neuropeptides and low grade inflammation. Neurogastroenterol Motil. 2012;24(4):318–e163. https://doi.org/10.1111/j.1365-2982.2011.01863.x.
49. Clemens CH, Samsom M, Roelofs J, van Berge Henegouwen GP, Smout AJ. Colorectal visceral perception in diverticular disease. Gut. 2004;53(5):717–22. https://doi.org/10.1136/gut.2003.018093.
50. Bassotti G, Villanacci V. Colonic diverticular disease: abnormalities of neuromuscular function. Dig Dis. 2012;30(1):24–8. https://doi.org/10.1159/000335702.
51. Smith JK, Marciani L, Humes DJ, Francis ST, Gowland P, Spiller RC. Anticipation of thermal pain in diverticular disease. Neurogastroenterol Motil. 2016;28(6):900–13. https://doi.org/10.1111/nmo.12790.

52. Spiller R. Is it diverticular disease or is it irritable bowel syndrome? Dig Dis. 2012;30(1):64–9. https://doi.org/10.1159/000335721.
53. Annibale B, Lahner E, Maconi G, Usai P, Marchi S, Bassotti G, et al. Clinical features of symptomatic uncomplicated diverticular disease: a multicenter Italian survey. Int J Color Dis. 2012;27(9):1151–9. https://doi.org/10.1007/s00384-012-1488-5.
54. Barbara G, Stanghellini V, De Giorgio R, Cremon C, Cottrell GS, Santini D, et al. Activated mast cells in proximity to colonic nerves correlate with abdominal pain in irritable bowel syndrome. Gastroenterology. 2004;126(3):693–702. https://doi.org/10.1053/j.gastro.2003.11.055.
55. Tursi A, Elisei W, Picchio M, Giorgetti GM, Brandimarte G. Moderate to severe and prolonged left lower-abdominal pain is the best symptom characterizing symptomatic uncomplicated diverticular disease of the colon: a comparison with fecal calprotectin in clinical setting. J Clin Gastroenterol. 2015;49(3):218–21. https://doi.org/10.1097/mcg.0000000000000094.
56. Barbaro MR, Cremon C, Fuschi D, Scaioli E, Veneziano A, Marasco G, et al. Nerve fiber overgrowth in patients with symptomatic diverticular disease. Neurogastroenterol Motil. 2019;31(9):e13575. https://doi.org/10.1111/nmo.13575.
57. De Simone V, van Baarle L, Matteoli G. Neurite outgrowth in symptomatic uncomplicated diverticular disease. Neurogastroenterol Motil. 2019;31(9):e13680. https://doi.org/10.1111/nmo.13680.
58. Collins SM. The immunomodulation of enteric neuromuscular function: implications for motility and inflammatory disorders. Gastroenterology. 1996;111(6):1683–99. https://doi.org/10.1016/s0016-5085(96)70034-3.
59. Spisani S, Traniello S, Martuccio C, Rizzuti O, Cellai L. Rifamycins inhibit human neutrophil functions: new derivatives with potential antiinflammatory activity. Inflammation. 1997;21(4):391–400. https://doi.org/10.1023/a:1027314419843.
60. Caruso I. Twenty years of experience with intra-articular rifamycin for chronic arthritides. J Int Med Res. 1997;25(6):307–17. https://doi.org/10.1177/030006059702500601.
61. Rosette C, Buendia-Laysa F Jr, Patkar S, Moro L, Celasco G, Bozzella R, et al. Anti-inflammatory and immunomodulatory activities of rifamycin SV. Int J Antimicrob Agents. 2013;42(2):182–6. https://doi.org/10.1016/j.ijantimicag.2013.04.020.
62. Scarpignato C, Pelosini I. Rifaximin, a poorly absorbed antibiotic: pharmacology and clinical potential. Chemotherapy. 2005;51(Suppl 1):36–66. https://doi.org/10.1159/000081990.
63. Ojetti V, Lauritano EC, Barbaro F, Migneco A, Ainora ME, Fontana L, et al. Rifaximin pharmacology and clinical implications. Expert Opin Drug Metab Toxicol. 2009;5(6):675–82. https://doi.org/10.1517/17425250902973695.
64. Scarpignato C, Pelosini I. Experimental and clinical pharmacology of rifaximin, a gastrointestinal selective antibiotic. Digestion. 2006;73(Suppl 1):13–27. https://doi.org/10.1159/000089776.
65. Gatta L, Scarpignato C. Systematic review with meta-analysis: rifaximin is effective and safe for the treatment of small intestine bacterial overgrowth. Aliment Pharmacol Ther. 2017;45(5):604–16. https://doi.org/10.1111/apt.13928.
66. Soldi S, Vasileiadis S, Uggeri F, Campanale M, Morelli L, Fogli MV, et al. Modulation of the gut microbiota composition by rifaximin in non-constipated irritable bowel syndrome patients: a molecular approach. Clin Exp Gastroenterol. 2015;8:309–25. https://doi.org/10.2147/CEG.S89999.
67. Ponziani FR, Scaldaferri F, Petito V, Paroni Sterbini F, Pecere S, Lopetuso LR, et al. The role of antibiotics in gut microbiota modulation: the Eubiotic effects of Rifaximin. Dig Dis. 2016;34(3):269–78. https://doi.org/10.1159/000443361.
68. Ponziani FR, Scaldaferri F, De Siena M, Mangiola F, Matteo MV, Pecere S, et al. Increased *Faecalibacterium* abundance is associated with clinical improvement in patients receiving rifaximin treatment. Benef Microbes. 2020;11(6):519–25. https://doi.org/10.3920/bm2019.0171.
69. Ferreira-Halder CV, Faria AVS, Andrade SS. Action and function of *Faecalibacterium prausnitzii* in health and disease. Best Pract Res Clin Gastroenterol. 2017;31(6):643–8. https://doi.org/10.1016/j.bpg.2017.09.011.

70. Tursi A, Scarpignato C, Brandimarte G, Di Mario F, Lanas A. Rifaximin for the management of colonic diverticular disease: far beyond a simple antibiotic. J Gastrointestin Liver Dis. 2018;27(4):351–5. https://doi.org/10.15403/jgld.2014.1121.274.rif.
71. Mencarelli A, Renga B, Palladino G, Claudio D, Ricci P, Distrutti E, et al. Inhibition of NF-κB by a PXR-dependent pathway mediates counter-regulatory activities of rifaximin on innate immunity in intestinal epithelial cells. Eur J Pharmacol. 2011;668(1–2):317–24. https://doi.org/10.1016/j.ejphar.2011.06.058.
72. Ma X, Shah YM, Guo GL, Wang T, Krausz KW, Idle JR, et al. Rifaximin is a gut-specific human pregnane X receptor activator. J Pharmacol Exp Ther. 2007;322(1):391–8. https://doi.org/10.1124/jpet.107.121913.
73. Mencarelli A, Migliorati M, Barbanti M, Cipriani S, Palladino G, Distrutti E, et al. Pregnane-X-receptor mediates the anti-inflammatory activities of rifaximin on detoxification pathways in intestinal epithelial cells. Biochem Pharmacol. 2010;80(11):1700–7. https://doi.org/10.1016/j.bcp.2010.08.022.
74. Cheng J, Shah YM, Ma X, Pang X, Tanaka T, Kodama T, et al. Therapeutic role of rifaximin in inflammatory bowel disease: clinical implication of human pregnane X receptor activation. J Pharmacol Exp Ther. 2010;335(1):32–41. https://doi.org/10.1124/jpet.110.170225.
75. Colucci R, Pellegrini C, Fornai M, Tirotta E, Antonioli L, Renzulli C, et al. Pathophysiology of NSAID-associated intestinal lesions in the rat: luminal bacteria and mucosal inflammation as targets for prevention. Front Pharmacol. 2018;9:1340. https://doi.org/10.3389/fphar.2018.01340.
76. Riva S, Silvestri LG. Rifamycins: a general view. Annu Rev Microbiol. 1972;26:199–224. https://doi.org/10.1146/annurev.mi.26.100172.001215.
77. Nardelli S, Pisani LF, Tontini GE, Vecchi M, Pastorelli L. MMX™ technology and its applications in gastrointestinal diseases. Ther Adv Gastroenterol. 2017;10(7):545–52. https://doi.org/10.1177/1756283x17709974.
78. Hoy SM, Rifamycin SV MMX™: a review in the treatment of Traveller's diarrhoea. Clin Drug Investig. 2019;39(7):691–7. https://doi.org/10.1007/s40261-019-00808-2.
79. Rosette C, Agan FJ, Rosette N, Moro L, Mazzetti A, Hassan C, et al. Rifamycin SV exhibits strong anti-inflammatory in vitro activity through pregnane X receptor stimulation and NFκB inhibition. Drug Metab Pharmacokinet. 2019;34(3):172–80. https://doi.org/10.1016/j.dmpk.2019.01.002.
80. Di Stefano AF, Rusca A, Loprete L, Dröge MJ, Moro L, Assandri A. Systemic absorption of rifamycin SV MMX administered as modified-release tablets in healthy volunteers. Antimicrob Agents Chemother. 2011;55(5):2122–8. https://doi.org/10.1128/aac.01504-10.
81. Kruis W, Poškus T, Böhm G, Bunganic I, Rácz I, Fratila O, et al. Rifamycin vs placebo for the treatment of acute uncomplicated diverticulitis: a randomised, double-blind study. GastroHep. 2020;2:295–308. https://doi.org/10.1002/ygh2.426.
82. Papi C, Ciaco A, Koch M, Capurso L. Efficacy of rifaximin on symptoms of uncomplicated diverticular disease of the colon. A pilot multicentre open trial. Diverticular disease study group. Ital J Gastroenterol. 1992;24(8):452–6.
83. Papi C, Ciaco A, Koch M, Capurso L. Efficacy of rifaximin in the treatment of symptomatic diverticular disease of the colon. A multicentre double-blind placebo-controlled trial. Aliment Pharmacol Ther. 1995;9(1):33–9. https://doi.org/10.1111/j.1365-2036.1995.tb00348.x.
84. Kasturi KS, Mummadi RR, Jaganmohan S. Cyclical Rifaximin for symptomatic, uncomplicated diverticular disease: a meta-analysis. Gastroenterology. 2008;134(Suppl 1):A-399.
85. Behera SS, Ray RC. Konjac glucomannan, a promising polysaccharide of *Amorphophallus konjac* K. Koch in health care. Int J Biol Macromol. 2016;92:942–56. https://doi.org/10.1016/j.ijbiomac.2016.07.098.
86. Stallinger S, Eller N, Hogenauer C. Non-interventional study evaluating efficacy and tolerability of rifaximin for treatment of uncomplicated diverticular disease. Wien Klin Wochenschr. 2014;126(1–2):9–14. https://doi.org/10.1007/s00508-013-0447-7.

87. Moniuszko A, Rydzewska G. The effect of cyclic rifaximin therapy on symptoms of diverticular disease from the perspective of the gastroenterology outpatient clinic: a "real-life" study. Prz Gastroenterol. 2017;12(2):145–51. https://doi.org/10.5114/pg.2017.68167.
88. De Bastiani R, Sanna G, Bertolusso L, Casella G, De Polo M, Zamparella M, et al. General practitioners' management of symptomatic uncomplicated diverticular disease of the colon by using rifaximin, a non-adsorbable antibiotic. Eur Rev Med Pharmacol Sci. 2021;25(1):423–30. https://doi.org/10.26355/eurrev_202101_24410.
89. Colecchia A, Vestito A, Pasqui F, Mazzella G, Roda E, Pistoia F, et al. Efficacy of long term cyclic administration of the poorly absorbed antibiotic rifaximin in symptomatic, uncomplicated colonic diverticular disease. World J Gastroenterol. 2007;13(2):264–9. https://doi.org/10.3748/wjg.v13.i2.264.
90. Bijkerk CJ, Muris JW, Knottnerus JA, Hoes AW, de Wit NJ. Systematic review: the role of different types of fibre in the treatment of irritable bowel syndrome. Aliment Pharmacol Ther. 2004;19(3):245–51. https://doi.org/10.1111/j.0269-2813.2004.01862.x.
91. Nagarajan N, Morden A, Bischof D, King EA, Kosztowski M, Wick EC, et al. The role of fiber supplementation in the treatment of irritable bowel syndrome: a systematic review and meta-analysis. Eur J Gastroenterol Hepatol. 2015;27(9):1002–10. https://doi.org/10.1097/meg.0000000000000425.
92. Di Mario F, Miraglia C, Cambie G, Violi A, Nouvenne A, Franceschi M, et al. Long-term efficacy of rifaximin to manage the symptomatic uncomplicated diverticular disease of the colon. J Investig Med. 2019;67(4):767–70. https://doi.org/10.1136/jim-2018-000901.
93. Lauritano EC, Gabrielli M, Scarpellini E, Lupascu A, Novi M, Sottili S, et al. Small intestinal bacterial overgrowth recurrence after antibiotic therapy. Am J Gastroenterol. 2008;103(8):2031–5. https://doi.org/10.1111/j.1572-0241.2008.02030.x.
94. Pietrzak AM, Dziki A, Banasiewicz T, Reguła J. Cyclic rifaximin therapy effectively prevents the recurrence of symptoms after exacerbation of symptomatic uncomplicated diverticular disease: a retrospective study. Prz Gastroenterol. 2019;14(1):69–78. https://doi.org/10.5114/pg.2019.83428.
95. Cuomo R, Barbara G, Pace F, Annese V, Bassotti G, Binda GA, et al. Italian consensus conference for colonic diverticulosis and diverticular disease. United European Gastroenterol J. 2014;2(5):413–42. https://doi.org/10.1177/2050640614547068.
96. Binda GA, Cuomo R, Laghi A, Nascimbeni R, Serventi A, Bellini D, et al. Practice parameters for the treatment of colonic diverticular disease: Italian Society of Colon and Rectal Surgery (SICCR) guidelines. Tech Coloproctol. 2015;19(10):615–26. https://doi.org/10.1007/s10151-015-1370-x.
97. Rana-Garibay R, Salgado-Nesme N, Carmona-Sanchez R, Remes-Troche JM, Aguilera-Carrera J, Alonso-Sanchez L, et al. The Mexican consensus on the diagnosis and treatment of diverticular disease of the colon. Rev Gastroenterol Mex. 2019;84(2):220–40. https://doi.org/10.1016/j.rgmx.2019.01.002.
98. Andersen JC, Bundgaard L, Elbrond H, Laurberg S, Walker LR, Stovring J. Danish national guidelines for treatment of diverticular disease. Dan Med J. 2012;59(5):C4453.
99. Pietrzak A, Bartnik W, Szczepkowski M, Krokowicz P, Dziki A, Regula J, et al. Polish interdisciplinary consensus on diagnostics and treatment of colonic diverticulosis (2015). Pol Przegl Chir. 2015;87(4):203–20. https://doi.org/10.1515/pjs-2015-0045.
100. Trifan A, Gheorghe C, Marica Sabo C, Diculescu M, Nedelcu L, Singeap AM, et al. Diagnosis and treatment of colonic diverticular disease: position paper of the Romanian Society of Gastroenterology and Hepatology. J Gastrointestin Liver Dis. 2018;27(4):449–57. https://doi.org/10.15403/jgld.2014.1121.274.rom.
101. Kruis W, Germer CT, Leifeld L, German Society for Gastroenterology, Digestive and Metabolic Diseases and The German Society for General and Visceral Surgery. Diverticular disease: guidelines of the German society for gastroenterology, digestive and metabolic diseases and the German society for general and visceral surgery. Digestion. 2014;90(3):190–207. https://doi.org/10.1159/000367625.

102. Copaci I, Constantinescu G, Mihăilă M, Micu L, Franculescu-Bertea A. Efficacy of Rifaximin-α vs dietary fiber on the evolution of uncomplicated colonic diverticular disease. Surg Gastroenterol Oncol. 2019;24(5):233–40. https://doi.org/10.21614/sgo-24-5-233.
103. Pietrzak AM, Banasiewicz T, Skoczylas K, Dziki A, Szczepkowski M. Combined therapy: rifaximin-α and arabinogalactan with lactoferrin combination effectively prevents recurrences of symptomatic uncomplicated diverticular disease. Pol Przegl Chir. 2020;92(2):22–8. https://doi.org/10.5604/01.3001.0014.0946.
104. Tursi A, Brandimarte G, Elisei W, Picchio M, Forti G, Pianese G, et al. Randomised clinical trial: mesalazine and/or probiotics in maintaining remission of symptomatic uncomplicated diverticular disease - a double-blind, randomised, placebo-controlled study. Aliment Pharmacol Ther. 2013;38(7):741–51. https://doi.org/10.1111/apt.12463.
105. Hill C, Guarner F, Reid G, Gibson GR, Merenstein DJ, Pot B, et al. Expert consensus document. The international scientific Association for Probiotics and Prebiotics consensus statement on the scope and appropriate use of the term probiotic. Nat Rev Gastroenterol Hepatol. 2014;11(8):506–14. https://doi.org/10.1038/nrgastro.2014.66.
106. Di Pierro F, Pane M. *Bifidobacterium longum* W11: uniqueness and individual or combined clinical use in association with rifaximin. Clin Nutr ESPEN. 2021;42:15–21. https://doi.org/10.1016/j.clnesp.2020.12.025.
107. Graziano T, Amoruso A, Nicola S, Deidda F, Allesina S, Pane M, et al. The possible innovative use of *Bifidobacterium longum W11* in association with Rifaximin: a new horizon for combined approach? J Clin Gastroenterol. 2016;50(Suppl 2):S153–s6. https://doi.org/10.1097/mcg.0000000000000683.
108. Di Pierro F, Bertuccioli A, Pane M, Ivaldi L. Effects of rifaximin-resistant *Bifidobacterium longum W11* in subjects with symptomatic uncomplicated diverticular disease treated with rifaximin. Minerva Gastroenterol Dietol. 2019;65(4):259–64. https://doi.org/10.23736/s1121-421x.19.02622-9.
109. Giaccari S, Tronci S, Falconieri M, Ferrieri A. Long-term treatment with rifaximin and lactobacilli in post-diverticulitic stenoses of the colon. Riv Eur Sci Med Farmacol. 1993;15(1):29–34.
110. Ponziani FR, Zocco MA, D'Aversa F, Pompili M, Gasbarrini A. Eubiotic properties of rifaximin: disruption of the traditional concepts in gut microbiota modulation. World J Gastroenterol. 2017;23(25):4491–9. https://doi.org/10.3748/wjg.v23.i25.4491.
111. Wieërs G, Verbelen V, Van Den Driessche M, Melnik E, Vanheule G, Marot JC, et al. Do probiotics during in-hospital antibiotic treatment prevent colonization of gut microbiota with multi-drug-resistant bacteria? A randomized placebo-controlled trial comparing *Saccharomyces* to a mixture of *Lactobacillus*, *Bifidobacterium*, and *Saccharomyces*. Front Public Health. 2020;8:578089. https://doi.org/10.3389/fpubh.2020.578089.
112. Pimentel M, Cash BD, Lembo A, Wolf RA, Israel RJ, Schoenfeld P. Repeat Rifaximin for irritable bowel syndrome: no clinically significant changes in stool microbial antibiotic sensitivity. Dig Dis Sci. 2017;62(9):2455–63. https://doi.org/10.1007/s10620-017-4598-7.
113. Nielsen OH, Munck LK. Drug insight: aminosalicylates for the treatment of IBD. Nat Clin Pract Gastroenterol Hepatol. 2007;4(3):160–70. https://doi.org/10.1038/ncpgasthep0696.
114. Olaisen M, Spigset O, Flatberg A, Granlund AVB, Brede WR, Albrektsen G, et al. Mucosal 5-aminosalicylic acid concentration, drug formulation and mucosal microbiome in patients with quiescent ulcerative colitis. Aliment Pharmacol Ther. 2019;49(10):1301–13. https://doi.org/10.1111/apt.15227.
115. Brandimarte G, Tursi A. Rifaximin plus mesalazine followed by mesalazine alone is highly effective in obtaining remission of symptomatic uncomplicated diverticular disease. Med Sci Monit. 2004;10(5):Pi70-3.
116. Salem TA, Molloy RG, O'Dwyer PJ. Prospective, five-year follow-up study of patients with symptomatic uncomplicated diverticular disease. Dis Colon Rectum. 2007;50(9):1460–4. https://doi.org/10.1007/s10350-007-0226-5.

117. Spiegel BM, Reid MW, Bolus R, Whitman CB, Talley J, Dea S, et al. Development and validation of a disease-targeted quality of life instrument for chronic diverticular disease: the DV-QOL. Qual Life Res. 2015;24(1):163–79. https://doi.org/10.1007/s11136-014-0753-1.
118. Chabok A, Pahlman L, Hjern F, Haapaniemi S, Smedh K. Randomized clinical trial of antibiotics in acute uncomplicated diverticulitis. Br J Surg. 2012;99(4):532–9. https://doi.org/10.1002/bjs.8688.
119. Cohen E, Fuller G, Bolus R, Modi R, Vu M, Shahedi K, et al. Increased risk for irritable bowel syndrome after acute diverticulitis. Clin Gastroenterol Hepatol. 2013;11(12):1614–9. https://doi.org/10.1016/j.cgh.2013.03.007.
120. Barbara G, Grover M, Bercik P, Corsetti M, Ghoshal UC, Ohman L, et al. Rome foundation working team report on post-infection irritable bowel syndrome. Gastroenterology. 2019;156(1):46–58.e7. https://doi.org/10.1053/j.gastro.2018.07.011.
121. Hall JF, Roberts PL, Ricciardi R, Read T, Scheirey C, Wald C, et al. Long-term follow-up after an initial episode of diverticulitis: what are the predictors of recurrence? Dis Colon Rectum. 2011;54(3):283–8. https://doi.org/10.1007/DCR.0b013e3182028576.
122. Eglinton T, Nguyen T, Raniga S, Dixon L, Dobbs B, Frizelle FA. Patterns of recurrence in patients with acute diverticulitis. Br J Surg. 2010;97(6):952–7. https://doi.org/10.1002/bjs.7035.
123. Lanas A, Ponce J, Bignamini A, Mearin F. One year intermittent rifaximin plus fibre supplementation vs. fibre supplementation alone to prevent diverticulitis recurrence: a proof-of-concept study. Dig Liver Dis. 2013;45(2):104–9. https://doi.org/10.1016/j.dld.2012.09.006.
124. Festa V, Spila Alegiani S, Chiesara F, Moretti A, Bianchi M, Dezi A, et al. Retrospective comparison of long-term ten-day/month rifaximin or mesalazine in prevention of relapse in acute diverticulitis. Eur Rev Med Pharmacol Sci. 2017;21(6):1397–404.
125. US National Library of Medicine. Rifaximin delayed release for the prevention of recurrent acute diverticulitis and diverticular complications (ROAD). https://clinicaltrials.gov/ct2/show/NCT03469050?term=NCT03469050&draw=2&rank=1. 2019.
126. Tursi A, Brandimarte G, Daffina R. Long-term treatment with mesalazine and rifaximin versus rifaximin alone for patients with recurrent attacks of acute diverticulitis of colon. Dig Liver Dis. 2002;34(7):510–5.
127. Stollman N, Smalley W, Hirano I, AGA Institute Clinical Guidelines Committee. American Gastroenterological Association Institute guideline on the management of acute diverticulitis. Gastroenterology. 2015;149(7):1944–9. https://doi.org/10.1053/j.gastro.2015.10.003.
128. Viscomi GC, Campana M, Barbanti M, Grepioni F, Polito M, Confortini D, et al. Crystal forms of rifaximin and their effect on pharmaceutical properties. CrystEngComm. 2008;10(8):1074–81. https://doi.org/10.1039/b717887e.
129. Ilfiker R. Polymorphysm in pharmaceutical industry. Wiley-VCH; 2006. p. 1–433.
130. Brittain HG. Polymorphism in pharmaceutical solids. 2nd ed. New York: Informa Healthcare; 2009. p. 1–640.
131. Blandizzi C, Viscomi GC, Scarpignato C. Impact of crystal polymorphism on the systemic bioavailability of rifaximin, an antibiotic acting locally in the gastrointestinal tract, in healthy volunteers. Drug Des Devel Ther. 2015;9:1–11. https://doi.org/10.2147/DDDT.S72572.
132. Blandizzi C, Viscomi GC, Marzo A, Scarpignato C. Is generic rifaximin still a poorly absorbed antibiotic? A comparison of branded and generic formulations in healthy volunteers. Pharmacol Res. 2014;85:39–44. https://doi.org/10.1016/j.phrs.2014.05.001.
133. DuPont HL. Rifaximin: an antibiotic with important biologic effects. Mini Rev Med Chem. 2015;16(3):200–5.
134. Snider DA, Addicks W, Owens W. Polymorphism in generic drug product development. Adv Drug Deliv Rev. 2004;56(3):391–5. https://doi.org/10.1016/j.addr.2003.10.010.
135. FDA. Draft guidance on rifaximin. https://www.accessdata.fda.gov/drugsatfda_docs/psg/Rifaximin_oral%20tablet_NDA%20022554%20and%20021361_RV03-17.pdf. Recommended Nov 2011, Feb 2012; revised March 2017.

Anti-inflammatory Agents 19

Wolfgang Kruis and Mauro Bafutto

19.1 Background

Among the options available for treating diverticular disease, anti-inflammatory agents have been widely established. The pharmacological armamentarium comprises directly acting compounds such as mesalazine (5-aminosalicylic acid) and indirectly acting strategies including changes in the intestinal microbiome by antimicrobial agents, probiotics, prebiotics, and diets. The focus of this chapter is on mesalazine for the treatment of uncomplicated diverticular disease and diverticulitis.

The emphasis is on appropriate indications of mesalazine in the complex field of diverticular disease with regard to the ongoing discussion on varying definitions and types. Another aspect addressed here is the question regarding which type of anti-inflammatory therapy with mesalazine is supposed to be implemented. Although other chapters of this book describe the pathogenesis in more detail, the following section makes a clear point on two types of inflammation in diverticular disease, which may be targeted by mesalazine application, overt (macroscopic) inflammation in diverticulitis, and "low-grade inflammation" in symptomatic uncomplicated diverticular disease (SUDD), which cannot be diagnosed with colonoscopy but only with molecular and histological methods.

W. Kruis (✉)
Em. Ev. Krankenhaus Kalk, Köln, University of Cologne, Pulheim-Freimersdorf, Germany
e-mail: Wolfgang.Kruis@googlemail.com

M. Bafutto
Department of Internal Medicine, Division of Gastroenterology,
Universidade Federal de Goiás, Goiânia, Brazil
e-mail: maurobafutto@yahoo.com.br

© The Author(s), under exclusive license to Springer Nature Switzerland AG 2022

A. Tursi et al. (eds.), *Colonic Diverticular Disease*,
https://doi.org/10.1007/978-3-030-93761-4_19

19.2 Inflammation in Diverticular Disease

By definition, asymptomatic diverticulosis is unrelated to any signs of inflammation. In this context, no signs of inflammation should be detected, both at endoscopic and also at histological assessments. Overt mucosal inflammation associated with diverticula may occur and is defined as segmental colitis associated with diverticulosis (SCAD). In fact, on a microscopic/molecular level, a study of more than 600 individuals undergoing screening colonoscopies with biopsies found no association between diverticulosis and levels of immune markers or cytokines implicated in inflammatory processes [1]. To conclude, diverticulosis does not show inflammation.

A different scenario may be observed in patients with diverticular disease defined as symptoms and/or complications in the presence of diverticula [2]. While overt inflammation is well defined in both uncomplicated and complicated diverticulitis, SUDD is still a matter of debate. SUDD is characterized by nonspecific symptomatic attacks, mainly abdominal pain, but no macroscopic evidence of an inflammatory process exists. Several authors refer to SUDD as "IBS with diverticulosis." However, these studies did not investigate whether patients who later developed diverticulitis or recurrent diverticulitis had subclinical mucosal or systemic inflammation.

Others are convinced that IBS and SUDD are different clinical entities, as shown by clinical data currently available. IBS and SUDD do not share the same epidemiology, but share a part of their clinical features, and patients with SUDD do not generally fulfill the (Rome) IBS criteria. Moreover, abdominal pain (left lower abdominal pain) lasting for more than 24 h characterizes SUDD and diffuse and short-lived abdominal pain characterizes IBS, and this discriminates patients with SUDD from those with IBS [3].

How low-grade inflammation in symptomatic diverticular disease develops is still an unresolved question. Dysbiosis has been hypothesized to be a trigger of symptoms in people with diverticulosis. Alterations in the microbial ecosystem have been described. Moreover, pilot studies found that SUDD patients have dysbiosis when compared with patients with simple diverticulosis, and this dysbiosis also seems to influence the host metabolome [3].

Many of the risk factors for diverticulitis, such as a low-fiber diet, high red meat consumption, obesity, smoking, and physical inactivity, which are also risk factors for both cardiovascular diseases and diabetes mellitus, are found to alter the intestinal microbiota and thus to be associated with chronic, low-grade inflammation. Thus, chronic inflammation might be the underlying mechanistic link between diet and lifestyle factors and diverticulitis [4].

Nearly 20 years ago, Narayan and Floch found a significant inflammatory infiltrate in SUDD patients compared with healthy controls [5]. Tursi and Elisei assessed both neutrophilic and lymphocytic infiltrates in SUDD, acute uncomplicated diverticulitis (AUD), and healthy controls. While the neutrophilic inflammatory infiltrate was found only in AUD, the mean lymphocytic cell density was significantly higher in SUDD than in asymptomatic diverticulosis and controls [6].

An enhanced expression of TNF-α, a proinflammatory cytokine, plays a key role in the pathophysiology of chronic inflammatory diseases including IBD and rheumatoid arthritis. Mucosal expression of TNF-α was higher compared to healthy controls not only in patients suffering from acute uncomplicated diverticular disease but also in those suffering from SUDD. These results were confirmed by others who, in addition, found TNF-α expression to be significantly higher in SUDD than in asymptomatic diverticulosis. Surprisingly, several research groups demonstrated higher expression of IL-10, an anti-inflammatory cytokine. It was hypothesized that this unexpected activation of an anti-inflammatory reaction might be an attempt by the immune system to control the low-grade inflammation. This finding matches well with the inverse expression of prostaglandin E2 in the colonic mucosa between acute diverticulitis and IBD. Prostaglandin E2 is the dominant prostaglandin in the colon, is associated with colonic inflammation, and also exhibits a protective mechanism in the mucosa of the gastrointestinal tract. Lower prostaglandin E2 levels may decrease the normal protection of the mucosa, which makes it more susceptible to luminal insults, thus creating a permissive environment for the development of acute diverticulitis [7].

These research results indicate that SUDD may be associated with "low-grade inflammation" in macroscopically unaltered colonic mucosa. Thus, currently, there is growing evidence for a differentiation between asymptomatic diverticulosis, IBS, and SUDD. The challenge is to present a clinical biomarker, which can be used as a real-world marker for diagnosis.

Fecal calprotectin (FC) has been shown in early studies to be a useful marker of inflammatory activity in IBD. FC is a cytoplasmic antimicrobial compound. It is released from intestinal granulocytes, monocytes, and macrophages during cell activation or death. Investigations, including a case–control study have described higher FC values in AUD and SUDD than in healthy controls and patients with IBS.

In conclusion, FC may be a useful tool in the detection of "low-grade inflammation" in the colon harboring diverticula, thus distinguishing between symptoms originating from diverticular inflammation and IBS overlapping diverticulosis [7]. However, additional studies are certainly needed.

19.3 Mode of Action of Mesalazine

The story of 5-aminosaliciylic acid (5-ASA) starts with Nana Svartz who published anti-inflammatory effects in rheumatoid arthritis late in the 30s in the previous century. While 5-ASA was initially only applied as a double molecule linked to sulfapyridine (sulfasalazine), it was not earlier than 1979 that Azad Khan and Truelove described the anti-inflammatory effects of 5-ASA monotherapy to treat IBD, and thereafter 5-ASA was referred to as mesalazine (Amer. mesalamine).

Mesalazine is a mainstay of anti-inflammatory therapy in IBD. Although the clinical effects of mesalazine in diseases with overt mucosal inflammation of the intestines are well known, a specific mode of pharmacological action has not yet

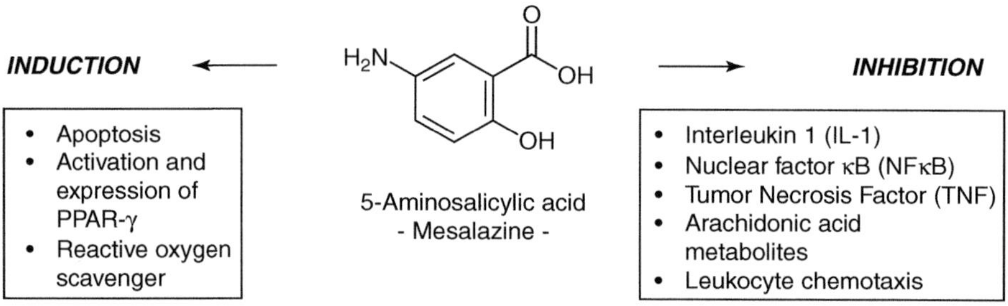

Fig. 19.1 Proposed mechanism of action of mesalazine at the colonic mucosa [mod 8]

been identified. Plurality of described effects have posed the hypothesis that mesalazine acts rather via a network of unspecific activities than through single effects.

Well-confirmed pharmacological actions comprise inhibition of cyclooxygenase and lipoxygenase pathways, targeting the peroxisome proliferator-activated receptor-g, and antioxidative properties [8] (Fig. 19.1). Other mechanisms that may be particularly related to the status of low-grade inflammation include interference with proinflammatory cytokines via decreasing the activity of nuclear factorκB (NF-κB) and inhibition of tumor necrosis factor (TNF), as well as effects on cellular functions of mucosal lymphocytes, macrophages, and natural killer cells [9].

In addition to its established anti-inflammatory properties, mesalazine is discussed to have a variety of alternative effects, such as antineoplastic, microbial, and pain-alleviating activities. A placebo-controlled proof-of-concept study analysis of mucosa biopsies from patients under mesalazine showed inhibition of histamine and tryptase mediators, which play a key role in visceral pain perception. These molecular findings were related to improvements in the general well-being and reduction of abdominal pain [10]. A placebo-controlled trial in acute uncomplicated diverticular disease revealed significant beneficial effects on pain [11].

In summary, possible effects on the pathophysiology of low-grade inflammation and on pain make mesalazine a promising candidate for treatment of symptomatic uncomplicated diverticular disease (SUDD).

19.4 Clinical Evidence of Therapeutic Effects of Mesalazine in Uncomplicated Diverticular Disease, SUDD, and Uncomplicated Diverticulitis

The aims of therapy with mesalazine are to alleviate symptoms in acute uncomplicated diverticular disease and SUDD. Asymptomatic disease should be maintained by preventing the occurrence of new symptomatic episodes and progression toward diverticulitis.

19.5 Symptom Improvement in (Sub) Acute Uncomplicated Diverticular Disease

Several open-label studies have shown the beneficial effects of mesalazine in SUDD [12]. One of the first publications about its use in SUDD was a case series by Brandimarte and Tursi (2004) who studied 90 consecutive patients with SUDD. The patients were treated with 800 mg/day of rifaximin plus 2.4 g/day of mesalazine for 10 days, and then with 1.6 g/day of mesalazine for 8 weeks. The results showed a statistically significant decrease in the symptom score and 77.78% of the patients were completely asymptomatic after the eighth week of treatment with mesalazine [13].

Moreover, three randomized controlled trials studied the improvement of symptoms in (sub) acute uncomplicated diverticular disease. A placebo-controlled 4-week study comparing mesalazine 1000 mg t.i.d. described favorable effects on pain [11]. Another RCT lasting for 12 weeks compared two doses of mesalazine with two doses of rifaximin. In all groups, favorable results were achieved. Results of mesalazine 1600 mg/day were significantly superior to rifaximin [14]. A trial with a similar design but longer follow-up confirmed these results. Again, mesalazine demonstrated superior effects over rifaximin [15].

19.6 Maintaining Long-Term Symptom Relief in Symptomatic Uncomplicated Diverticular Disease (SUDD)

Several systematic reviews and meta-analyses include trials that describe the maintenance of remission in patients with a diagnosis of SUDD [16–18]. Study end points were symptoms after at least 12 months and comparison of the symptoms with a control group.

Picchio et al. [16] conducted a systematic review seeking to identify only controlled and randomized studies in SUDD with mesalazine. They analyzed seven articles, of which four studies spanned at least a time between 12 and 48 months. A placebo-controlled study comprised four arms of cyclicity (10 days/month) that were administered mesalazine (1.6 g/day), or Lactobacillus casei subsp. DG (24 billion/day), or Lactobacillus casei subsp. DG (24 billion/day) plus mesalazine or placebo. After 12 months, relief from symptoms was achieved in 93.3% patients with mesalazine compared to 54.0% under placebo [19].

Ianonne et al. [18] systematically reviewed the evidence of mesalazine versus all other treatments in patients with diverticular disease. The analysis included 13 RCTs, of which 6 were related to the maintenance of SUDD. According to PRISMA and GRADE, they confirm the results of the study by Picchio et al. [16], thus concluding that mesalazine may improve quality of life in symptomatic uncomplicated diverticular disease (SUDD) and patients' symptoms in diverticular disease. Both meta-analyses indicate the problem of limited quality of the trials analyzed.

19.7 Preventing the Progression from SUDD to Diverticulitis

There are only few studies on the course of SUDD and the risk of developing acute diverticulitis. Outcomes of SUDD up to 5 years of follow-up are known from three studies [20]. It is most likely that extremely different methodological approaches generated a wide range of occurrences of diverticulitis in patients with SUDD, ranging from 1.7 to 10.4%.

A recent retrospective cohort study analyzing outcomes during the natural course of SUDD (not scheduled, but only sporadic treatments according to the discretion of the attending physicians) has included 185 SUDD patients as diagnosed by stringent criteria. The patients were followed up for a median time of 156 months (91–171). The follow-up identified 14 patients with acute diverticulitis; about half of them occurred between 2 and 4 years after the SUDD diagnosis. In all, 6 cases experienced uncomplicated disease and eight cases developed requiring surgical resection in six patients with an overall mortality of two cases (peritonitis) [20].

The meta-analysis [18] could not find a significant difference in the likelihood of developing acute diverticulitis in SUDD between mesalazine and control interventions, but the risk calculation was in favor of the active treatment (3 trials, 484 participants, RR = 0.26, 95% CI 0.06–1.20).

The results of a four-arm, placebo-controlled trial are particularly interesting [19]. Acute diverticulitis occurred in seven (3.1%) of the analyzed patients during 12 months of follow-up: six patients were in the placebo group, no patient under mesalazine developed diverticulitis, and one patient receiving placebo underwent surgery due to free perforation.

In conclusion, development of acute diverticulitis in patients suffering from SUDD is a rare event. Some results indicate that this risk may be prevented by therapy with mesalazine, but further studies are needed to provide reasons for any recommendations.

19.8 Mesalazine for Acute Uncomplicated Diverticulitis

The aims of treatment in this clinical situation are resolution of inflammation and its symptoms to avoid worsening toward complicated diverticulitis and to prevent surgical interventions. The background for the concept of treatment of diverticulitis with mesalazine is its undoubtedly beneficial effectiveness in other inflammatory diseases such as IBD.

Unfortunately, there is a paucity of trials. If only studies using stringent inclusion criteria are considered (e.g., imaging methods such as computed tomography or ultrasound), then two studies can be quoted. In a single-center, retrospective, controlled cohort study, patients admitted to the surgical department ($n = 50$) received mesalazine 3.2 g/day or standard treatment [21]. A nonsignificant trend for a faster decrease in CRP and a shorter hospital stay under mesalazine was observed.

A recent meta-analysis [18] has mentioned only one RCT [22]. This RCT [22] compared the effects of three treatments for 12 weeks: mesalazine, mesalazine plus probiotics, and placebo. The end point was the global symptom score. The trial failed to show significantly different effects after 10 days and 12 weeks between patient groups.

To conclude, on the basis of the currently available evidence, mesalazine cannot be recommended for treatment of acute uncomplicated diverticulitis.

19.9 Mesalazine for Prevention of Relapses of Acute Uncomplicated Diverticulitis

The rationale of 5-ASA therapy for the control of symptoms and prevention of the recurrence of diverticulitis could be because of the presence of mild chronic inflammation in diverticular disease, which may be the cause of diverticulitis and its recurrence. However, the results of studies on the use of mesalazine to prevent recurrence of AUD are conflicting. There are difficulties in reaching conclusions about this account of heterogeneous studies with differences in doses, formulations, time of use of medication, and association of drugs.

Qualified, double-blind, placebo-controlled studies were performed. Some studies have shown improvement in symptoms and quality of life. However, most studies have shown no statistically significant difference in the use of mesalazine compared to placebo [22–25] (Table 19.1).

Table 19.1 Double-blind, placebo-controlled studies for mesalazine in recurrent diverticulitis

		Results	Results
Authors	Intervention	Time; relapse rates	*p*
Parente [23]	Mesalazine retard tablets 800 mg b.i.d. Placebo	24 month: 13.3% /27.7 %	$p = 0.10$
Stollman [22]	Eudragit L 2.4 g od Placebo	3 month + 9 month follow 28.1%/31.0%	$p > 0.05$
Raskin [24]	MMX 1.2 *versus* placebo	24 month; <u>free of recurrence</u>	
		Prevent 1 (Prevent2)	
	Placebo	64.6% (67.6%)	
	1.2 g od	62.2% (62.8%)	$p = 0.78$ (0.36)
	2.4 g od	62.9% (59.2%)	$p = 0.74$ (0.15)
	4.8 g od	52.7% (69.1%)	$p = 0.04$ (0.77)
Kruis [25]	Mesalazine granules	SAG 37 (SAG 51)	
		12 month (24 month)	
	Placebo	11.9% (21.0%)	
	1.5 g od	– (17.2%)	– (0.36)
	3.0 g od	18.3% (20.0%)	0.69 (0.95)

A recent systematic review and meta-analysis has included eight randomized controlled trials with a variety of dosing regimens and the use of concomitant probiotics. 5-ASA compounds were not superior to controls for preventing recurrent attacks (RR 0.86, 95% CI 0.63–1.17) [26].

Therefore, to conclude based on these studies, mesalazine does not present evidence as an effective treatment for preventing the recurrence of acute uncomplicated diverticulitis.

19.10 Safety of Mesalazine

Mesalazine has been on the pharmacy market throughout the world for more than 30 years. Although it has been indicated on several occasions to treat various conditions, it is in the context of the treatment of inflammatory bowel disease that the data on safety are recorded.

5-ASA is generally well tolerated, and the most common side effects include headache, nausea, and abdominal pain [27]. A French pharmacovigilance study of mesalazine (Pentasa) reported between 6.6 and 9.0 adverse events per million treatment days over a 2-year period [28]. A British pharmacovigilance study of mesalazine (Asacol, Pentasa, or Salofalk) over an 8-year interval identified 393 adverse events per million prescriptions for mesalazine [29].

Loftus et al. published a systematic review about the short-term adverse events of 5-aminosalicylic acid agents in the treatment of ulcerative colitis. A total of 46 randomized trials of oral mesalazine, olsalazine, or balsalazide for the treatment of active disease or for the maintenance of remission were included. They concluded that all three 5-aminosalicylic acid agents are safe in the short term. In mesalazine-treated patients, the frequencies of adverse events or withdrawals due to adverse events were comparable with those in placebo-treated patients [30].

Seghal et al. (2018), in a systematic review, evaluated the safety of mesalazine in ulcerative colitis. An electronic search was performed without language restrictions using the PubMed database from inception up to 1 December 2017. A total of 91 articles were included, pointing to some adverse events that were not related to drug dosage but possibly linked to hypersensitivity: pancreatitis, cardiotoxicity, hepatotoxicity, musculoskeletal complaints, respiratory symptoms, nephropathies, and sexual dysfunction. The main concern was about renal adverse effects (interstitial nephritis 0–1%, renal failure 0–0.2%, and proteinuria 0.3%). They recommended checking creatinine levels prior to starting treatment and rechecking them yearly while on treatment.

In conclusion, they reported that patients on mesalazine should be monitored for worsening of ulcerative colitis and development of new-onset organ dysfunction. High-dose mesalazine seems to have similar safety profile as that of low dose and is not associated with greater risks of adverse events [31].

19.11 Summary and Conclusions

Anti-inflammatory activities and effects on symptoms like pain are the pharmacological properties of mesalazine, which promise therapeutic effectiveness in diverticular disease and diverticulitis. In fact, the current evidence confirms the favorable effects of mesalazine in inducing symptom relief in acute uncomplicated diverticular disease and in maintaining remission in SUDD. Owing to a lack of data on the prevention of development of diverticulitis in patients with SUDD, the clinical resolution of inflammation in acute diverticulitis cannot be properly analyzed. Long-term therapy with mesalazine is not able to prevent recurrences of diverticulitis.

References

1. Peery AF, Keku TO, Addamo C, McCoy AN, Martin CF, Galanko JA, et al. Colonic diverticula are not associated with mucosal inflammation or chronic gastrointestinal symptoms. Clin Gastroenterol Hepatol. 2018;16:884–91.
2. Kruis W, Germer CT, Leifeld L. German Society for Gastroenterology, digestive and metabolic diseases and the German Society for General and Visceral Surgery. Diverticular disease: guidelines of the german society for gastroenterology, digestive and metabolic diseases and the german society for general and visceral surgery. Digestion. 2014;90(3):190–207.
3. Elisei W, Tursi A. The pathophysiology of colonic diverticulosis: inflammation versus constipation? Inflamm Intest Dis. 2018;3(2):55–60.
4. Tursi A, Scarpignato C, Strate LL, Lanas A, Kruis W, Lahat A, Danese S. Colonic diverticular disease. Nat Rev Dis Primers. 2020;6(1):20.
5. Narayan R, Floch MH. Microscopic colitis as part of the the natural history of diverticular disease. Am J Gastroenterol. 2002;97(9):S112–3.
6. Tursi A, Elisei W. Role of inflammation in the pathogenesis of diverticular disease. Mediat Inflamm. 2019;2019:8328490. https://doi.org/10.1155/2019/8328490.
7. Strate LL, Morris AM. Epidemiology, pathophysiology, and treatment of diverticulitis. Gastroenterology. 2019;156(5):1282–98.
8. Ye B, van Langenberg DR. Mesalazine preparations for the treatment of ulcerative colitis: are all created equal? World J Gastrointest Pharmacol Ther. 2015;6(4):137–44.
9. Nakashima J. Preuss CV.Mesalamine (USAN). In: StatPearls. Treasure Island (FL): StatPearls Publishing; 2021. Bookshelf ID: NBK551714.
10. Corinaldesi R, Stranghellini V, Cremon C, Gargano L, Cogliandro RF, De Georgio R, Bartesaghi G, Canovi B, Barbara G. Effect of mesalazine on mucosal immune biomarkers in irritable bowel syndrome: a randomized controlled proof-of-conceptStudy. Aliment Pharmacol Ther. 2009;30(3):245–52.
11. Kruis W, Meier E, Schumacher M, et al. Randomised clinical trial: mesalazine (Salofalk granules) for uncomplicated diverticular disease of the colon–a placebo-controlled study. Aliment Pharmacol Ther. 2013;37:680–90.
12. Tursi A, Papa A, Danese S. Review article: the pathophysiology and medical management of diverticulosis and diverticular disease of the colon. Aliment Pharmacol Ther. 2015;42(6):664–84.
13. Brandimarte G, Tursi A. Rifaximin plus mesalazine followed by mesalazine alone is highly effective in obtaining remission of symptomatic uncomplicated diverticular disease. Med Sci Monit. 2004;10(5):70–3.
14. Di Mario F, Aragona G, Leandro G, Comparato G, Fanigliulo L, Cavallaro LG, Cavestro GM, Iori V, Maino M, Moussa AM, Gnocchi A, Mazzocchi G, Franze A. Efficacy of mesalazine in the treatment of symptomatic diverticular disease. Dig Dis Sci. 2005;50(3):581–6.

15. Comparato G, Fanigliulo L, Cavallaro LG, Aragona G, Cavestro GM, Iori V, Maino M, Mazzocchi G, Muzzetto P, Colla G, Sianesi M, Franzé A, Di Mario F. Prevention of complications and symptomatic recurrences in diverticular disease with mesalazine: a 12-month follow-up. Dig Dis Sci. 2007;52:2934–41.
16. Picchio M, Elisei W, Brandimarte G, et al. Mesalazine for the treatment of symptomatic uncomplicated diverticular disease of the colon and for primary prevention of diverticulitis: a systematic review of randomized clinical trials. J Clin Gastroenterol. 2016;50(Suppl 1):S64–9.
17. Picchio M, Elisei W, Tursi A. Mesalazine to treat symptomatic uncomplicated diverticular disease and to prevent acute diverticulitis occurrence. A systematic review with meta-analysis of randomized, placebo-controlled trials. J Gastrointestin Liver Dis. 2018;27(3):291–7.
18. Ianonne A, Ruospo M, Wong G, et al. Mesalazine for people with diverticular disease: a systematic review of randomized controlled trials. Can J Gastroenterol Hepatol. 2018;2018:5437135.
19. Tursi A, Brandimarte G, Elisei W, et al. Randomised clinical trial: mesalazine and/or probiotics in maintaining remission of symptomatic uncomplicated diverticular disease–a double-blind, randomised, placebo-controlled study. Aliment Pharmacol Ther. 2013;38:741–51.
20. Tursi A, Franceschi M, Elisei W, Picchio M, Di Mario F, Brandimarte G. The natural history of symptomatic uncomplicated diverticular disease: a long-term follow-up study. Ann Gastroenterol. 2021;34(2):208–13.
21. Nespoli L, Lo Bianco G, Uggeri F, Romano F, Nespoli A, Bernasconi DP, Gianotti L. Effect of oral mesalamine on inflammatory response in acute uncomplicated diverticulitis. World J Gastroenterol. 2015;21(27):8366–72.
22. Stollman N, Magowan S, Shanahan F, Quigley E. DIVA investigation group. A randomized controlled study of mesalamine after acute diverticulitis: results of the DIVA trial. J Clin Gastroenterol. 2013;47(7):621–9.
23. Parente F, Bargiggia S, Prada A, Bortoli A, Giacosa A, Germanà B, Ferrari A, Casella G, De Pretis G, Miori G. "Gismi study group". Intermittent treatment with mesalazine in the preventionof diverticulitis recurrence: a randomised multicentre pilotdouble-blind placebo-controlled study of 24-month duration. Int J Color Dis. 2013;28:1423–31.
24. Raskin JB, Kamm MA, Jamal MM, Márquez J, Melzer E, Schoen RE, Szalóki T, Barrett K, Streck P. Gastroenterology. 2014;147(4):793–802.
25. Kruis W, Kardalinos V, Eisenbach T, Lukas M, Vich T, Bunganic I, Pokrotnieks J, Derova J, Kondrackiene J, Safadi R, Tuculanu D, Tulassay Z, Banai J, Curtin A, Dorofeyev AE, Zakko SF, Ferreira N, Björck S, Diez Alonso MM, Mäkelä J, Talley NJ, Dilger K, Greinwald R, Mohrbacher R, Spiller R. Randomised clinical trial: mesalazine versus placebo in the prevention of diverticulitis recurrence. Aliment Pharmacol Ther. 2017;46:282–91.
26. Urushidani S, Kuriyama A, Matsumura M. 5-aminosalicylic acid agents for prevention of recurrent diverticulitis: a systematic review and meta-analysis. J Gastroenterol Hepatol. 2018;33(1):12–1.
27. Rao SS, Cann PA, Holdsworth CD. Clinical experience of the tolerance of mesalazine and olsalazine in patients intolerant of sulphasalazine. Scand J Gastroenterol. 1987;22(3):332–6.
28. Marteau P, Nelet F, Le Lu M, et al. Adverse events in patients treated with 5-aminosalicyclic acid: 1993–1994 pharmacovigilance report for Pentasa in France. Aliment Pharmacol Ther. 1996;10:949–56.
29. Ransford RA, Langman MJ. Sulphasalazine and mesalazine: serious adverse reactions re-evaluated on the basis of suspected adverse reaction reports to the committee on safety of medicines. Gut. 2002;51:536–9.
30. Loftus EV Jr, Kane SV, Bjorkman D. Systematic review: short-term adverse effects of 5-aminosalicylic acid agents in the treatment of ulcerative colitis. Aliment Pharmacol Ther. 2004;19:179–89.
31. Seghal P, Columbel JF, Aboubakr A, et al. Syatematic review: safety of mesalazine in ulcerative colitis. Aliment Pharmacol Ther. 2018;47(12):1597–609.

20 Probiotics

Edoardo Savarino, Veronica Ojetti, and Angela Saviano

20.1 Introduction: The Role of the *Gut Microbiota* in Colonic Diverticular Disease

Diverticular disease is a common gastrointestinal disorder in the Western world. The clinical manifestation ranges from asymptomatic diverticulosis to symptomatic diverticular disease, simple (SUDD) or complicated (acute diverticulitis). Most of the cases (80%) are asymptomatic diverticulosis of the colon with a prevalence that increases with age. Symptoms of the simple forms are often not so specific and comparable to irritable bowel syndrome [1]. Many factors can contribute to the development of patients' symptoms such as inflammation, changes in gut microbiota composition, visceral hypersensitivity, and impaired colon motility. The gut microbiota plays a fundamental role in every phase of diverticular disease, from the initial simple asymptomatic form to the complicated symptomatic one. In this context, probiotics can modify gut microbial homeostasis with health benefits [2]. In fact, probiotics can have anti-inflammatory properties, maintaining an adequate bacterial colonization of the gut, with promising effects in the treatment of diverticular disease. In the last three decades, the value of the gut microbiota as a determinant of human health and disease has progressively grown [3]. Alterations in gut microbiota composition have proved to be responsible for the pathogenesis of many gastrointestinal diseases, including simple symptomatic diverticular disease.

E. Savarino (✉)
Department of Surgery, Oncology and Gastroenterology—DiSCOG,
University of Padua—Azienda Ospedale Università di Padova, Padova, Italy
e-mail: edoardo.savarino@unipd.it

V. Ojetti · A. Saviano
Emergency Department, Fondazione Policlinico Universitario A. Gemelli IRCCS,
Università Cattolica del Sacro Cuore, Rome, Italy
e-mail: veronica.ojetti@gmail.com; saviange@libero.it

© The Author(s), under exclusive license to Springer Nature Switzerland AG 2022
A. Tursi et al. (eds.), *Colonic Diverticular Disease*,
https://doi.org/10.1007/978-3-030-93761-4_20

Probiotics can exert significant regulatory functions and provide relevant gut microbial rebalance, thus reducing the inflammatory state, improving self-defenses against pathogens, and inhibiting the bacterial proliferation of the colon and the metabolism of pathogenic bacteria. In clinical practice, probiotics are useful for symptom control, reduction of blood markers of inflammation, and a more effective response to treatment. However, there are currently no "strong" and "standardized" recommendations for the use of probiotics in diverticular disease [3, 4], but more studies are needed to confirm these results.

In addition to a genetic predisposition to the development of colic diverticula, the risk factors for diverticular disease include a diet rich in refined foods (simple sugars, fats, etc.) and low in water-soluble fiber (fruit, vegetables, etc.), obesity, smoking, and reduction of intestinal motility and fecal volume with chronic constipation. These factors contribute to substantial changes in gut microbiota composition, leading to "dysbiosis". The latter is characterized by a reduction of the "healthy" bacterial flora and an increase of the "pathogenic" one, with the production of toxic substances for the intestinal mucosa, a greater exposure to invasion by pathogenic bacteria, and bacterial overgrowth. Furthermore, the reduction in fiber intake, a nutritional element for the intestinal microbiota, reduces the production of short-chain fatty acids (acetic acid, propionic acid, and butyric acid) and the gut barrier defenses and has a negative impact on immune system modulation (both local and systemic) [1]. In addition, intestinal dysbiosis is associated with alterations in gut motility, increase in intestinal permeability, exposure of the luminal bacterial antigens, production of toxins, and activation of the immune system with release of proinflammatory cytokines.

Literature studies have tried to characterize the "dysbiosis" of patients affected by diverticular disease through microbiome genome-wide association studies, polymerase chain reaction (PCR), and analysis of colonic biopsies, showing alterations in gut microbiota composition with a prevalence of *Fusobacterium*, *Clostridium*, *Bacteroides*, *Streptococci*, and some strains of *Bifidobacterium* (such as *Bifidobacterium animalis* and *Bifidobacterium longum*) in patients' stool. The detection of *Bifidobacterium longum* in PCR analysis of colonic mucosal biopsies reveals the deep disruption of the gut mucosa since it normally has anti-inflammatory properties in murine models of colitis. Typically, the healthy human gut microbiota composition is made up of *Bacteroidetes*, *Proteobacteria*, *Firmicutes*, *Verrucomicrobia*, and *Actinobacteria*. These bacteria produce short-chain fatty acids, increase the mucosal barrier, and control the immune system. Patients with diverticular disease showed a depletion of some *Bacteroides* strains such as *Bacteroides fragilis*, a reduction of *Collinsella* (*Collinsella stercoris* and *Collinsella aerofaciens*) with an overrepresentation of *Enterobacteriaceae* (as *Pseudomonas*), and a consequential mucosal inflammation. Moreover, patients with diverticular disease showed a mild increase of *Comamonadaceae* (phylum *Proteobacteria*) and an overgrowth of *Akkermansia muciniphila*, but its significance has not yet been clarified. *Akkermansia muciniphila* is involved in mucus metabolism, and an overexpression in diverticular disease can explain the increased mucus production, a sign of colonic inflammation because mucus can act as a defense barrier of the colonic mucosa and mucin can act as a metabolic substrate. With regard to fungi, patients with complicated diverticular disease show an enrichment of *Microbacteriaceae* and *Ascomycota* in colonic biopsies, confirming that the diverticulum microbiota can be different from the gut microbiota of the remaining intestinal mucosa [2–4]. Many studies supported the idea that the gut microbiota is involved in the progression of asymptomatic diverticulosis to diverticular disease and acute diverticulitis but not in diverticular pathogenesis. Interestingly, a recent study has reported that in a few cases, after fecal microbiota transplantation for *Clostridium difficile* infection, patients developed acute diverticulitis. This indicated the pivotal role of gut microbiota composition in the development of acute phases of diverticular disease. On the contrary, *Helicobacter pylori* infection seems to be protective against the onset of diverticular disease from asymptomatic diverticulosis.

Based on these findings, it is a shared opinion that modulation of the gut microbiota (which affects the turnover of the gastrointestinal epithelium, production of mucin, peristaltic activity, digestion of nutrients, pH, intestinal secretions, metabolism of drugs, etc.) could be useful in a more effective prevention and treatment of symptomatic, simple, or complicated forms of diverticular disease [1, 2].

20.2 Probiotics: Which, When, and How

Probiotics are defined as "live" microorganisms that, when administered in adequate quantities, can determine human health benefits (WHO definition). They are classified as single strains, multiple strains, or mixed with other substances. Probiotics are able to modulate the gut microbiota with positive effects on the gastrointestinal system. They protect against the invasion of pathogenic strains (by increasing the release of mucin and the production of short-chain fatty acids, by reducing intraluminal pH, or by contributing to the release of bacteriocin and defensin antibacterial substances, etc.); some of them stimulate the formation of intercellular epithelial junctions and adhesions (increasing *zonuline*, *occludin*, *claudin-1*, components of tight junctions), decreasing intestinal permeability and preventing bacterial colonization through competition with the adhesion sites of pathogens and with toxin receptors. Furthermore, probiotics are able to modulate the host's inflammatory and immune responses. Literature studies have shown how the use of probiotics helps to stimulate T lymphocytes and natural killer cells, with the production of anti-inflammatory cytokines (for example, IL-10, TGF-beta) and with the reduction of proinflammatory cytokines (for example, IL-12, IL-14, TNF-alpha, INF-alpha etc.). Some probiotics modulate the immune response by inducing the development of T-regulatory lymphocytes (T-regs) and the secretion of IgA. There are several microorganisms currently used as probiotics. They are named starting from the genus (for example, *Lactobacillus*) and then from the species (for example, *casei*). It is possible to add the "strain" in the denomination, to be more specific. With regard to this, it is important to remember that the probiotic properties are characteristic of a single strain and cannot be extended to other bacteria even if they belong to the same species. Even more importantly, a specific probiotic is effective in a specific disease and/or symptom but it cannot perform beneficial functions for all the other kinds of diseases for which it is not specific. Most probiotics are made up of *Lactobacilli* and *Bifidobacteria*, which are capable of producing lactic acid from various substrates (hence the name "lactic ferments") [5, 6]. Yeasts such as *Saccharomyces boulardii* can also be a probiotic. Alternatively, some microorganisms, such as *Bacillus clausii*, can be administered in the form of spores. The authorization and the use of probiotics are now based on some criteria such as identification, safety, and efficacy profiles. Good probiotics have some requirements. For example, they must survive both gastric juice and bile, adhere to the intestinal mucosa and colonize it (for now, research on mucoadhesion molecules is limited only to *Lactobacilli* probiotics), be able to be well-defined in the strain and concentration, and there must be scientific evidence regarding the effective dose and therapeutic indications. Some probiotics for which beneficial properties have been recognized include *Lactobacillus casei Shirota* studied for the prevention of gastrointestinal disorders and the maintenance of a balanced intestinal bacterial flora; *Lactobacillus acidophilus NCF01748* for the treatment of constipation and the prevention of diarrhea associated with radiotherapy; *Lactobacillus johnsonii La1* for increasing immune defenses, easy adherence to human intestinal cells, rebalancing of the intestinal bacterial flora, and improvement of *Helicobacter pylori* gastritis; *Lactobacillus rhamnosus GG* for the prevention of antibiotic-associated diarrhea, the treatment and prevention of rotavirus diarrhea and acute diarrhea, the treatment of recurrent *Clostridium difficile* diarrhea, and the improvement of symptoms in Crohn's disease. It has been well studied for intestinal immunity; it increases the number of IgA and other immunoglobulins in the intestinal mucosa. Moreover, *Lactobacillus reuteri* is effective in attenuating human inflammatory gastrointestinal diseases (such as infantile colic or *Helicobacter pylori* infection) [7–9]. Other studied probiotics include *Bifidobacterium bifidum* for rotavirus diarrhea and the rebalancing of intestinal bacterial flora after viral diarrhea, and *Saccharomyces boulardii* approved for the prevention of traveler's diarrhea and *Clostridium difficile* diarrhea, i.e., a specific strain for a specific disease [3, 4]. With regard to diverticular disease, a systematic review of 11 studies collected data about the use of probiotics in different phases of diverticular disease and provided evidences on the efficacy of probiotics in symptom control and in the prevention of acute diverticulitis. This review includes many strains of probiotics such as *Escherichia coli strain Nissle*, *Streptococcus thermophilus DSM 24731*, *Bifidobacterium (longum DSM 24736, breve DSM 24732, infantis DSM 24737)*, and *Lactobacillus* (*helveticus*, *acidophilus DSM 24735, plantarum DSM 24730, paracasei DSM 24733, paracasei F19, bulgaricus DSM 24734*). Probiotics have also increasingly gained prominence for gut neuromodulation. As described above, neuromuscular gut alterations due to age and genetic factors represent risk factors for symptomatic diverticular disease. The increased intraluminal pressure due to constipation related to motor abnormalities is responsible for diverticula inflammation and abdominal pain. The probiotic *Lactobacillus rhamnosus JB-1* has an inhibitory effect on visceral pain, acting on GABA receptors in mice models, whereas *Lactobacillus reuteri (DSM 17938)* shows beneficial effects on chronic constipation, decreasing methane (CH_4)

production by *Methanobrevibacter smithii*, with positive health effects on gut motility. These probiotics could be safe and effective in preventing symptomatic diverticular disease, but more data are needed to draw definitive conclusions [6, 7, 9].

20.3 Probiotics for Symptom Relief in SUDD

One-fifth of subjects with colonic diverticula may present with abdominal symptoms, such as recurrent abdominal pain or discomfort, changes in bowel habits, and bloating, in the absence of macroscopical alterations other than diverticula. This condition is termed "symptomatic uncomplicated diverticular disease" (SUDD), and it mimics the clinical picture associated with irritable bowel syndrome (IBS), although the abdominal pain associated with SUDD is typically localized in left iliac fossa and patients with SUDD usually experience diarrhea instead of constipation [1]. Moreover, they have more frequently long-lasting symptoms (over 24 h) and do not report relief after defecation or flatulence as compared to IBS subjects.

The main purpose in the management of SUDD is relief from abdominal symptoms. A standard therapeutic approach has not yet been established, but several dietary and pharmacological strategies have been proposed. In particular, given the key pathogenetic role of the gut microbiota [2, 3], different probiotics are able to change the gut microbial balance, thus leading to the study of health benefits (Table 20.1). In general, these probiotics showed anti-inflammatory effects with the capability to enhance anti-inflammatory defenses by maintaining an adequate bacterial colonization in the gastrointestinal tract and by inhibiting colonic bacterial overgrowth and metabolism of pathogens.

In a prospective open-label trial, Fric et al. [11] evaluated the effects of *Escherichia coli Nissle* in 15 patients with SUDD, demonstrating that this strain, characterized by anti-inflammatory properties, significantly prolonged the remission time and improved abdominal symptoms, including abdominal pain, irregular defecation, bloating, and excessive flatulence. Notably, this strain can colonize the human intestine and persists in the gut for about 2 weeks after its discontinuation. In a pilot study, Annibale et al. [17] investigated the effects of a 6-month cyclic therapy (14 days/month for 6 months) with *Lactobacillus paracasei sub. Paracasei F19* associated with a high-fiber diet versus a high-fiber diet alone. With the high-fiber diet, they reported a significant beneficial effect on symptoms, such as abdominal bloating and prolonged abdominal pain and on the quality of life, whereas the high-fiber diet alone seemed to be clinically ineffective, without improving the quality of life of the patients. Furthermore, no safety issues were raised by a prolonged administration of the probiotic. Another prospective, open-label, uncontrolled, pilot study has been performed by Tursi et al. [12] in 12 consecutive patients affected by SUDD. These patients underwent treatment with 10 mg/day of beclomethasone dipropionate (BDP) for 4 weeks, accompanied by a mix of probiotics (2.5 g/day) for 15 consecutive days, including 450 billion viable lyophilized bacteria of 4 strains of Lactobacillus (*Lactobacillus casei, Lactobacillus plantarum, Lactobacillus acidophilus*, and *Lactobacillus delbrueckii subsp. Bulgaricus)*, 3 strains of bifidobacterium

Table 20.1 Characteristics of the studies evaluating the use of probiotics in diverticular diseases

First author	Year of publication	No. of patients treated	Study design	Number of arms and treatment per arm	Type of diverticular disease
Giaccari S. [10]	1993	79	Open-label	1: Rifaximin + lactobacillus (strain not specified)	SUDD in Remission
Fric P. [11]	2003	15	Open-label	1: Dichlorchinolinol 2: Dichlorchinolinol + *E. coli* Nissle	SUDD
Tursi A. [12]	2005	12	Open-label	1: Beclomethasone dipropionate + VSL#3	SUDD
Tursi A. [13]	2006	85	Open, randomized	1: Mesalazine 2: *L. casei* DG 3: Mesalazine + *L. casei* DG	SUDD in Remission
Tursi A. [14]	2007	30	Open, randomized	1: Balsalazide + VSL#3 2: VSL#3	AUD in Remission
Tursi A. [15]	2008	75	Open, randomized	1: Mesalazine 800 mg 2: Mesalazine 1.6 g 3: Mesalazine 800 mg + *L. casei* DG 4: Mesalazine 1.6 g + *L. casei* DG 5: *Lactobacillus casei* DG	SUDD in Remission
Lamiki P. [16]	2010	46	Open-label	1: SCM-III symbiotic mixture	SUDD in Remission
Annibale B. [17]	2011	50	Open, randomized	1: High-fiber diet alone 2: Genefilus F19 2/die + high-fiber diet 3: Genefilus F19 4/die + high-fiber diet	SUDD
Lahner E. [18]	2012	45	Open, randomized	1: Lactobacillus paracasei B21060 + High-fiber 2: High-fiber diet alone	SUDD
Stollman N. [19]	2013	117	Double-blind, placebo-controlled	1: Placebo 2: Mesalamine 3: Mesalamine + Bifidobacterium Infantis 35,624	AUD in Remission

Tursi A. [20]	2013	210	Double-blind, placebo-controlled	1: Mesalazine 1.6 g + placebo 2: *L. casei* DG + placebo 3: *L. casei* DG 24 + mesalazine 4: Placebo	SUDD in Remission
Ojetti V. [5]	2016	20	Open, randomized	1: Ciprofloxacin + metronidazole + Probiotic mixture 2: Ciprofloxacin + metronidazole	AUD
Kvasnovsky [21]	2017	143	Double-blind, placebo-controlled	1: Probiotic mixture 2: Placebo	SUDD
Petruzziello C. [6]	2019	88	Double-blind, placebo-controlled	1: Ciprofloxacin + metronidazole + *L. reuteri* 4659 2: Ciprofloxacin + metronidazole + placebo	AUD
Petruzziello C. [22]	2019	84	Open-label, controlled trial	1: Ciprofloxacin + metronidazole + Bifidobacterium lactis LA 304, lactobacillus salivarius LA 302, lactobacillus acidophilus LA 201 2: Ciprofloxacin + metronidazole	AUD

(*Bifidobacterium longum*, *Bifidobacterium breve*, and *Bifidobacterium infantis*), and 1 strain of *Streptococcus salivarius subsp. Thermophilus*. In addition, patients were further treated with a half dosage of BDP for another 4 weeks and the mix of probiotics for another 15 days. In all, 11 of 12 (91.66%) patients completed the treatment, with 10 patients (per-protocol, 90.90%; on intention-to-treat, 83.33%) being asymptomatic already at the fourth and at the eighth week of treatment. It is of particular interest that endoscopic and histological scores also improved. A multicenter, 6-month, randomized, controlled, parallel-group intervention study by Lahner et al. [18] in 2012 investigated the efficacy of a symbiotic preparation containing *Lactobacillus paracasei B21060* in association with a high-fiber diet compared to a high-fiber diet alone, on abdominal symptoms in patients with SUDD. A total of 45 consecutive outpatients with SUDD were enrolled and randomized to two treatment arms. The main results showed that a high-fiber diet alone was effective on some abdominal symptoms, but the combination with a symbiotic preparation containing *Lactobacillus paracasei B21060* allowed a significant improvement of the therapeutic response after 3 and 6 months of treatment. Again, a significant regression of prolonged abdominal pain was found with the high-fiber diet alone, but this therapeutic response was greater with the combined treatment strategy. Finally, abdominal bloating was significantly reduced only in patients supplemented with the symbiotic treatment. A randomized, double-blind, placebo-controlled trial of a multistrain probiotic was conducted by Kvasnovsky et al. [21] in 143 patients suffering from SUDD. They were randomized to two arms, one with the supplementation of *Lactobacillus rhamnosus*, *Escherichia faecium*, *Lactobacillus acidophilus*, and *Lactobacillus plantarum* (1 mL/kg/day) and the other with placebo for 3 months. As a result, a significant decrease of some symptoms, including constipation, diarrhea, mucorrhea, and back pain, was found only in the group supplemented with probiotics, whereas abdominal pain was decreased in both groups without any significant difference.

In conclusion, supplementation with specific probiotic strains that have an anti-inflammatory effect could be useful for providing symptom relief in patients with SUDD, but more robust data are required to draw firm conclusions.

20.4 Probiotics for Maintaining Remission in SUDD

As for acute treatment of SUDD, data for maintaining remission in SUDD are limited and controversial. The main goal of therapy is to relieve symptoms and avoid progression to acute diverticulitis. To achieve this, the most commonly used drugs are represented by poorly absorbable antibiotics and/or mesalamine. However, recent studies have suggested that only 50% of the subjects taking these drugs are free of symptoms. Indeed, other pathophysiological factors, including visceral hypersensitivity, abnormal colonic motility, and/or altered intestinal microbiota concur in the development of gastrointestinal complaints in patients with SUDD. In particular, Tursi et al. conducted a prospective study evaluating the efficacy of mesalazine (1.6 g/die) and/or *Lactobacillus casei* (24 billion/die) in preventing recurrence of abdominal symptoms in 85 patients with SUDD, during a 12-month period of follow-up [20]. The authors observed that both mesalazine and *Lactobacillus casei* were effective in preventing the recurrence of SUDD, but their association seemed to be even stronger. In particular, *Lactobacillus casei* alone was able to maintain an excellent remission rate (76.7%) after 12 months of cyclic administration, but the combination of both mesalazine and *Lactobacillus casei* was superior (100%) than mesalazine (76.7%) or *Lactobacillus casei* alone (76.7%). The authors justified this high rate of success to the downregulation of the inflammatory cascade by the inhibition of several proinflammatory factors induced by mesalazine, whereas *Lactobacillus casei* acted by maintaining a balanced colonization in the gastrointestinal tract. Lamiki et al. conducted a prospective, randomized, open-label study evaluating the safety and effectiveness of a symbiotic mixture in preventing the recurrence of constipation related abdominal pain in patients with uncomplicated diverticular disease of the colon [16]. They also verified their survivability through genomic techniques. A total of 46 consecutive patients with SUDD completed the 6-month follow-up study, reporting, at different time points, the occurrence of constipation, diarrhea, and abdominal pain using a validated quantitative scale. After recruitment, patients were assigned to a treatment consisting of *Lactobacillus acidophilus*, *Lactobacillus helveticus*, and *Bifidobacterium spp.* together with a medium containing Urtica dioica, Ribes nigrum, Vaccinium myrtillus, Taraxacum officinale leaves and roots, Daucus carota, and Echinacea purpurea leaves and roots in a 10 mL liquid formulation, three times a day. The main result was that 68% of patients were completely free of symptoms 6 months after treatment start, and 78% of the patients reported that the treatment was "effective" or "very effective". The microbiological study showed that, as compared to baseline, this symbiotic mixture was able to achieve a significant increase in the Lactobacilli and Bifidobacteria count and a decrease in Clostridia in the faces. Genomic analysis confirmed the survivability of the ingested strain during the treatment period. Another study by Tursi et al. was conducted to assess the effectiveness of mesalazine and/or probiotics in maintaining remission in SUDD [13]. In this multicenter, double-blind, placebo-controlled trial, mesalazine (1.6 g/die) and/or probiotics (*Lactobacillus casei DG* 24 billion/die) were administered to 210 patients with SUDD for 10 days each month for 12 months. For comparison, a placebo group was also included. The authors found that *Lactobacillus casei DG* was significantly better than placebo for maintaining SUDD remission, but the combination of mesalazine and probiotics was even superior. Moreover, both treatments, alone or in combination, were significantly better than placebo for preventing the occurrence of acute diverticulitis. Furthermore, Tursi et al., in an open-label, pilot trial published in 2007, enrolled 30 patients with SUDD and randomized them to receive balsalazide 2.25 g daily for 10 days every month plus a mixture of *Streptococcus thermophilus*, *Bifidobacterium breve*, *Bifidobacterium longum*, *Bifidobacterium infantis*, *Lactobacillus acidophilus*, *Lactobacillus plantarum*, *Lactobacillus paracasei*, and *Lactobacillus delbrueckii*, 450 billion/day for 15 days every month or the mixture of probiotics alone, 450 billion/day for 15 days every month [14]. The primary end point was the maintenance of remission after an episode of acute diverticulitis throughout a 12-month follow-up. The main result was that more than half of the patients in both groups were free of abdominal symptoms at the end of follow-up and that probiotics alone determined the complete disappearance of gastrointestinal symptoms in 60% of the patients. In contrast, in 2013, Stollman et al. [19] performed a randomized, controlled study using mesalamine and *Bifidobacterium infantis 35,624* for 12 weeks. They enrolled 117 patients divided into 3 arms: (1) probiotics plus mesalamine (2.4 daily); (2) mesalamine alone (2.4 g daily); and (3) placebo. Overall, mesalamine alone showed a trend in reducing symptoms, but adding probiotics did not result in a significant clinical benefit.

In conclusion, the use of probiotics with an anti-inflammatory effect alone or in association with anti-inflammatory drugs such as mesalazine or balsalazide seems to be effective in favoring the maintenance of remission in patients with SUDD.

20.5 Probiotics and Acute Diverticulitis

Acute diverticulitis (AD) is an inflammatory condition affecting at least one colonic diverticulum, often associated with pericolonic inflammation. Abdominal pain in the left lower quadrant, fever, and leukocytosis are the main symptoms. Contrast-enhanced computerized tomography (CT) is considered as the gold standard since it offers a more comprehensive evaluation of the uncomplicated and complicated forms according to the modified Hinchey's criteria [1]. The most important risk factors associated with the development of diverticulitis are smoking, reduction of physical activity, dietary habits, and, especially, fiber consumption. In the past few years, antibiotics were considered mandatory in the treatment of AD, even in mild cases, because of its belief that diverticulitis was due to obstruction of a diverticulum leading to mucosal abrasions, microperforation, and bacterial translocation [23]. Recent hypotheses have highlighted that AD may be due to an inflammatory process rather than an infectious condition. Recent studies on acute uncomplicated diverticulitis (AUD) have demonstrated the presence of an altered composition of the gut microbiota, with a reduction of taxa with anti-inflammatory activity, such as *Clostridium cluster IV*, *Lactobacilli*, and *Bacteroides* and an increase in *Enterobacteriaceae* and *Streptococcus*. This "dysbiosis" could be linked to the development of mucosal inflammation, altered activation of gastroenteric nerve fibers, and consequent alteration in intestinal motility with development of abdominal symptoms.

Moreover, the "dysmotility" is connected to the "bacterial translocation" from the diverticular lumen to the perivisceral area with a possible activation of cellular Toll-like receptors (TLRs) and tissue inflammation. The intestinal microbiota has a key role in regulating immune/anti-inflammatory activity, improving immune tolerance, and stimulating the expression of T-regulatory cells (T-regs), lymphocyte regulators of immunity [1]. This regulatory activity has been mainly observed in *Bacteroides fragilis* and in some species of *Clostridium*. The reduction of these microbial species with anti-inflammatory activity may be responsible, together with other factors (the presence of diverticula, diet, genetic predisposition, connective alterations, fecal stasis), for the development of symptomatic diverticular diseases. Restoration of a more balanced composition of the intestinal microbiota, with a "renewed" bacterial colonization obtained with the use of probiotic strains, can potentially have beneficial effects on health [2]. A meta-analysis published in 2015 showed that probiotics are effective in treating irritable bowel syndrome with remission of abdominal symptoms [24]. In simple symptomatic diverticular disease, the number of studies is lower yet compared to those in irritable bowel syndrome. A review of the literature that collected 11 articles (in a time period of 20 years) for a total of 760 patients with abdominal diverticular disease symptoms failed to draw conclusions about the efficacy of the use of probiotics due to the heterogeneity of the studies, in which different probiotic bacterial strains with different dosages and for different treatment periods had been used. In addition, patients were often treated with antibiotics and/or anti-inflammatory agents [7]. The most frequently used strain was *Lactobacilli*; meanwhile, *Bifidobacteria* or other probiotic strains were less used. Knowing the mechanisms through which the gut microbiota has a role in determining the "health status", it is easier to understand the potential beneficial effect of some probiotic strains. The gut microbiota, for example, modulates the immune response through the production of short-chain fatty acids (SCFAs). In fact, when fibers are ingested and digested, bacteria produce a wide range of short-chain fatty acids, such as butyrate, which is able to modulate the expression of histone deacetylase directly, thereby increasing the expression of T-reg lymphocytes. Moreover, the gut microbiota acts as a physical barrier against pathogens and as a "chemical" barrier (for the production of antimicrobial substances), thus preventing them from overcoming the intestinal mucosa and from spreading at a systemic level. In addition, beneficial bacterial species compete for nutrients by reducing the growth of other pathogenic microorganisms [2, 3]. This microbial diversity may be responsible for the onset of diverticular disease symptoms, but how the microbiota can determine diverticular inflammation is not entirely clear. However, patients with recurrent episodes of symptomatic diverticular disease not susceptible to surgery have been treated successfully with microbiota transplantation. In addition, rifaximin, which has a positive effect on reducing excessive growth of *Roseburia*, *Veillonella*, *Streptococcus*, and *Haemophilus* and on increasing other species such as *Akkermansia*, has been successfully used in some studies on diverticular disease. Some specific probiotics such as *Lactobacillus salivarius*, *Lactobacillus acidophilus*, *Bifidobacterium lactis*, and *Lactobacillus reuteri 4659* have been proven to have an important anti-inflammatory effect in vitro, thus suggesting a possible role in AD [3]. *Lactobacillus reuteri* is one of the most studied probiotics in humans. There are different strains on the market with specific characteristics of action. Strain 4659 has been shown to have a powerful anti-inflammatory action on inhibiting experimental colitis, by modulating TLR-4 and NF-κB. It also reduces the levels of proinflammatory cytokines such as tumor necrosis factor alpha (TNF-α). This indicates the therapeutic potential of *Lactobacillus reuteri strain 4659* in inflammatory diseases of the intestine. In 2019, Ojetti et al. [6] published a double-blind, randomized, controlled trial on the efficacy of *Lactobacillus reuteri 4659* supplementations during an acute attack of uncomplicated diverticulitis. The 88 patients who met the inclusion criteria were randomly assigned to 2 groups; the first one received standard antibiotic therapy, consisting of ciprofloxacin 400 mg twice a day and metronidazole 500 mg three times a day for 7 days, with supplementation of the probiotic *Lactobacillus reuteri* 4659 twice a day for 10 days. The other group received the same standard antibiotic therapy and a matching placebo for the same periods. They showed for the first time in real life that the use of this particular strain of *Lactobacillus reuteri* is able to significantly reduce the CRP values compared with placebo after 3 days of treatment. This also led to a significant reduction in abdominal pain. In particular, the mean delta reduction in abdominal pain from day 1 to day 3 was 4.5 VAS points in the *Lactobacillus reuteri* group, compared with 2.3 in the placebo group ($p < 0.0001$). With the early reduction in the inflammatory index and reduction in abdominal pain, patients were quickly discharged from hospital [6]. The possible mechanism underlying this phenomenon could be, on one side, the expression of mucus adhesins that exert this specific strain and, on the other side, the immunoregulatory effects in the gut through modulating the Th1-promoting capacity of dendritic cells upon interaction with C-type lectins. These mucus adhesins also mediate both anti-inflammatory and proinflammatory effects by induction of interleukin-10 (IL-10), TNF-α, IL-1β, IL-6, and IL-12 cytokines. To confirm these data, the same authors tested the efficacy of a mix of three probiotic strains (*Bifidobacterium lactis LA 304*, *Lactobacillus salivarius LA 302*, and *Lactobacillus acidophilus LA 201*) [22] administered in association with conventional antibiotics for the treatment of AUD compared to conventional antibiotics used alone. The interventional group was treated with ciprofloxacin 400 mg twice a day and metronidazole 500 mg three times a day for 1 week and was simultaneously supplemented with the probiotic mix, 1 sachet twice a day for 10 days. The control group received the same antibiotic treatment without the probiotic mix. With regard to abdominal pain, the group who received the supplementation showed a significant decrease of 4.06 points (51.4%) in the VAS score on day 3, compared to a decrease of 2.79 points (34.9%) in the other group. With regard to inflammation, the supplemented group showed a decrease in CRP value of 64%, compared to a decrease of only 35% in the other. This led to a significantly shorter hospitalization (89 h; 3.7 days) of the supplemented group compared to 101 h (4.2 days) of the other group ($p = 0.03$) [22].

In IBD patients, Foligne et al. [25] proved that *Lactobacillus salivarius Ls33* and *Lactobacillus acidophilus NCF* are two of the three best-performing probiotics in terms of increased induction of the anti-inflammatory cytokine IL-10 and reduced induction of the pro-inflammatory cytokine IL-12. The same strains both in vitro and in vivo improve the recovery of inflamed tissues in a rat colitis model. Moreover, the combination of the two strains had better properties than those of the strains taken separately when it came to modulating TLR-2-mediated NF-κB and MAPK signaling pathways involved in IBD-related inflammation. Abdominal pain is the main symptom in patients with AUD, and it seems to be related to visceral hypersensitivity. Recent studies have reported that the gut microbiota influences the visceral perception of pain, thus suggesting a new approach for the treatment of this condition. It has been speculated that some probiotics may have an impact on the gut epithelial cells' expression of receptors that locally modulate the transmission of nociception to the intestinal nervous system. *Lactobacillus acidophilus* and

Lactobacillus salivarius strains were able to induce a higher in vitro expression of opioid and cannabinoid receptors, respectively, on gut epithelial cells, thus indicating that they are better strains for facilitating pain relief. Moreover, in a murine model, these strains showed an analgesic effect similar to that of morphine. Based on these considerations on the beneficial immunomodulatory effects and potentially analgesic properties, it is easy to understand why the authors chose this combination. It would therefore seem that restoring the use of probiotics in "beneficial" microbial species can maintain and restore gastrointestinal homeostasis, with functions of the "barrier" against pathogens and reduction of inflammation. The latter seems to be the key point; in particular, probiotic species such as *Bifidobacterium adolescentis*, *Phascolarctobacterium*, and *Akkermansia muciniphila* are capable of reducing the level of C-reactive protein, IL-6, and tumor necrosis factor (TNF), the direct damage caused by the activation of inflammasomes, and the production of proinflammatory interleukins IL-1 and IL-18 [8, 9]. Moreover, some cell wall components of *Lactobacilli* and *Bifidobacteria*, like lipoteichoic acid, stimulate the synthesis of nitric oxide, which is fundamental in the mechanisms regulating cell death after pathogen infection. In addition, nitric oxide acts on some TLRs that are involved in phagocytosis. Probiotics have also been shown to interact with enterocytes, Th1, Th2, T-regs, and intestinal dendritic cells, thus regulating the adaptive immunity in the attack against pathogens that can damage the intestinal mucosa and cause local inflammation. In animal models of rat colitis, the administration of *Lactobacillus salivarius Ls33* produced positive results in the recovery of local tissue inflammation, with increased anti-inflammatory cytokines such as IL-10 and the decrease of proinflammatory ones such as IL-12 [25]. When the intestinal barrier is damaged, it itself produces proinflammatory cytokines of "alarm" that contribute to local inflammation. In conclusion, supplementation with specific probiotic strains that exhibit an anti-inflammatory effect is useful during an acute attack of uncomplicated diverticulitis accelerating the reduction of the CRP level and gastrointestinal symptoms, thus reducing the length of hospital stay with a huge impact on the overall cost reduction.

20.6 Conclusions

Colonic diverticular disease is an extremely common acquired condition in which several pathogenic factors may be implicated, including dysbiosis. Changes in microbiota composition with a reduction of taxa with anti-inflammatory activity and an increase in proinflammatory bacteria have been observed during the acute phase of inflammation. A vicious cycle could start from mucosal inflammation to dysbiosis at the same time. Translocation of bacteria to perivisceral fat activates the TLRs with a subsequent inflammatory reaction at the level of the perivisceral tissues.

Moreover, an alteration in the gut microbiota can lead to an altered activation of nerve fibers and subsequent neuronal and muscular dysfunction, thus favoring abdominal symptom development. It is easy to understand how the use of probiotics could be useful for restoring a healthy colonic microenvironment in patients with

DD. In this chapter, we analyze data on the efficacy of probiotic therapies in different phases of DD, such as SUDD, and maintenance of remission in SUDD and AUD. Probiotics [4, 7, 9], in this context, could contribute to "strengthen" the intestinal barrier (also through the stimulation of cell adhesion proteins), reducing the damage and risk of complications (microperforation) in diverticular disease. In addition, intestinal bacterial flora mediates the interaction and communication between immunity and the intestinal barrier, thus restoring a healthy microenvironment in the colon, which on the contrary, is often altered in uncomplicated symptomatic diverticular disease. Supplementation with specific probiotic strains that have an anti-inflammatory effect could be useful for providing symptom relief in patients with SUDD, but more robust data are required to draw firm conclusions. The use of probiotics alone or in association with anti-inflammatory drugs such as mesalazine or balsalazide seems to be effective in maintaining remission in patients with SUDD. During an acute attack of uncomplicated diverticulitis, supplementation with specific probiotic strains that exhibit an anti-inflammatory effect is useful in accelerating the reduction of the CRP level and gastrointestinal symptoms, thus reducing the length of hospital stay with a huge impact on the overall cost reduction. In conclusion, despite the importance of the results obtained, the role of probiotics in different phases of DD is still to be fully understood, in particular, whether a beneficial effect of a specific probiotic therapy is related to a definite change in the gut microbiota composition. For these reasons, new randomized, controlled placebo studies including a larger number of patients are now needed to unequivocally demonstrate the actual role of each probiotic strain in different manifestations of DD.

References

1. Tursi A, Scarpignato C, Strate LL, et al. Colonic diverticular disease. Nat Rev Dis Primers. 2020;6:20.
2. Ticinesi A, Nouvenne A, Corrente V, et al. Diverticular disease: a gut microbiota perspective. J Gastrointestin Liver Dis. 2019;3:327–37.
3. Piccioni A, Franza L, et al. Gut microbiota and acute diverticulitis: role of probiotics in Management of this Delicate Pathophysiological Balance. J Pers Med. 2021;11:298.
4. Lahner E, Annibale B. Probiotics and diverticular disease evidence based? J Clin Gastroenterol. 2016;50:S159–60.
5. Ojetti V, Petruzziello C, Sinatti D, et al. The efficacy of Lactibiane IKI (BifidobacteriumLactis LA 304, lactobacillus Salivarius LA 302, lactobacillus acidophilus LA 201) in reducing abdominal symptoms and inflammatory biomarkers in acute uncomplicated. Diverticulitis J Clin Gastroenterol. 2016;50:S110.
6. Petruzziello C, Migneco A, Cardone S, et al. Supplementation with lactobacillus reuteri ATCC PTA 4659 in patients affected by acute uncomplicated diverticulitis: a randomized double-blind placebo-controlled trial. Int J Color Dis. 2019;34:1087.
7. Lahner E, Bellisario C, Hassan C, et al. Probiotics in the treatment of diverticular disease. A systematic review. J Gastrointestin Liver Dis. 2016;25:79–86.
8. Carabotti M, Annibale B. Treatment of diverticular disease: an update on latest evidence and clinical implications. Drugs in Context. 2018;7:212526.
9. Ojetti V, Petruzziello C, Cardone S, et al. The use of probiotics in different phases of diverticular disease. Rev Recent Clin Trials. 2018;13:89–96.

10. Giaccari S, Tronci S, Falconieri M, et al. Long-term treatment with rifaximin and lactobacilli in post-diverticulitic stenoses of the colon. Riv Eur Sci Med Farmacol. 1993;15:29–34.
11. Fric P, Zavoral M. The effect of non-pathogenic Escherichia coli in symptomatic uncomplicated diverticular disease of the colon. Eur J Gastroenterol Hepatol. 2003;15:313–5.
12. Tursi A, Brandimarte G, Giorgetti GM, et al. Beclomethasone dipropionate plus VSL#3 for the treatment of mild to moderate diverticular colitis: an open, pilot study. J Clin Gastroenterol. 2005;39:644–5.
13. Tursi A, Giorgetti GM, Brandimarte G, et al. Beclomethasone dipropionate for the treatment of mild-to-moderate Crohn's disease: an open-label, budesonide-controlled, randomized study. Med Sci Monit. 2006;12:PI29–32.
14. Tursi A, Brandimarte G, Giorgetti GM, et al. Balsalazide and/or high-potency probiotic mixture (VSL#3) in maintaining remission after attack of acute, uncomplicated diverticulitis of the colon. Int J Colorectal Dis. 2007;22:1103–8.
15. Tursi A, Brandimarte G, Giorgetti GM, et al. Mesalazine and/or Lactobacillus casei in maintaining long-term remission of symptomatic uncomplicated diverticular disease of the colon. Hepatogastroenterology. 2008;55(84):916–20.
16. Lamiki P, Tsuchiya J, Pathak S, et al. Probiotics in diverticular disease of the colon: an open label study. J Gastrointestin Liver Dis. 2010;19:31–6.
17. Annibale B, Maconi G, Lahner E, et al. Efficacy of Lactobacillus paracasei sub. paracasei F19 on abdominal symptoms in patients with symptomatic uncomplicated diverticular disease: a pilot study. Minerva Gastroenterol Dietol. 2011;57:13–22.
18. Lahner E, Esposito G, Zullo A, et al. High-fibre diet and Lactobacillus paracasei B21060 in symptomatic uncomplicated diverticular disease. World J Gastroenterol. 2012;18:5918–24.
19. Stollman N, Magowan S, Shanahan F, et al. A randomized controlled study of mesalamine after acute diverticulitis: results of the DIVA trial. J Clin Gastroenterol. 2013;47(7):621–9.
20. Tursi A, Brandimarte G, Elisei W, et al. Randomised clinical trial: mesalazine and/or probiotics in maintaining remission of symptomatic uncomplicated diverticular disease--a double-blind, randomised, placebo-controlled study. Aliment Pharmacol Ther. 2013;38:741–51.
21. Kvasnovsky CL, Bjarnason I, Donaldson AN, et al. A randomized double-blind placebo-controlled trial of a multi-strain probiotic in treatment of symptomatic uncomplicated diverticular disease. Inflammopharmacology. 2017.
22. Petruzziello C, Marannino M, Migneco A, et al. The efficacy of a mix of three probiotic strains in reducing abdominal pain and inflammatory biomarkers in acute uncomplicated diverticulitis.Eur Rev Med Pharmacol Sci. 2019;23:9126–33.
23. Peery AF, Shaukat A, Strate LL. AGA Clinical Practice Update on Medical Management of Colonic Diverticulitis: Expert Review. Gastroenterology. 2021;160:906-911.
24. Didari T, Mozaffari S, Nikfar S, et al. Effectiveness of probiotics in irritable bowel syndrome: Updated systematic review with meta-analysis. World J Gastroenterol. 2015;21:3072–84.
25. Foligne, Nutten, Grangette, et al. Correlation between in vitro and in vivo immunomodulatory properties of lactic acid bacteria. World J Gastroenterol. 2007;13:236–43.

Other Treatments

21

Akira Mizuki, Alexandre Ferreira Bafutto, and Eduardo Ferreira Bafutto

Diverticulosis of the colon is the most frequent anatomical alteration of the colon in developed countries, and the highest rates occur in the United States and Europe. Approximately 60% of individuals over the age of 60 living in industrialized countries will develop colonic diverticula [1]. When diverticulosis becomes symptomatic, it is called "diverticular disease" (DD), a term generally including symptomatic uncomplicated diverticular disease (SUDD) and acute diverticulitis (AD) [2, 3].

DD is likely to occur in 10–25% of that population [4]. Complications of diverticulitis can be serious and life-threatening, including bowel perforation, abscess, fistula, bleeding, and stricture leading to obstruction. Surgical intervention may be warranted and can range from endoscopic or percutaneous procedures to laparoscopic and open surgery. At present, this condition ranks as the fifth most important gastrointestinal disease in terms of direct and indirect costs [5, 6].

Although the pathogenesis and management of diverticulosis and DD remain uncertain, new hypotheses and observations are changing the pharmacological and surgical management of DD. Developing an effective method of diagnosis, treatment, and prevention of DD, SUDD, and diverticulitis could lead to a significant reduction in morbidity, mortality, and also medical burden.

A. Mizuki (✉)
Department of Internal Medicine, Tokyo Sea Fort Square Clinic, Tokyo, Japan
e-mail: amizuki2@yahoo.co.jp

A. F. Bafutto
Department of Surgery, Hospital da Santa Casa de Misericórdia de São Paulo, São Paulo, Brazil
e-mail: abafutto@gmail.com

E. F. Bafutto
Department of Internal Medicine, Division of Gastroenterology and Endoscopy, Hospital Estadual Geral de Goiânia Dr. Alberto Rassi, Goiânia, Brazil
e-mail: eduardobafutto@outlook.com

© The Author(s), under exclusive license to Springer Nature Switzerland AG 2022

A. Tursi et al. (eds.), *Colonic Diverticular Disease*,
https://doi.org/10.1007/978-3-030-93761-4_21

SUDD is defined as the concomitant presence of diverticula accompanied by symptoms of abdominal pain and bloating, bowel habit changes that include diarrhea and constipation, or a mixed bowel habit, in the absence of macroscopic inflammation [7, 8]. The severity and frequency of symptoms may have an impact on daily activities and severely affect quality of life [9], which can be assessed with the DD-specific DV-QOL survey [10]. Whereas the exact etiology is not certain, a number of aspects of this condition have been investigated.

Treatments of SUDD by a high-fiber diet, anti-inflammatory agents, and probiotics have been discussed in a previous chapter. In this chapter, we discuss the probability of other treatments, (traditional herbal medicines, butyrate, curcuma, etc.) for SUDD and also DD.

21.1 Traditional Herbal Medicines

Worldwide, modern health-care systems are increasingly putting the spotlight on integrative health-care modalities that incorporate ancient wisdom. This movement started in both the United Kingdom and the United States as "alternative medicine." As alternative health-care modalities became more prevalent, the descriptive term changed to "complementary medicine" or "complementary and alternative medicine" (CAM). Now, due to further incorporation of such practices, the more frequently used term is "integrative medicine." Kampo medicine or Japanese traditional medicine is integrative as it has been used by Western physicians in addition to conventional medicine.

After ancient Chinese medicine was introduced in Japan about 1500 years ago, it fused with the natural features and culture of Japan, traced a unique course of development that was free of interference from other countries, and became accepted among the people of Japan as "Japanese herbal medicine" (JHM) or "Kampo medicine." An emerging therapeutic target for this class of medicine is colonic diverticular disease. Since conventional pharmacology has been either poorly effective or associated with adverse events, the use of complementary and alternative medicine (CAM) including herbal medicines is gaining appeal for use in clinical practice.

Worldwide, many traditional medicine systems (TMSs) are used, including the Chinese traditional medicine, Indian Ayurvedic medicine, and the popular Unani medicine of Arab cultures. Many other indigenous traditional medicine systems have also been developed in the past by African, Asian, Arabic, Pacific, American, and also some other cultures. The theory and application of these traditional medicine systems differ significantly from those of well-developed allopathic medicines [11]. Today, the increasing demands for use of traditional herbal therapies, more likely based on the good past experiences of the effectiveness and safety of these herbal medicines, still require positive research evidence, and, so, recent developments in the biological and analytical sciences, along with innovations in proteomics and genomics, surely can play a dominant role in the validation of traditional herbal medicines, to further improve their quality, safety, and efficacy with clinic-based evidence [12, 13].

Misawa et al. [14] conducted a well-designed randomized trial ($n = 10$) to determine the efficacy of daiobotampito extracts for treating AD.

They conducted a single-center, open-label, prospective study. In all, 10 patients who suffered from diverticulitis of the colon were recruited. The patients were treated with fasting, antibacterial agents, and daiobotampito extracts (TJ-33; Tsumura & Co, Tokyo, Japan) for 10 days in or out of hospital. The patients individually recorded their body temperature, grade of abdominal pain, number of times that analgesics were used, and number of stools daily. They checked whether the patients had adverse reactions such as abdominal pain or diarrhea. No patients experienced serious adverse reactions. One patient had moderate abdominal pain and diarrhea soon after daiobotampito intake. This patient discontinued daiobotampito on day 4, and the pain and diarrhea quickly resolved. The abdominal pain of this patient was worse 6 days before treatment, and the pain was almost relieved with initial daiobotampito treatment. Daiobotampito seems to be a safe treatment option for early-stage AD.

Both diverticular bleeding (DB) and AD show high recurrence rates [15, 16]. The establishment of optimal strategies that prevent the recurrence of DB and AD is a major concern among gastroenterologists.

Mizuki et al. [17] conducted a large (n = 161) and well-designed randomized trial to determine the efficacy of burdock tea for the prevention of DB and AD recurrences.

Newly diagnosed patients with DB (n = 91) or AD (n = 70) were randomly assigned to two groups. The experimental group received 1.5 g of burdock tea three times a day (burdock tea 1.5 g, t.i.d.; Ahjikan, Co., Ltd., Hiroshima, Japan), whereas the control group did not receive any treatment. The median (interquartile) range of observation for the recurrence of DB or AD was 22.0 (14.1) and 30.3 (18.6) months, respectively. The burdock tea treatment showed significant preventive effects on recurrence of AD. A lower AD recurrence rate (5/47 (10.6%) vs. 14/44 (31.8%)) and longer recurrence-free duration was observed in the burdock tea group (59.3 months (95% CI 54.0–64.7) vs. 45.1 months (95% CI 37.1–53.0) by the Kaplan–Meier analysis; p = 0.012 by log-rank test) than in the control group, although there were no significant preventive effects on the DB recurrence. This randomized clinical trial demonstrated that daily intake of burdock tea could be an effective strategy for prevention of AD recurrence but not for CDB recurrence.

Burdock (scientific name: Arctium lappa) is a plant, which is widely used in Asian medicine as a diuretic antipyretic tea that assists in treating hypertension, gout, hepatitis, and other inflammatory disorders [18, 19]. Pharmacological studies have indicated that burdock roots promote antimicrobial, anti-inflammatory, and free radical scavenging activity as they contain multiple polyphenols [18–20]. Recently, Lee et al. [21] have reported that burdock roasting tea has high antioxidant properties. In addition, tea is the easiest way to consume health-promoting components from whole foods, containing a combination of multiple polyphenols [22]. This study showed that all participants demonstrate high compliance (more than 95%), indicating that consumption of burdock tea is possible in the long term. Thus, burdock tea could actually be a potent strategy for prevention against recurrence of AD (Table 21.1).

Table 21.1 Treatment of diverticular disease

Traditional herbal medicines may be able to treat diverticulitis and prevent diverticular recurrence
Microencapsulated sodium butyrate may prevent diverticular recurrence
Curcumin and Boswellia phytosome extracts may provide relief from SUDD pain
Nutraceutical formulation may provide relief from SUDD pain and bloating

21.2 Microencapsulated Sodium Butyrate (MSB)

Krokowicz et al. [23] conducted a well-designed randomized trial ($n = 52$) to determine the efficacy of microencapsulated sodium butyrate (MSB) for the prevention of AD.

A total of 73 patients with diverticulosis (diagnosed at colonoscopy and/or barium enema and/or CT colonography) were recruited for the study and randomized. The investigated group was administered MSB 300 mg daily, and the control group was administered placebo. After 12 months, a total of 52 patients (30 subjects and 22 controls) completed the study and were subjected to analysis. During the study, the number of episodes of diverticulitis (symptomatic diagnosis with acute pain, fever, and leukocytosis), hospitalizations, and surgery performed for diverticulitis were recorded. Additionally, a questionnaire regarding the subjective improvement of symptoms reflected the changes in quality of life during the analysis. After 12 months, the study group noted a significantly decreased number of diverticulitis episodes in comparison to those in the control group. The subjective quality of life in the study group was higher than that in the control group. There were no side effects of MSB during the therapy.

MSB reduces the frequency of diverticulitis episodes, is safe, and improves the quality of life. It can play a role in the prevention of diverticulitis. Although there is no certainty as to what renders sodium butyrate (SB) to be so beneficial in such a wide range of colonic diseases, it has been established that SB can act as a regulator of the intestinal environment. It is a preferred energy substrate for colonocytes, can moderate intestinal permeability, reduce oxidative stress, and reinforce the colonic defense barrier, leading to decreased inflammation of the mucosa, increased cell regeneration rate, and promote healing [24–26]. What prompted the authors to study the efficacy of SB for diverticulitis was the lack of side effects of SB [27, 28] and the similarities between diverticulitis and irritable bowel syndrome for which SB has been shown to be effective, such as the presence of abnormal colonic motility, visceral hypersensitivity, the presence of low-grade inflammation, and increased circulating levels of either substance P or vasoactive intestinal polypeptide [29, 30]. They utilized a microencapsulated form of SB to maximize the biological effect on the colon. Unprotected forms of SB induce fast absorption in the small bowel, thus preventing its passage to the large intestine where local release of SB seems to be of most benefit. They utilized a unique lipid membrane microencapsulation, designed to release SB distal from the ileocecal region and used successfully in previous studies [31]. Other formulas to release SB in the colon have been used, including hydroxypropyl methylcellulose and shellac coating [32] (Table 21.1).

21.3 Curcumin and Boswellia Phytosome (CBP) Extracts

The efficacy of Boswellia extracts in the treatment of SUDD symptoms was previously hypothesized by Tursi et al. They positively treated a group of patients with an association of natural active ingredients, including B. serrata, inulin, niacin, cranberry, vitamins B1, B2, B6, and B12, zinc, and folic acid [33]. The anti-inflammatory effect of the association of curcumin and Boswellia extracts supplemented as CBP would mimic the anti-inflammatory activity revealed for mesalazine that has been shown to be better than placebo in reducing symptoms in patients with SUDD [34].

Giacosa al [35]. conducted a well-designed randomized trial ($n = 52$) to determine the efficacy of curcumin and Boswellia phytosome (CBP) extracts for the treatment of symptomatic SUDD.

In a 30-day, one-group longitudinal explanatory study, patients (men and women) were treated with an innovative association of CBP-standardized extracts (500 mg b.i.d.). Treatment of SUDD with the association of CBP was followed by a significant decrease in abdominal pain ($p < 0.0001$). The study group showed that the CBP supplementation was efficacious within 10 days and that the efficacy was maintained almost constantly until the 30th day of intervention.

A phytosome of curcumin and Boswellia extracts may be useful in relief from SUDD pain. However, controlled studies should be conducted for final conclusions to be drawn. Bafutto et al. [36] treated 12 patients with SUDD with 2 g of curcumin for 30 days with a significant reduction in the abdominal pain intensity. Moreover, these authors showed a reduction in abdominal distension and in fecal calprotectin levels.

C. longa L. is a perennial herb plant widespread in Southeast Asia and is extensively cultivated in China, India, Indonesia, and Thailand. The active components of the roots are three curcuminoids: curcumin, demethoxycurcumin, and bisdemethoxycurcumin. These curcuminoids are linked to the important physiological and biological effects of curcumin, acting as effective anti-inflammatory agents with multiple activities, including antioxidant and metabolic modulation. The effects of curcumin have been well demonstrated in several clinical studies, showing effectiveness in inflammatory bowel disease (IBD), arthritis, prediabetes, and in the early stages of some cancers [37]. A recent meta-analysis on 15 randomized clinical trials has shown that curcumin downregulates inflammation and oxidation products by decreasing the levels of IL-6, high-sensitivity C-reactive protein, and malondialdehyde [38]. Experimental studies in animal models of IBD demonstrated that treatment with curcumin may decrease TNF-α, an inflammatory cytokine associated with IBD as well as with diverticular disease and acute diverticulitis [39, 40]. It is well known that curcumin has a low human bioavailability, and, to explore its clinical potential effects and overcome this issue, several formulations have been developed, including the application of food-grade phytosome technology. Comparison studies have shown that a curcumin phytosome significantly ameliorates the bioavailability of curcuminoids in the plasma and in the intestinal mucosa [41, 42]. In addition, curcumin phytosome administration also shows a protective effect toward gastrointestinal barrier damage [43].

Oleo gum resins from B. serrata Roxb. ex Colebr have been used in traditional medicines in India and Africa as a remedy to cure various inflammatory diseases [44]. Preclinical and clinical studies showed interesting data on the effects of B. serrata extracts and their active components, boswellic acids [45–47]. However, pharmacokinetic studies revealed low and erratic systemic absorption of boswellic acids in animals and humans. To improve the bioavailability of Boswellia, a lecithin-based (phytosome) delivery form of standardized B. serrata extracts has been developed, showing the optimization of boswellic acid delivery in healthy volunteers [48]. The Boswellia phytosome was shown to be effective and safe in the management of gut discomforts such as IBS and in attenuating symptoms associated with mild ulcerative colitis in remission, thereby reducing the need for drugs and medical consultations [49–51]. In combination with curcumin, Boswellia was shown to inhibit the production of inflammatory cytokines, IL-6, IL-8, TNF-α, and reactive oxygen species in vitro [27] in a clinical study for joint health [52] (Table 21.1).

21.4 Nutraceutical Formulation

D'Amico et al. [53] conducted a large ($n = 101$) and well-designed trial to determine the efficacy of a new nutraceutical formulation, DIVER-100®, for SUDD symptoms.

A prospective observational study was conducted to evaluate the efficacy of DIVER-100® in consecutive patients with SUDD, confirmed by radiology or endoscopy. All patients were treated with DIVER-100®, 2 capsules/day, 10 days a month for 3 months. The primary end point was the clinical remission rate, defined as the reduction of abdominal pain and bloating, improvement of bowel habits, and prevention of acute diverticulitis (AD). The secondary end point was the rate of adverse events. A total of 101 patients were consecutively enrolled at the Internal Medicine and Gastroenterology Unit, Sant'Orsola Hospital, Bologna, Italy. DIVER-100® was effective in inducing remission of symptoms in 12 patients (11.9%) at 3 months and in 10 patients (9.9%) at 6 months. DIVER-100® significantly reduced abdominal pain and bloating in 45.5 and 57.4% of patients, respectively ($p < 0.001$) after 3 months. No episodes of AD and no adverse events related to DIVER-100® were recorded at 6 months in the study population. DIVER-100® is a safe and effective nutraceutical compound in obtaining remission and symptom relief in SUDD patients. Further randomized, placebo-controlled clinical trials are needed to confirm these preliminary data.

The efficacy and safety of this nutraceutical compound could be explained by the combination of the various ingredients that compose it. Boswellia serrata and zinc, as investigated in vitro and in animal experimental models of intestinal inflammation, can preserve the intestinal epithelial barrier and function and can protect from oxidative and inflammatory damages [54, 55]. Cranberries, reducing the production of biofilms and the adhesion capacity of microorganisms, have an anti-inflammatory effect [56]. Prebiotics such as inulin are nondigestible food ingredients, which are fermented at the level of the colon, causing changes in the intestinal microbiota and resulting in beneficial effects [57]. Probiotics competing with pathogenic microorganisms could lead to health benefits, reducing colonization and bacterial overgrowth of the gastrointestinal tract and favoring the balance of the gut microbiota [58]. Moreover, recently, a 12-month, prospective pilot study, including 15 patients with SUDD (14 DICA 1 patients and 1 DICA 2 patient), has shown that DIVER-100® was effective in reducing abdominal pain, meteorism, constipation, and diarrhea. No adverse event was reported during the 12-month follow-up [59]. Despite these promising preliminary data, further randomized and placebo-controlled clinical trials are needed to confirm the efficacy and safety of DIVER-100® and to rule out a possible placebo effect related to its intake (Table 21.1).

21.5 Conclusions

Traditional herbal medicines may be useful in the treatment and prevention of AD. Moreover, butyrate may play a role in the prevention of AD. Curcumin and nutraceutical formulations may be useful in relief from SUDD pain. However, additional and controlled studies need to be conducted to draw final conclusions.

References

1. Parks TG. Natural history of diverticular disease of the colon. Clin Gastroenterol. 1975;4:3–21.
2. Strate LL, Modi R, Cohen E, Spiegel BM. Diverticular disease as a chronic illness: evolving epidemiologic and clinical insights. Am J Gastroenterol. 2012;107:1486–93.
3. Papa A, Papa V. The economic burden of diverticular disease. J Clin Gastroenterol. 2016;50(Suppl 1):S2–3.
4. Floch MH, Bina I. The natural history of diverticulitis: fact and theory. J Clin Gastroenterol. 2004;38:S2–7.
5. Kruis W, Germer CT, Leifeld L. German Society for Gastroenterology, digestive and metabolic diseases and The German Society for General and Visceral Surgery. Diverticular disease: guidelines of the german society for gastroenterology, digestive and metabolic diseases and the german society for general and visceral surgery. Digestion. 2014;90:190–207.
6. Stollman N, Smalley W, Hirano I. AGA Institute clinical guidelines committee. American Gastroenterological Association Institute guideline on the Management of Acute Diverticulitis. Gastroenterology. 2015;149:1944–9.
7. Cuomo R, Barbara G, Pace F, et al. Italian consensus conference for colonic diverticulosis and diverticular disease. United European Gastroenterol J. 2014;2:413–42.
8. Spiller R. Diverticular disease and IBS: overlapping or misunderstanding? J Clin Gastroenterol. 2016;50(Suppl 1):S29–32.
9. Comparato G, Fanigliulo L, Aragona G, et al. Quality of life in uncomplicated symptomatic diverticular disease: is it another good reason for treatment? Dig Dis. 2007;25:252–9.
10. Spiegel BM, Reid MW, Bolus R, et al. Development and validation of a disease-targeted quality of life instrument for chronic diverticular disease: the DV-QOL. Qual Life Res. 2015;24:163–79.
11. European Colorectal Cancer Screening Guidelines Working Group. European guidelines for quality assurance in colorectal cancer screening and diagnosis: overview and introduction to the full supplement publication. Endoscopy. 2013;45:51–9.
12. Kovacic K. Current concepts in functional gastrointestinal disorders. Curr Opin Pediatr. 2015;27:619–24.
13. Hobson KG, Roberts PL. Etiology and pathophysiology of diverticular disease. Clin Colon Rectal Surg. 2004;17:147–53.

14. Misawa S, Kuwabara S, Sato Y, et al. Japanese Eculizumab trial for GBS (JET-GBS) study group. Safety of Daiobotampito in the Treatment of Acute Diverticulitis of the Colon: A Single-Center, Open-Label, Prospective Trial. Lancet Neurol. 2018;17:519–29.
15. Mizuki A, Nagata H, Tatemichi M, et al. The out-patient management of patients with acute mild-to-moderate colonic diverticulitis. Aliment Pharmacol Ther. 2005;21:889–97.
16. Mizuki A, Tatemichi M, Nakazawa A, et al. Long-term clinical course after conservative and endoscopic treatment of colonic diverticular bleeding. Digestion. 2016;94:186–91.
17. Mizuki A, Tatemichi M, Nakazawa A, et al. Effects of burdock tea on recurrence of colonic diverticulitis and diverticular bleeding: an open-labelled randomized clinical trial. Sci Rep. 2019;9:6793.
18. Shimura S, et al. Effects of roasted burdock powder on simple chronic constipation-a pilot study. Shimane J Med Sci. 2012;29:31–6.
19. Ashour ML, Youssef FS, Gad HA, Wink M. Inhibition of cytochrome P450 (CYP3A4) activity by extracts from 57 plants used in traditional Chinese medicine (TCM). Pharmacogn Mag. 2017;13:300–8.
20. Predes FS, Ruiz AL, Carvalho JE, Foglio MA, Dolder H. Antioxidative and in vitro antiproliferative activity of Arctium lappa root extracts. BMC Complement Altern Med. 2011;11:25.
21. Lee D, Kim CY. Influence of roasting treatment on the antioxidant activities and color of burdock root tea. Prev Nutr Food Sci. 2017;22:21–9.
22. Jamal Talabani A, Lydersen S, Ness-Jensen E, Endreseth BH, Edna TH. Risk factors of admission for acute colonic diverticulitis in a population-based cohort study: the north Trondelag health study. Norway World J Gastroenterol. 2016;22:10663–72.
23. Krokowicz L, Stojcev Z, Kaczmarek BF, et al. Microencapsulated sodium butyrate administered to patients with diverticulosis decreases incidence of diverticulitis--a prospective randomized study. Int J Color Dis. 2014;29:387–93.
24. Vernia P, Annese V, Bresci G, d'Albasio G, D'Incà R. Giaccari S topical butyrate improves efficacy of 5-ASA in refractory distal ulcerative colitis: results of a multicentre trial. Eur J Clin Investig. 2003;33:244–8.
25. Hamer HM, Jonkers D, Venema K, Vanhoutvin S, Troost FJ. Brummer RJ review article: the role of butyrate on colonic function. Aliment Pharmacol Ther. 2008;27:104–19.
26. Topping DL. Clifton PM short-chain fatty acids and human colonic function: roles of resistant starch and nonstarch polysaccharides. Physiol Rev. 2001;81:1031–64.
27. Canani RB, Terrin G, Cirillo P, et al. Butyrate as an effective treatment of congenital chloride diarrhea. Gastroenterology. 2004;127:630–4.
28. Schmitt MG Jr, Soergel KH. Wood CM absorption of short chain fatty acids from the human jejunum. Gastroenterology. 1976;70:211–5.
29. Clemens CH, Samsom M, Roelofs J, van Berge Henegouwen GP. Smout AJ colorectal visceral perception in diverticular disease. Gut. 2004;53:717–22.
30. Petruzziello L, Iacopini F, Bulajic M, Shah S. Costamanga G review article: uncomplicated diverticular disease of the colon. Aliment Pharmacol Ther. 2006;23:1379–91.
31. Banasiewicz T, Krokowicz L, Stojcev Z, et al. Microencapsulated sodiumbutyrate reduces the frequency of abdominal pain in patients with irritable bowel syndrome. Color Dis. 2013;15:204–9.
32. Roda A, Simoni P, Magliulo M, et al. A new oral formulation for the release of sodium butyrate in the ileo-cecal region and colon. World J Gastroenterol. 2007;13:1079–108.
33. Tursi A, Brandimarte G, Di MF, Elisei W, Picchio M. Efficacy and safety of a new nutraceutical formulation in managing patients with symptomatic uncomplicated diverticular disease: a 12-month, prospective, pilot study. J Gastrointest Liver Dis. 2018;27:201–5.
34. Picchio M, Elisei W, Brandimarte G, et al. Mesalazine for the treatment of symptomatic uncomplicated diverticular disease of the colon and for primary prevention of diverticulitis: a systematic review of randomized clinical trials. J Clin Gastroenterol. 2016;50:S64–9.

35. Giacosa A, Riva A, Petrangolini G, et al. Symptomatic uncomplicated diverticular disease management: an innovative food-grade formulation of Curcuma longa and Boswellia serrata extracts. Drugs Context. 2020;9:2020-9-2.
36. Bafutto M, Cherubin D, Cruvinel Dionis MV, et al. Evaluation showed of curcumin in the treatment of symptomatic uncomplicated diverticular disease. J Gastrointest Liver Dis. 2019;28:67–8.
37. Perrone D, Ardito F, Giannatempo G, et al. Biological and therapeutic activities, and anticancer properties of curcumin (review). Exp Ther Med. 2015;10:1615–23.
38. Tabrizi R, Vakili S, Akbari M, et al. The effects of curcumin-containing supplements on biomarkers of inflammation and oxidative stress: a systematic review and meta-analysis of randomized controlled trials. Phyther Res. 2019;33(2):253–62.
39. Tursi A, Elisei W, Brandimarte G, et al. Musosal tumour necrosis factor α in diverticular disease of the colon is overexpressed with disease severity. Color Dis. 2012;14:e258–63.
40. Tursi A, Elisei W, Giorgetti GM, et al. Expression of basic fibroblastic growth factor, syndecan 1 and tumour necrosis factor α in resected acute colonic diverticulitis. Color Dis. 2014;16:O98–103.
41. Cuomo J, Appendino G, Dern AS, et al. Comparative absorption of a standardized curcuminoid mixture and its lecithin formulation. J Nat Prod. 2011;74:664–9.
42. Asher GN, Xie Y, Moaddel R, et al. Randomized pharmacokinetic crossover study comparing 2 curcumin preparations in plasma and rectal tissue of healthy human volunteers. J Clin Pharmacol. 2017;57:185–93.
43. Szymanski MC, Gillum TL, Gould LM, Morin DS, Kuennen MR. Short-term dietary curcumin supplementation reduces gastrointestinal barrier damage and physiological strain responses during exertional heat stress. J Appl Physiol. 2018;124:330–40.
44. Siddiqui MZ. *Boswellia serrata*, a potential antiinflammatory agent: an overview. Indian J Pharm Sci. 2011;73:255–61.
45. Abdel-Tawab M, Werz O, Schubert-Zsilavecz M. Boswellia serrata: an overall assessment of in vitro, preclinical, pharmacokinetic and clinical data. Clin Pharmacokinet. 2011;50:349–69.
46. Banno N, Akihisa T, Yasukawa K, et al. Anti-inflammatory activities of the triterpene acids from the resin of Boswellia carteri. J Ethnopharmacol. 2006;107:249–53.
47. Poeckel D, Werz O. Boswellic acids: biological actions and molecular targets. Curr Med Chem. 2006;13:3359–69.
48. Riva A, Morazzoni P, Artaria C, et al. A single-dose, randomized, cross-over, two-way, open-label study for comparing the absorption of boswellic acids and its lecithin formulation. Phytomedicine. 2016;23:1375–82.
49. Pellegrini L, Milano E, Franceschi F, et al. Managing ulcerative colitis in remission phase: usefulness of Casperome®, an innovative lecithin-based delivery system of Boswellia serrata extract. Eur Rev Med Pharmacol Sci. 2016;20:2695–700.
50. Belacaro G, Gizzi G, Pellegrini L, et al. Supplementation with a lecithin-based delivery form of Boswellia serrata extract (Casperome®) controls symptoms of mild irritable bowel syndrome. Eur Rev Med Pharmacol Sci. 2017;21:2249–54.
51. Riva A, Giacomelli L, Togni S, et al. Oral administration of a lecithin-based delivery form of boswellic acids (Casperome®) for the prevention of symptoms of irritable bowel syndrome: a randomized clinical study. Minerva Gastroenterol Dietol. 2019;65:30–5.
52. Kizhakkedath R. Clinical evaluation of a formulation containing Curcuma longa and Boswellia serrata extracts in the management of knee osteoarthritis. Mol Med Rep. 2013;8:1542–8.
53. D'Amico F, Fiorini G, Tursi A, et al. Efficacy of a new nutraceutical formulation in patients with symptomatic uncomplicated diverticular disease (SUDD): a prospective observational study. J Gastrointestin Liver Dis. 2019;28(suppl. 4):49–52.
54. Catanzaro D, Rancan S, Orso G, et al. Boswellia serrata preserves intestinal epithelial barrier from oxidative and inflammatory damage. PLoS One. 2015;10:e0125375.
55. Sturniolo GC, Fries W, Mazzon E, Di Leo V, Barollo M, D'inca R. Effect of zinc supplementation on intestinal permeability in experimental colitis. J Lab Clin Med. 2002;139:311–5.

56. Blumberg JB, Basu A, Krueger CG, et al. Impact of cranberries on gut microbiota and Cardiometabolic health: proceedings of the cranberry Health Research conference 2015. Adv Nutr. 2016;7:759S–70S.
57. Akram W, Garud N, Joshi R. Role of inulin as prebiotics on inflammatory bowel disease. Drug Discov Ther. 2019;13:1–8.
58. Sullivan A, Nord CE. Probiotics and gastrointestinal diseases. J Intern Med. 2005;257:78–92.
59. Tursi A, Brandimarte G, Di Mario F, Elisei W, Picchio M. Efficacy and safety of a new nutraceutical formulation in managing patients with symptomatic uncomplicated diverticular disease: a 12-month, prospective, pilot study. J Gastrointestin Liver Dis. 2018;27:201–2.

Part VI

Medical Treatment of Acute Diverticulitis

Treatment for Uncomplicated Acute Diverticulitis

22

Sebastiano Biondo, Dmitry Bordin, and Thomas Golda

22.1 Definition

Diverticulosis is an common age-related anatomical condition. Individuals who develop chronic gastrointestinal symptoms or complications are referred to as having diverticular disease [1].

The risk of developing diverticulitis (inflammation of one or a few diverticula and the surrounding colon) and diverticular bleeding (acute bleeding from a nutrient vessel in a diverticulum) is widespread among these individuals. They may also develop chronic gastrointestinal symptoms (abdominal pain, bloating, or changes in bowel habits), which is symptomatic uncomplicated diverticular disease (SUDD) [2]. The main characteristic of SUDD of the colon is left lower quadrant pain lasting

S. Biondo (✉)
Department of General and Digestive Surgery, Bellvitge University Hospital, University of Barcelona, Barcelona, Spain
e-mail: sbn.biondo@gmail.com

D. Bordin
Department of Pancreatic, Biliary and Upper Digestive Tract Disorders, A. S. Loginov Moscow Clinical Scientific Center, Moscow, Russia

Department of Outpatient Therapy And Family Medicine, Tver State Medical University, Tver, Russian Federation

Department of Propaedeutic of Internal Diseases and Gastroenterology, A.I. Yevdokimov Moscow State University of Medicine and Dentistry, Moscow, Russia
e-mail: d.bordin@mknc.ru

T. Golda
Colorectal Unit—Department of General and Digestive Surgery, Bellvitge University Hospital, University of Barcelona, Barcelona, Spain
e-mail: tgolda@bellvitgehospital.cat

© The Author(s), under exclusive license to Springer Nature Switzerland AG 2022
A. Tursi et al. (eds.), *Colonic Diverticular Disease*,
https://doi.org/10.1007/978-3-030-93761-4_22

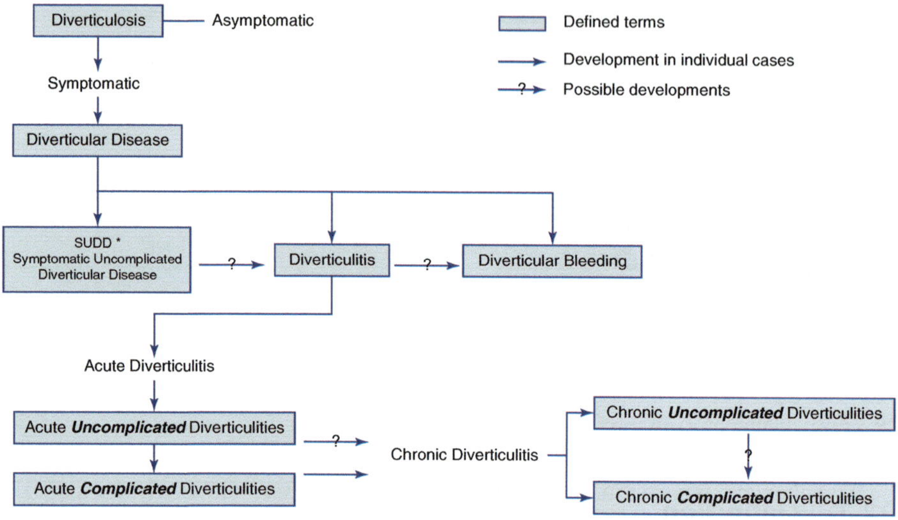

Fig. 22.1 List of terms and stages used in the guidelines of the European Society of Coloproctology [4]. The flowchart shows the different stages of diverticulosis and diverticular disease. It should be noted that although diverticulosis is conditio sine qua non for the other stages, the different stages are not part of a continuous development and may appear independently in individual cases. *The term "SUDD" is controversial, as it remains unclear whether it is a disease or whether it represents the coexistence of irritable bowel syndrome and diverticulosis

>24 h, not fulfilling the criteria for irritable bowel syndrome diagnosis, and associated with increased levels of fecal calprotectin, occurring in about 20% of people with diverticulosis [3].

There is generally no accepted classification yet due to a lack of reliable validation. The ESCP Guideline Committee (2020) proposed definitions based on evidence with some overlap with existing classifications (Fig. 22.1) [4] .

Diverticulosis of the colon develops in the majority of individuals in Western countries with increasing age and usually remains asymptomatic. Therefore, diverticulosis per se should not be considered a disease. The term "diverticular disease (DD)" implies that there are symptoms related to the diverticula.

It is a matter of dispute whether diverticula can lead to symptoms in the absence of inflammation or bleeding [5, 6]. Symptomatic uncomplicated diverticulosis is the most common clinical problem with recurring symptoms associated with diverticula (abdominal pain, irregular stools, bloating). Inflammatory marker levels are not elevated, and there are no abnormalities on imaging, which makes this condition distinct from diverticulitis [7]. So, the term "***symptomatic uncomplicated diverticular disease (SUDD)***" is used in some countries for patients with diverticula who experience abdominal symptoms and changes in bowel habits (e.g., diarrhea, constipation, or alternating bowel habits) in the absence of inflammation [1]. However, the term has not gained general acceptance, and a uniform definition does not exist. A major difficulty is the differential diagnosis between irritable bowel syndrome (IBS) and SUDD as there is an overlap between the two (Table 22.1). Epidemiological studies have shown that IBS-like symptoms may develop after a bout of acute

Table 22.1 Differential features between irritable bowel syndrome and symptomatic uncomplicated diverticular disease [1]

	IBS	SUDD
Age	Young	Older
Gender	Females predominant	Males predominant
Structural changes in the colon	No	Yes
Rome III criteria	100%	15%
Pain pattern	Short length and frequent recurrences	Extended pain episodes (>24 h) with long remissions
Pain location	Diffuse	Left lower quadrant
Bowel changes	Diarrhea and/or constipation	Diarrhea predominant
Fecal calprotectin level	Usually normal	Usually increased

diverticulitis [8]. The overlap between IBS and SUDD has also been highlighted in a study from the Mayo clinic [9], which points out that age is a critical factor.

Diverticulitis (acute uncomplicated diverticulitis) is associated with systemic inflammatory response, which clinically presents as chills, fever, and abnormal laboratory results (increased ESR, CRP, calprotectin), and with diagnostic imaging (ultrasound, computed tomography—as the 'gold standard'), which presents thickening of the intestinal wall and the inflammatory infiltrate in the surrounding adipose tissue [7].

The term "diverticulitis" describes a peridiverticular inflammation of the bowel wall and usually the surrounding tissue. It can be acute or chronic and complicated or uncomplicated with different possible complications including abscess, perforation, fistula, obstruction, and bleeding. The best ways to determine the severity of acute diverticulitis are mainly those by cross-sectional imaging (CT scan, ultrasound) and laboratory tests (C-reactive protein). In general, uncomplicated acute diverticulitis is differentiated from complicated acute diverticulitis. The boundary between the two terms lies in the degree of inflammation. ***Acute uncomplicated diverticulitis*** is inflammation in a diverticula-bearing bowel segment and the surrounding tissue without signs of perforation (extraluminal air) or abscess formation. Chronic diverticulitis can develop if acute diverticulitis does not resolve completely. Wall thickening or chronic mucosal inflammation in the absence of stenosis is called ***chronic uncomplicated diverticulitis***. Complicated chronic diverticulitis includes both stenotic disease, which may lead to acute bowel obstruction, and fistulation most common to the urinary tract.

22.2 Investigations to Diagnose Acute Uncomplicated Diverticulitis

C-reactive protein (CRP) has an important predictive value in defining the presence and severity of acute diverticulitis. The CRP cutoff value of 149.5 mg/l significantly discriminates acute uncomplicated diverticulitis from complicated diverticulitis (specificity 65%, sensitivity 85%). In a multivariate analysis, a CRP value of more than 150 mg/l and old age were independent risk factors for acute complicated diverticulitis. The mean CRP value was significantly higher in patients who died (207 mg/l) than in those who survived (139 mg/l). In addition, a CRP value of more than 150 mg/l and free abdominal fluid in CT were independent variables, indicating a high probability of postoperative mortality [10].

Fecal calprotectin (FC) may be useful in differentiating between SUDD and IBS. There was no difference between asymptomatic diverticulosis, healthy controls, and IBS patients. Higher FC values were found in acute uncomplicated diverticulitis and in symptomatic uncomplicated DD than in healthy controls and in IBS patients. In addition, FC values correlated with the inflammatory infiltrate and decreased to normal values after treatment both in acute uncomplicated diverticulitis and in symptomatic uncomplicated DD [11]. Consequently, fecal calprotectin might be useful in distinguishing symptomatic uncomplicated diverticular disease from irritable bowel syndrome, but a cutoff level needs to be identified.

Possible modalities that have been studied as tools to identify and classify diverticulitis include computed tomography (CT), ultrasound, and magnetic resonance imaging (MRI). CT has a high sensitivity (93–97%) and specificity (100%) in the diagnosis of acute diverticulitis [12, 13].

A well-performed abdominal ultrasound has a high diagnostic accuracy and also has the advantages of avoiding ionizing radiation and easy repetition if needed and thus can be useful in pregnancy. A systematic review and meta-analysis of the accuracy of CT and ultrasound in diagnosing acute diverticulitis has shown that summary sensitivity estimates were 92% for ultrasound versus 94% for CT. Summary specificity estimates were 90% for ultrasound versus 99% for CT. For the identification of alternative diseases, sensitivity ranged between 33 and 78% for ultrasound and between 50 and 100% for CT. Therefore, both ultrasound and CT can be used as initial diagnostic tools. However, CT is more likely to identify alternative diseases [14].

MRI is highly sensitive (94%) and specific (88%) in the differential diagnoses of diverticulitis with positive likelihood ratios of more than 7.5 and negative likelihood ratios of less than 0.07 [15]. However, as it is both time-consuming and less available than CT, it has not gained wide acceptance. MRI is an alternative when ultrasound is inconclusive in pregnant women as well as after the acute phase to assist in differential diagnoses.

An International Consensus on Diverticulosis and Diverticular Disease published in 2019 [16] recommended contrast-enhanced computer tomography (CE-CT) as the first-line colonic examination since it offers a more comprehensive evaluation of both uncomplicated and complicated forms. CE-CT can also be used in therapeutic interventions. Ultrasound has slightly lower sensitivity and specificity compared to those of CT in the assessment of acute diverticulitis, and its use as a first-line diagnostic procedure—followed by a CT scan in the case of inconclusive sonographic findings—may spare the use of CT in more than 50% of cases. Ultrasound is useful in monitoring patients after acute diverticulitis and in particular the lesions treated conservatively.

The DICA endoscopic classification seems to have a predictive value on the outcome of the disease [16].

22.3 Antibiotics in the Treatment of Uncomplicated Acute Diverticulitis

Treatment of diverticular disease is based on the intake of fibers and dietary fiber supplements and, more recently, has been relying on the poorly absorbed antibiotic rifaximin, mesalazine, and probiotics, alone or in combination.

Mild-to-moderate diverticulitis can be treated in an outpatient setting, and therapeutic recommendations include liquid and easily digestible diet, analgesics, proper hydration, antipyretics, and antispasmodics. No significant differences were observed between patients receiving and those not receiving antibiotics, and, hence, systemic antibiotic therapy should be reserved for patients with severe disease conditions admitted to the hospital [17], for patients from high-risk groups, e.g., with immunodeficiency (HIV, AIDS, on immunosuppressant drugs, steroids) and comorbidities (e.g., chronic kidney disease, chronic obstructive pulmonary disease), or for elderly patients [18].

Probably the most prescribed oral treatment is the combination of ciprofloxacin and metronidazole [19]. However, recent studies have found no support for the routine use of antibiotics [20]. A systematic review and meta-analysis concluded that antibiotic use is not associated with reductions in the rates of major complications, disease recurrence rates, or surgical resection, although it may be associated with a significantly shorter duration of hospital stay [21].

Two randomized clinical trials (AVOD [22] and DIABOLO [23]) were conducted comparing antibiotic and nonantibiotic treatments in immunocompetent and nonseptic patients with uncomplicated acute diverticulitis. There were no differences in time to recovery from the initial episode or in the duration of hospital stay [24]. Furthermore, no differences were observed in the two trials regarding the rates of complicated diverticulitis and the need for sigmoid resection after the initial diverticulitis episode and in the long term, in the rates of recurrent diverticulitis. In the AVOD study, a total of 556 of 623 patients (89.2%) were followed up for a median of 11 years. There were no differences between the nonantibiotic and antibiotic groups in recurrences, complications, and surgery for diverticulitis or colorectal cancer, thus leading to the conclusion that treatment of uncomplicated acute diverticulitis without antibiotics is feasible, safe, and effective. Recently, a published meta-analysis has shown that treatment of uncomplicated acute diverticulitis without antibiotics is associated with a significantly shorter hospital stay. In this study, there was no significant difference in the percentage of patients requiring additional treatment or intervention to settle during the initial episode, the rate of readmission or deferred admission, the need for surgical or radiological intervention, recurrence, and complications [25].

These findings prove that antibiotics in patients with uncomplicated acute diverticulitis should not be used routinely, with selective use reserved for the treatment of those patients with complicated disease, severe infection/sepsis, or significant comorbidities. This is reflected in treatment recommendations in the current European [4], Dutch [26], Italian [27], German [28], and US [29] guidelines.

Mesalazine has been used in patients with SUDD. The justification for the use of aminosalicylates is based on the assumption of low-grade inflammation in SUDD and symptom generation, whereas overt inflammation may induce diverticulitis [30]. After oral or rectal administration, mesalazine is absorbed by colonic epithelial cells and its efficacy is related to its mucosal concentration. The main anti-inflammatory mechanisms of mesalazine are not completely understood.

In a systematic review, symptom relief with mesalazine was better than that with placebo, high-fiber diet, and low-dose rifaximin. The incidence of diverticulitis with mesalazine was lower only when compared with placebo [31]. Everyday mesalazine may be better than cyclic administration to prevent relapse [32]. The combination of cyclic mesalazine and Lactobacillus casei DG seems to be better than placebo for maintaining remission of SUDD, but the small size of the study requires confirmation [33]. In addition, two randomized, double-blind, placebo-controlled multicenter trials [34, 35] and one meta-analysis [36] failed to show a positive effect with mesalazine.

The rationale for the use of antibiotics with high intraluminal availability is based on the evidence that diverticula are pouches of the colonic wall that, in predisposed individuals, favor fecal entrapment, bacterial overgrowth, and potential breakdown of the epithelial lining involved in bacterial translocation, mucosal inflammation, and complications [37]. This assumption is supported by data showing the presence of dysbiosis in patients with diverticular disease [38]. Rifaximin is effective in the treatment of small intestinal bacterial overgrowth (SIBO) and related (organic and functional) gastrointestinal disorders [39].

Rifaximin is a nonaminoglycoside, semisynthetic, nonsystemic antibiotic. Use of rifaximin (400 mg b.d. for 7 days every month for a year) aims to prevent diverticulitis and its complications, which not only eliminates pathogenic intestinal flora but also prevents its excessive growth. In vitro and in vivo, it shows a strong activity against Gram-positive and Gram-negative bacteria, both aerobes and anaerobes [40]. Rifaximin has shown eubiotic effects since it stimulates the growth of beneficial bacterial species, including Lactobacilli and Bifidobacteria [41, 42]. In addition, Rifaximin has also shown good anti-inflammatory properties [40]. The safety profile of rifaximin is excellent, and adverse events have been rarely reported in the many trials conducted, with a number needed to harm (NNH) of 9871 [43, 44].

Both rifaximin and mesalazine have been studied to evaluate their ability in preventing recurrent diverticulitis or persistent symptoms after an episode of acute diverticulitis. A systematic review showed a lower likelihood of disease recurrence with mesalazine than controls in symptomatic uncomplicated diverticular disease but not in acute uncomplicated diverticulitis. There was no difference in the likelihood of developing acute diverticulitis in symptomatic uncomplicated diverticular disease between the two groups. However, there was a higher global symptom score reduction with mesalazine than controls in acute uncomplicated diverticulitis [44].

The effect of rifaximin 7 days per month was assessed in a randomized clinical trial (3.5 g of high-fiber supplementation b.d. with or without 1 week per month of the nonabsorbable antibiotic rifaximin (400 mg b.d.) for 12 months) [45]. Recurrences occurred in 10.4% of patients administered rifaximin plus fibers vs. 19.3% of patients receiving fibers alone. Patients receiving rifaximin for diverticulitis diagnosed since ≥1 year also had a lower incidence of recurrences. However, the number needed to treat is high and it is hence not clinically useful. On the other hand, rifaximin has been found to be effective in treating SUDD symptoms. In particular, a meta-analysis found that rifaximin was significantly better than some control therapies (fiber, placebo) to treat symptoms, with an excellent number needed to treat [18].

The two observational studies comparing the effects of 7–10 days per month rifaximin and mesalazine found opposing results—one was in favor of rifaximin [46] and the other was in favor of mesalazine [47].

A newly published review pointed out discrepant evidence regarding the efficacy of 5-ASA treatment in the prevention of diverticulitis and has shown the necessity of further RCTs [48].

Even though the use of antibiotics remains a disputable issue in the management of complicated cases, recent guidelines have revealed that antibiotics can be used selectively, rather than routinely, in uncomplicated AD. Regarding the treatment of primary and secondary prophylaxis of AD, the efficacy of rifaximin and mesalazine was suggested, although the recommendations among the guidelines do not coincide [49].

Thus, we must conclude that the available data are inconsistent and do not adequately demonstrate the positive effect of these drugs on complications and recurrence.

22.4 Outpatient Treatment

The vast majority (>70%) of acute presentations of diverticulitis are uncomplicated (modified Hinchey classification 0 and Ia by Wasvary), with high success rates of conservative management (>90%) [26, 50]. This group of patients contrasts with acute diverticulitis associated with an abscess (modified Hinchey Ib/II, reported in up to 15–25%) and is already a part of the wide range of complicated diverticulitis [50–52].

The treatment of uncomplicated acute diverticulitis has notably evolved since the initial report of the practice parameters by the ASCRS in 1995 with intravenous antibiotics and fluids, bowel rest, and hospitalization [53]. Whether the treatment can be managed in an outpatient or an inpatient setting depends on the health-care setup, the presentation, and the severity of symptoms. Nevertheless, three aspects are critical for an adequate inpatient or outpatient management of an episode of uncomplicated acute diverticulitis: precise diagnosis, tolerance of oral medication, and clinical assessment of the patient [54].

Contrast-enhanced computed tomography (CE-CT) as the gold standard of cross-sectional imaging enables precisely and reliably to distinguish complicated acute diverticulitis (with perforation or abscess) from uncomplicated acute diverticulitis [55]. This has changed the thinking about (fear of missing an alternative pathology or difficulty in establishing a diagnosis), and also the management of, uncomplicated acute diverticulitis [56]. The diagnosis of uncomplicated acute diverticulitis by CT applying the modified Hinchey classification by Wasvary is now standard in clinical practice and investigation (Hinchey I subdivided as Ia when inflammation is restricted to a pericolic area and as Ib when a pericolic abscess is identified) [54]. In the treatment of uncomplicated acute diverticulitis, not only are established guidelines advocating antibiotics questioned but also hospitalization for uncomplicated acute diverticulitis in selected patients is challenged [57, 58].

Generally, clinical improvement in patients affected by uncomplicated acute diverticulitis is observed within 3–4 days. In hospitalized patients, following the change from intravenous to oral treatment, the patient usually can be discharged to finish another 7–10 days treatment course [59–61]. However, various studies have questioned this standard of hospitalization.

Two recent meta-analyses have identified 19 and 21 studies including 2303 and 1781 ambulatory-treated patients, respectively, and have investigated outpatient treatment versus hospitalization for uncomplicated diverticulitis of the left colon [62, 63]. Of these studies, one is a randomized multicenter study, the DIVER trial [64].

Patients with comorbidities (diabetes, heart failure, renal insufficiency, or obstructive pulmonary disorder) were excluded from outpatient management in some studies [65–67], whereas, in others (including DIVER), these patients were included regardless. A systematic review identified a Charlson score of 3 or greater as an independent risk factor for complications [65]. However, in other studies [63], neither a Charlson score of 3 or greater nor the presence of diabetes could be demonstrated to predict the need for surgery, prolonged admission, or readmission [68, 69]. Due to these literature findings, the comorbidity score is not considered an absolute contraindication for the outpatient management of uncomplicated acute diverticulitis, but clinical judgment should be applied [65].

Based on the exclusion criteria used in the above studies, several international guidelines and various meta-analyses emphasize that ambulatory treatment is only applicable in patients who tolerate oral diet, have an adequate social network, and do not suffer from associated severe comorbidities or immunosuppression [63, 70]. All these criteria ensure that the patient is able to fulfill the prescribed oral antibiotic treatment, understand the situation and warning signs, does not suffer from an increased vulnerability to infectious complications, and realizes when to ask for help in case of not being able to fend for oneself.

In the randomized DIVER trial, the treatment in both management groups failed in a total of 7 out of 132 patients. Of these, four patients (6.1%) from the hospitalization group and three patients (4.5%) from the outpatient group required readmittance to the hospital. No differences were found between both groups with respect to the primary objective, i.e., readmission to the hospital. Reported readmission rates from other studies on outpatient treatment ranged from 0 to 14.3%. In comparison, the incidence of readmission after discharge for the hospitalized group ranged from 0 to 33% [64].

One of the aforementioned meta-analysis performed a pooled analysis of the incidence of readmission on all outpatient treatments, finding a readmission rate of 7%. After outpatient treatment, the rate of readmission and drainage of a diverticular abscess was 0.2% (2 of 1082 patients) and the rate of urgent surgery was 0.2% (2 of 1288 patients) [62]. In the DIVER study, neither percutaneous drainage nor urgent surgery was necessary. There was no related mortality within 60 days of the diagnosis [64].

Readmission is necessary in the majority of cases for persisting abdominal pain or vomiting and thus the inability to take oral medication but in the absence of any diverticular complications. Several systematic reviews show that even if readmission is needed for parenteral treatment or pain control, the risk of a worsened clinical picture and the need for aggressive measures is low [71, 72]. Most studies compare outpatient treatment to a reference group fulfilling one or more exclusion criteria for outpatient treatment and thus are not strictly comparable due to selection bias [73–78]. A recent meta-analysis has commented on pooled rates including 21 studies showing an overall failure rate of 4.3%, defining failure as emergency admission to the hospital within 60 days for acute diverticulitis [63].

These findings demonstrate the safety of outpatient treatment for a selected group of patients with uncomplicated acute diverticulitis.

Clinical control in outpatient management varies essentially between the different studies from one visit in outpatient clinics 4–7 days after diagnosis [66] to a daily visit at home by a medical team or a sort of outpatient hospitalization including parenteral antibiotic treatment at home [77]. The daily follow-up telephone call within the DIVER trial to control temperature, general conditions, and pain and to adjust diet and analgesia was abandoned in the routine practice after completion of the DIVER study. There is just one appointment in the outpatient clinic scheduled 10–15 days after diagnosis. Nevertheless, the threshold to repeat the diagnostic workup with clinical exploration, blood analysis, and computed tomography should be low for the patient presenting again at the emergency department with worsening of the clinical condition or increase of pain. However, there are no studies or recommendations on the diagnostic workup if treatment failure is suspected. A great number of studies have assessed the risk of treatment failure for complicated diverticulitis, but the literature is scarce for uncomplicated diverticulitis.

The DIVER trial also assessed the quality of life at day 14 and at day 60 after diagnosis. An improvement in the quality of life could be measured between 14 and 60 days of follow-up without differences between the hospitalized and ambulatory patients [64].

Finally, it has been shown that outpatient treatment significantly reduces the costs of treating uncomplicated acute diverticulitis. Five studies refer to the costs of the two treatments [64, 74, 79–81]. The cost reduction of ambulatory treatment ranges between 42 and 82%. In the DIVER trial, the costs were three times lower for ambulatory treatment than those for hospitalization (average hospital stay of

3 days), with a saving of € 1124.70 (67%) for each patient treated on an outpatient basis.

All guidelines and consensus conferences on diverticulitis of the main national and international associations of colorectal surgery and gastroenterology published in the last 5 years recommend outpatient treatment for uncomplicated diverticulitis in selected patients (specified, e.g., in the guidelines of the European Society of Coloproctology as an adequate social network, tolerating oral intake and the absence of sepsis, significant comorbidity, and immunosuppression) [4].

The recently published guidelines of the Japan Gastroenterological Association [82] and the Clinical Practice Guidelines Committee of the American Society of Colon and Rectal Surgeons have not even dedicated an individual paragraph to the outpatient treatment of uncomplicated diverticulitis, but the ASCRS goes even further with the statement that "Antibiotic treatment alone for abscesses smaller than 3 cm is typically successful and, in stable patients, treatment can usually be administered in the outpatient setting" [54].

A recent systematic review has supported the outpatient treatment approach, suggesting that 97% of uncomplicated cases could be treated as outpatients with a substantial cost-saving effect. [83].

The most typical regimen for outpatient treatment published to date comprises antibiotics in most protocols and starts on a liquid-only diet, which is gradually progressed over the following days. The most commonly prescribed antibiotics are amoxicillin–clavulanic acid or ciprofloxacin and metronidazole in penicillin-allergic patients. The duration of antibiotic therapy ranges from 7 to 14 days in those who received antibiotics. [64–66, 74, 84–87].

The acceptance of ambulatory treatment in uncomplicated diverticulitis is reflected in a decline in hospital admissions from 58.0% in 2006 to 47.1% in 2013 in the USA, although diverticulitis-related emergency department visits rose from 89.8 to 113.9 visits per 100,000 population between 2006 and 2013 [88]. The combination of an aging population and the increased prevalence of diverticular disease will also drive an increase in presentations of acute diverticulitis and may put pressure on limited inpatient systems [65].

Concerning the risk of recurrence, 3 studies including 240 patients on outpatient treatment reported a follow-up of about 1 year. These studies reported an acute diverticulitis recurrence rate of 13.0% in the outpatient group versus 12.1% in the hospitalization group [66, 74, 89]; so, ambulatory treatment does not influence disease recurrence.

22.5 Diet

Upon diagnosis of uncomplicated acute diverticulitis, short-term food deprivation or low dietary fiber intake—generally defined as less than 10 g/day—is traditionally recommended [90].

Bowel rest is usually used in clinical routines as it is believed that a less-active bowel reduces colonic irritation and reinflammation [91]. Conceptually, this dogma would be based on a low-fiber diet theoretically reducing the frequency and the volume of stools to favor passage through the inflamed segment, thus allowing the inflammation to improve more quickly [65].

This low-residue diet regimen is normally administered in an inpatient setting, but it is also recommended in outpatient care. Although there is a lack of studies advocating dietary restrictions and supporting that bowel rest is required for resolution of an acute episode of uncomplicated cases, traditional practice and some guidelines advise a low-fiber diet [17, 59]. However, the Dutch guidelines of 2012 abandoned this advice [26].

Evidence, however scarce, with a lack of high-quality interventional research and risk of bias [92], demonstrated an unrestricted diet in uncomplicated acute diverticulitis with shorter hospitalization to be equal to a restricted diet for the outcomes of recovery, gastrointestinal symptoms, and complications; moreover, a liberalized diet tends to have lower health-care use and costs. A prospective study found a complication rate of 8.1%, leaving patients with an unrestrictive diet in a first episode of acute uncomplicated diverticulitis [93], which is similar to the literature data on diet restriction [62, 64]. These data were confirmed in a retrospective study and a randomized trial, showing no differences in complications but a shorter hospital stay in the groups of less-restricted diets [58, 94].

Beyond that, there are data suggesting that bowel rest in acute diseases of the colon is ineffective in reducing inflammation, risk of infection, and other complications [95]. Based on a systematic literature review, a liberalized diet is recommended for patients with uncomplicated diverticulitis (i.e., allowing consumption of solid food). There seems to be no evident difference for treatment failures between liberalized and restricted diets, recurrence or patient symptoms; on the other hand, liberalized diets may decrease the length of hospital stay and prevent restriction of essential nutrient intake [92].

Similar to outpatient treatment of uncomplicated acute diverticulitis, the majority of patients would probably prefer food autonomy having a low risk of harm and likely benefits to patients and the health-care system. In many units, the opposite strategy, i.e., gentle bowel stimulation and cleansing with small aliquots of magnesium citrate, might help reduce the stool load to promote resolution of symptoms and—if surgery should be needed—increase the chances for a primary anastomosis [50].

22.6 Controversies in Uncomplicated Diverticulitis: Semi-Urgent Surgery in Radiologically Uncomplicated Diverticulitis

Although uncomplicated acute diverticulitis has a benign disease course, a few patients are at increased risk of short-term complications including the need for emergent surgery. Identification of these patients may favor the selection of treatment strategies such as outpatient treatment or antibiotic treatment.

It is logical, and some authors strongly recommend the clinical routine to set a time frame for benchmarks expected to be attained. For example, within 72 h after initiation of an appropriate treatment, symptoms and objective parameters (pain, fever, leukocytosis, systemic inflammatory response syndrome (SIRS), etc.) need to completely resolve or at least improve. Failure to achieve this goal should prompt either (1) repeat imaging to discern whether a drainable abscess has formed or (2) a necessity for surgical intervention.

It is poorly understood why a 1–5% fraction of patients with seemingly uncomplicated diverticulitis on initial imaging do not respond to standard conservative management and ultimately require a semi-emergent surgical intervention, but the literature on this is scarce [50, 51, 96].

A recent observational study has analyzed 1087 patients with initially CT-proven uncomplicated diverticulitis and found that 4.9% (53/1087) developed complicated diverticulitis within 3 months, with colonic obstruction (2.1%), perforation (1.2%), abscess (0.7%), and fistula (0.8%). However, most perforations and abscesses (76%) with need for semi-urgent surgery occurred during the first 10 days after diagnosis [97].

Other retrospective studies found the same complications (perforation, abscess, colonic obstruction, or fistula) in initially uncomplicated diverticulitis in 2.0–2.7% of patients within 1 month from diagnosis [98, 99]. Two retrospective cohort studies on uncomplicated diverticulitis just reported rates of inpatient semi-urgent interventions for diverticular complications, which occurred in 3.5 [100] and 7.1%, and the latter study also reported 0% of postoperative complications in these patients [51]. In our own retrospective study on acute diverticulitis in patients under 50 years, we found the need for a semi-urgent surgical intervention in 7% of patients [101].

Another observational study analyzed a subgroup of uncomplicated acute diverticulitis (Hinchey 1a), but with free air within 5 cm of the inflamed segment and found a rate of 9% for semi-urgent surgery within a median of 6 days after initial diagnosis [102].

As independent risk factors for the transition from uncomplicated to complicated diverticulitis contribute the American Society of Anesthesiologists (ASA) classification III/IV, duration of symptoms longer than 5 days before diagnosis, vomiting, and C-reactive protein (CRP) above 140 mg/L [97].

However, the most recent recommendations of the ASCRS comment on this problem, without any reference to the literature, are scarce: "*patients who do not significantly improve from a clinical standpoint with medical therapy or continue with significant abdominal pain or the inability to tolerate enteral nutrition are typically recommended to undergo colectomy. … Clinical judgment ultimately determines the need for definitive surgical treatment in this setting*" [54].

Conflict of interest No conflicts of interest are declared.

References

1. Scarpignato C, Barbara G, Lanas A, Strate LL. Management of colonic diverticular disease in the third millennium: highlights from a symposium held during the united European gastroenterology week 2017. Ther Adv Gastroenterol. 2018;11:1756284818771305.

2. Spiller RC, Humes DJ, Campbell E, Hastings M, Neal KR, Dukes GE, et al. The patient health questionnaire 12 somatic symptom scale as a predictor of symptom severity and consulting behaviour in patients with irritable bowel syndrome and symptomatic diverticular disease. Aliment Pharmacol Ther. 2010;32(6):811–20.
3. Di Mario F, Miraglia C, Cambiè G, Violi A, Nouvenne A, Franceschi M, et al. Long-term efficacy of rifaximin to manage the symptomatic uncomplicated diverticular disease of the colon. J Investig Med. 2019;67(4):767–70.
4. Schultz JK, Azhar N, Binda GA, Barbara G, Biondo S, Boermeester MA, et al. European Society of Coloproctology: guidelines for the management of diverticular disease of the colon. Color Dis. 2020;22(Suppl 2):5–28.
5. Peery AF, Keku TO, Addamo C, McCoy AN, Martin CF, Galanko JA, et al. Colonic diverticula are not associated with mucosal inflammation or chronic gastrointestinal symptoms. Clin Gastroenterol Hepatol. 2018;16(6):884–891.e1.
6. Tursi A, Scarpignato C. Symptomatic uncomplicated diverticular disease: chronic abdominal pain in diverticulosis is not enough to make the diagnosis. Clin Gastroenterol Hepatol. 2018;16(12):2001–2.
7. Banasiewicz T, Francuzik W, Bobkiewicz A, Krokowicz Ł, Borejsza-Wysocki M, Paszkowski J, et al. The influence of rifaximin on diverticulitis rate and quality of life in patients with diverticulosis. Pol Przegl Chir. 2017;89(1):22–31.
8. Cohen E, Fuller G, Bolus R, Modi R, Vu M, Shahedi K, et al. Increased risk for irritable bowel syndrome after acute diverticulitis. Clin Gastroenterol Hepatol. 2013;11(12):1614–9.
9. Jung H-K, Choung RS, Locke GR, Schleck CD, Zinsmeister AR, Talley NJ. Diarrhea-predominant irritable bowel syndrome is associated with diverticular disease: a population-based study. Am J Gastroenterol. 2010;105(3):652–61.
10. Mäkelä JT, Klintrup K, Takala H, Rautio T. The role of C-reactive protein in prediction of the severity of acute diverticulitis in an emergency unit. Scand J Gastroenterol. 2015;50(5):536–41.
11. Tursi A, Brandimarte G, Elisei W, Giorgetti GM, Inchingolo CD, Aiello F. Faecal calprotectin in colonic diverticular disease: a case-control study. Int J Color Dis. 2009;24(1):49–55.
12. Ambrosetti P, Grossholz M, Becker C, Terrier F, Morel P. Computed tomography in acute left colonic diverticulitis. Br J Surg. 1997;84(4):532–4.
13. Cho KC, Morehouse HT, Alterman DD, Thornhill BA. Sigmoid diverticulitis: diagnostic role of CT--comparison with barium enema studies. Radiology. 1990;176(1):111–5.
14. Laméris W, van Randen A, Bipat S, Bossuyt PMM, Boermeester MA, Stoker J. Graded compression ultrasonography and computed tomography in acute colonic diverticulitis: meta-analysis of test accuracy. Eur Radiol. 2008;18(11):2498–511.
15. Heverhagen JT, Sitter H, Zielke A, Klose KJ. Prospective evaluation of the value of magnetic resonance imaging in suspected acute sigmoid diverticulitis. Dis Colon Rectum. 2008;51(12):1810–5.
16. Tursi A, Brandimarte G, Di Mario F, Lanas A, Scarpignato C, Bafutto M, et al. International consensus on diverticulosis and diverticular disease. Statements from the 3rd international symposium on diverticular disease. J Gastrointestin Liver Dis. 2019;28(suppl. 4):57–66.
17. Pietrzak A, Bartnik W, Szczepkowski M, Krokowicz P, Dziki A, Reguła J, et al. Polish interdisciplinary consensus on diagnostics and treatment of colonic diverticulosis (2015). Pol Przegl Chir. 2015;87(4):203–20.
18. Bianchi M, Festa V, Moretti A, Ciaco A, Mangone M, Tornatore V, et al. Meta-analysis: long-term therapy with rifaximin in the management of uncomplicated diverticular disease. Aliment Pharmacol Ther. 2011;33(8):902–10.
19. Tursi A, Papa A, Danese S. Review article: the pathophysiology and medical management of diverticulosis and diverticular disease of the colon. Aliment Pharmacol Ther. 2015;42(6):664–84.
20. Tandon A, Fretwell VL, Nunes QM, Rooney PS. Antibiotics versus no antibiotics in the treatment of acute uncomplicated diverticulitis—a systematic review and meta-analysis. Color Dis. 2019;62(8):1005–12.

21. Mocanu V, Dang JT, Switzer N, Tavakoli I, Tian C, Gara C de et al. The role of antibiotics in acute uncomplicated diverticulitis: a systematic review and meta-analysis. Am J Surg 2018; 216(3):604–609.
22. Isacson D, Smedh K, Nikberg M, Chabok A. Long-term follow-up of the AVOD randomized trial of antibiotic avoidance in uncomplicated diverticulitis. Br J Surg. 2019;106(11):1542–8.
23. van Dijk ST, Daniels L, Ünlü Ç, de Korte N, van Dieren S, Stockmann HB, et al. Long-term effects of omitting antibiotics in uncomplicated acute diverticulitis. Am J Gastroenterol. 2018;113(7):1045–52.
24. Chabok A, Påhlman L, Hjern F, Haapaniemi S, Smedh K. Randomized clinical trial of antibiotics in acute uncomplicated diverticulitis. Br J Surg. 2012;99(4):532–9.
25. Au S, Aly EH. Treatment of uncomplicated acute diverticulitis without antibiotics: a systematic review and meta-analysis. Dis Colon Rectum. 2019;62(12):1533–47.
26. Andeweg CS, Mulder IM, Felt-Bersma RJF, Verbon A, van der Wilt GJ, van Goor H, et al. Guidelines of diagnostics and treatment of acute left-sided colonic diverticulitis. Dig Surg. 2013;30(4–6):278–92.
27. Cuomo R, Barbara G, Pace F, Annese V, Bassotti G, Binda GA, et al. Italian consensus conference for colonic diverticulosis and diverticular disease. United European Gastroenterol J. 2014;2(5):413–42.
28. Kruis W, Germer C-T, Leifeld L. Diverticular disease: guidelines of the german society for gastroenterology, digestive and metabolic diseases and the german society for general and visceral surgery. Digestion. 2014;90(3):190–207.
29. Stollman N, Smalley W, Hirano I. American Gastroenterological Association Institute guideline on the management of acute diverticulitis. Gastroenterology. 2015;149(7):1944–9.
30. Barbara G, Cremon C, Barbaro MR, Bellacosa L, Stanghellini V. Treatment of diverticular disease with Aminosalicylates: the evidence. J Clin Gastroenterol. 2016;50(Suppl 1):S60–3.
31. Picchio M, Elisei W, Brandimarte G, Di Mario F, Malfertheiner P, Scarpignato C, et al. Mesalazine for the treatment of symptomatic uncomplicated diverticular disease of the colon and for primary prevention of diverticulitis: a systematic review of randomized clinical trials. J Clin Gastroenterol. 2016;50(Suppl 1):S64–9.
32. Tursi A, Di Mario F, Brandimarte G, Elisei W, Picchio M, Loperfido S, et al. Tu1181 intermittent versus every-day Mesalazine therapy in preventing complications of diverticular disease: a long-term follow-up study. Gastroenterology. 2013;144(5):S-782–3.
33. Tursi A, Brandimarte G, Elisei W, Picchio M, Forti G, Pianese G, et al. Randomised clinical trial: mesalazine and/or probiotics in maintaining remission of symptomatic uncomplicated diverticular disease--a double-blind, randomised, placebo-controlled study. Aliment Pharmacol Ther. 2013;38(7):741–51.
34. Raskin JB, Kamm MA, Jamal MM, Márquez J, Melzer E, Schoen RE, et al. Mesalamine did not prevent recurrent diverticulitis in phase 3 controlled trials. Gastroenterology. 2014;147(4):793–802.
35. Kruis W, Kardalinos V, Eisenbach T, Lukas M, Vich T, Bunganic I, et al. Randomised clinical trial: mesalazine versus placebo in the prevention of diverticulitis recurrence. Aliment Pharmacol Ther. 2017;46(3):282–91.
36. Khan RMA, Ali B, Hajibandeh S. Effect of mesalazine on recurrence of diverticulitis in patients with symptomatic uncomplicated diverticular disease: a meta-analysis with trial sequential analysis of randomized controlled trials. Color Dis. 2018;20(6):469–78.
37. Humes DJ, Spiller RC. Review article: the pathogenesis and management of acute colonic diverticulitis. Aliment Pharmacol Ther. 2014;39(4):359–70.
38. Barbara G, Scaioli E, Barbaro MR, Biagi E, Laghi L, Cremon C, et al. Gut microbiota, metabolome and immune signatures in patients with uncomplicated diverticular disease. Gut. 2017;66(7):1252–61.
39. Cuomo R, Barbara G, Annibale B. Rifaximin and diverticular disease: position paper of the Italian Society of Gastroenterology (SIGE). Dig Liver Dis. 2017;49(6):595–603.
40. Scarpignato C, Pelosini I. Experimental and clinical pharmacology of rifaximin, a gastrointestinal selective antibiotic. Digestion. 2006;73(Suppl 1):13–27.

41. Soldi S, Vasileiadis S, Uggeri F, Campanale M, Morelli L, Fogli MV, et al. Modulation of the gut microbiota composition by rifaximin in non-constipated irritable bowel syndrome patients: a molecular approach. Clin Exp Gastroenterol. 2015;8:309–25.
42. Ponziani FR, Scaldaferri F, Petito V, Paroni Sterbini F, Pecere S, Lopetuso LR, et al. The role of antibiotics in gut microbiota modulation: the Eubiotic effects of Rifaximin. Dig Dis. 2016;34(3):269–78.
43. Gatta L, Scarpignato C. Systematic review with meta-analysis: rifaximin is effective and safe for the treatment of small intestine bacterial overgrowth. Aliment Pharmacol Ther. 2017;45(5):604–16.
44. Iannone A, Ruospo M, Wong G, Barone M, Principi M, Di Leo A, et al. Mesalazine for people with diverticular disease: a systematic review of randomized controlled trials. Can J Gastroenterol Hepatol. 2018;2018:5437135.
45. Lanas A, Ponce J, Bignamini A, Mearin F. One year intermittent rifaximin plus fibre supplementation vs. fibre supplementation alone to prevent diverticulitis recurrence: a proof-of-concept study. Dig Liver Dis. 2013;45(2):104–9.
46. Festa V, Spila Alegiani S, Chiesara F, Moretti A, Bianchi M, Dezi A, Traversa G, Koch M. Retrospective comparison of long-term ten-day/month rifaximin or mesalazine in prevention of relapse in acute diverticulitis. Eur Rev Med Pharmacol Sci. 2017;21:6.
47. Tursi A, Elisei W, Giorgetti GM, Inchingolo CD, Nenna R, Picchio M, Maiorano M, Penna A, Lecca PG, Brandimarte G. Effectiveness of different therapeutic strategies in preventing diverticulitis recurrence. Eur Rev Med Pharmacol Sci. 2013;17:342–8.
48. Stefanelli G, Viscido A, Valvano M, Vernia F, Frieri G, Ashktorab H, et al. Is mesalazine treatment effective in the prevention of diverticulitis? A review. Eur Rev Med Pharmacol Sci. 2020;24(15):8164–76.
49. Carabotti M, Annibale B. Treatment of diverticular disease: an update on latest evidence and clinical implications. Drugs Context. 2018;7:212526.
50. Hanna MH, Kaiser AM. Update on the management of sigmoid diverticulitis. World J Gastroenterol. 2021;27(9):760–81.
51. Kaiser AM, Jiang J-K, Lake JP, Ault G, Artinyan A, Gonzalez-Ruiz C, et al. The management of complicated diverticulitis and the role of computed tomography. Am J Gastroenterol. 2005;100(4):910–7.
52. Devaraj B, Liu W, Tatum J, Cologne K, Kaiser AM. Medically treated diverticular abscess associated with high risk of recurrence and disease complications. Dis Colon Rectum. 2016;59(3):208–15.
53. Roberts P, Abel M, Rosen L, Cirocco W, Fleshman J, Leff E, et al. Practice parameters for sigmoid diverticulitis. The standards task force American Society of Colon and Rectal Surgeons. Dis Colon Rectum. 1995;38(2):125–32.
54. Hall J, Hardiman K, Lee S, Lightner A, Stocchi L, Paquette IM, et al. The American Society of Colon and Rectal Surgeons clinical practice guidelines for the treatment of left-sided colonic diverticulitis. Dis Colon Rectum. 2020;63(6):728–47.
55. Ambrosetti P, Becker C, Terrier F. Colonic diverticulitis: impact of imaging on surgical management -- a prospective study of 542 patients. Eur Radiol. 2002;12(5):1145–9.
56. Morris AM, Regenbogen SE, Hardiman KM, Hendren S. Sigmoid diverticulitis: a systematic review. JAMA. 2014;311(3):287–97.
57. Hjern F, Josephson T, Altman D, Holmström B, Mellgren A, Pollack J, et al. Conservative treatment of acute colonic diverticulitis: are antibiotics always mandatory? Scand J Gastroenterol. 2007;42(1):41–7.
58. Ridgway PF, Latif A, Shabbir J, Ofriokuma F, Hurley MJ, Evoy D, et al. Randomized controlled trial of oral vs intravenous therapy for the clinically diagnosed acute uncomplicated diverticulitis. Color Dis. 2009;11(9):941–6.
59. Köhler L, Sauerland S, Neugebauer E. Diagnosis and treatment of diverticular disease: results of a consensus development conference. The scientific Committee of the European Association for endoscopic surgery. Surg Endosc. 1999;13(4):430–6.
60. Stollman N, Raskin JB. Diverticular disease of the colon. Lancet. 2004;363(9409):631–9.

61. Tursi A. Diverticulosis today: unfashionable and still under-researched. Ther Adv Gastroenterol. 2016;9(2):213–28.
62. van Dijk ST, Bos K, de MGJ B, Draaisma WA, van Enst WA, Felt RJF, et al. A systematic review and meta-analysis of outpatient treatment for acute diverticulitis. Int J Color Dis. 2018;33(5):505–12.
63. Cirocchi R, Randolph JJ, Binda GA, Gioia S, Henry BM, Tomaszewski KA, et al. Is the outpatient management of acute diverticulitis safe and effective? A systematic review and meta-analysis. Tech Coloproctol. 2019;23(2):87–100.
64. Biondo S, Golda T, Kreisler E, Espin E, Vallribera F, Oteiza F, et al. Outpatient versus hospitalization management for uncomplicated diverticulitis: a prospective, multicenter randomized clinical trial (DIVER trial). Ann Surg. 2014;259(1):38–44.
65. Hawkins AT, Wise PE, Chan T, Lee JT, Glyn T, Wood V, et al. Diverticulitis: an update from the age old paradigm. Curr Probl Surg. 2020;57(10):100862.
66. Alonso S, Pera M, Parés D, Pascual M, Gil MJ, Courtier R, et al. Outpatient treatment of patients with uncomplicated acute diverticulitis. Color Dis. 2010;12(10 Online):e278–82.
67. Rueda JC, Jimenez A, Caro A, Feliu F, Escuder J, Gris F, et al. Home treatment of uncomplicated acute diverticulitis. Int Surg. 2012;97(3):203–9.
68. Young-Fadok TM. Diverticulitis. N Engl J Med. 2018;379(17):1635–42.
69. Yoo T, Yang KH, Kim J, Park I, Cho H, Gwak G, et al. Predictive factors affecting the clinical course of patients with diverticulitis: who needs hospital management? Ann Coloproctol. 2018;34(1):23–8.
70. Estrada Ferrer O, Ruiz Edo N, Hidalgo Grau L-A, Abadal Prades M, Del Bas RM, Garcia Torralbo EM, et al. Selective non-antibiotic treatment in sigmoid diverticulitis: is it time to change the traditional approach? Tech Coloproctol. 2016;20(5):309–15.
71. van Dijk ST, Rottier SJ, van Geloven AAW, Boermeester MA. Conservative treatment of acute colonic diverticulitis. Curr Infect Dis Rep. 2017;19(11):44.
72. Balasubramanian I, Fleming C, Mohan HM, Schmidt K, Haglind E, Des WC. Out-patient Management of Mild or uncomplicated diverticulitis: a systematic review. Dig Surg. 2017;34(2):151–60.
73. Ünlü Ç, Gunadi PM, Gerhards MF, Boermeester MA, Vrouenraets BC. Outpatient treatment for acute uncomplicated diverticulitis. Eur J Gastroenterol Hepatol. 2013;25(9):1038–43.
74. Moya P, Arroyo A, Pérez-Legaz J, Serrano P, Candela F, Soriano-Irigaray L, et al. Applicability, safety and efficiency of outpatient treatment in uncomplicated diverticulitis. Tech Coloproctol. 2012;16(4):301–7.
75. Sirany A-ME, Gaertner WB, Madoff RD, Kwaan MR. Diverticulitis diagnosed in the emergency room: is it safe to discharge home? J Am Coll Surg. 2017;225(1):21–5.
76. Joliat G-R, Emery J, Demartines N, Hübner M, Yersin B, Hahnloser D. Antibiotic treatment for uncomplicated and mild complicated diverticulitis: outpatient treatment for everyone. Int J Color Dis. 2017;32(9):1313–9.
77. Mora López L, Flores Clotet R, Serra Aracil X, Montes Ortega N, Navarro SS. The use of the modified Neff classification in the management of acute diverticulitis. Rev Esp Enferm Dig. 2017;109(5):328–34.
78. Mali JP, Mentula PJ, Leppäniemi AK, Sallinen VJ. Symptomatic treatment for uncomplicated acute diverticulitis: a prospective cohort study. Dis Colon Rectum. 2016;59(6):529–34.
79. Lorente L, Cots F, Alonso S, Pascual M, Salvans S, Courtier R, et al. Tratamiento ambulatorio de la diverticulitis aguda no complicada: impacto sobre los costes sanitarios. Cir Esp. 2013;91(8):504–9.
80. Martín Gil J, Serralta De Colsa D, García Marín A, Vaquero Rodríguez A, Rey Valcárcel C, Pérez Díaz MD, et al. Eficiencia y seguridad del tratamiento ambulatorio de la diverticulitis aguda. Gastroenterol Hepatol. 2009;32(2):83–7.
81. Rodríguez-Cerrillo M, Poza-Montoro A, Fernandez-Diaz E, Romero AI. Patients with uncomplicated diverticulitis and comorbidity can be treated at home. Eur J Intern Med. 2010;21(6):553–4.

82. Nagata N, Ishii N, Manabe N, Tomizawa K, Urita Y, Funabiki T, et al. Guidelines for colonic diverticular bleeding and colonic diverticulitis: Japan gastroenterological association. Digestion. 2019;99(Suppl 1):1–26.
83. Jackson JD, Hammond T. Systematic review: outpatient management of acute uncomplicated diverticulitis. Int J Color Dis. 2014;29(7):775–81.
84. Ünlü Ç, van de Wall BJ, Gerhards MF, Wiezer M, Draaisma WA, Consten EC, et al. Influence of age on clinical outcome of acute diverticulitis. J Gastrointest Surg. 2013;17(9):1651–6.
85. Sánchez-Velázquez P, Grande L, Pera M. Outpatient treatment of uncomplicated diverticulitis: a systematic review. Eur J Gastroenterol Hepatol. 2016;28(6):622–7.
86. Swanson SM, Strate LL. Acute Colonic Diverticulitis. Ann Intern Med. 2018;168(9):ITC65–80.
87. You H, Sweeny A, Cooper ML, von Papen M, Innes J. The management of diverticulitis: a review of the guidelines. Med J Aust. 2019;211(9):421–7.
88. Bollom A, Austrie J, Hirsch W, Nee J, Friedlander D, Ellingson K, et al. Emergency department burden of diverticulitis in the USA, 2006-2013. Dig Dis Sci. 2017;62(10):2694–703.
89. Peláez N, Pera M, Courtiera R, Sánchez J, José Gil M, Parés D, et al. Aplicabilidad, seguridad y eficacia de un protocolo de tratamiento ambulatorio de la diverticulitis aguda no complicada. Cir Esp. 2006;80(6):369–72.
90. Lijoi D, Ferrero S, Mistrangelo E, Della Casa I, Crosa M, Remorgida V, et al. Bowel preparation before laparoscopic gynaecological surgery in benign conditions using a 1-week low fibre diet: a surgeon blind, randomized and controlled trial. Arch Gynecol Obstet. 2009;280(5):713–8.
91. de Korte N, Klarenbeek BR, Kuyvenhoven JP, Roumen RMH, Cuesta MA, Stockmann HBAC. Management of diverticulitis: results of a survey among gastroenterologists and surgeons. Color Dis. 2011;13(12):e411–7.
92. Dahl C, Crichton M, Jenkins J, Nucera R, Mahoney S, Marx W, et al. Evidence for dietary fibre modification in the recovery and prevention of reoccurrence of acute, uncomplicated diverticulitis: a systematic literature review. Nutrients. 2018;10(2)
93. Stam MAW, Draaisma WA, van de Wall BJM, Bolkenstein HE, Consten ECJ, Broeders IAMJ. An unrestricted diet for uncomplicated diverticulitis is safe: results of a prospective diverticulitis diet study. Color Dis. 2017;19(4):372–7.
94. van de Wall BJM, Draaisma WA, van Iersel JJ, van der Kaaij R, Consten ECJ, Broeders IAMJ. Dietary restrictions for acute diverticulitis: evidence-based or expert opinion? Int J Color Dis. 2013;28(9):1287–93.
95. Mattei P, Rombeau JL. Review of the pathophysiology and management of postoperative ileus. World J Surg. 2006;30(8):1382–91.
96. Peery AF. Management of colonic diverticulitis. BMJ. 2021;372:n72.
97. Rottier SJ, van Dijk ST, Ünlü Ç, van Geloven AAW, Schreurs WH, Boermeester MA. Complicated disease course in initially computed tomography-proven uncomplicated acute diverticulitis. Surg Infect. 2019;20(6):453–9.
98. Chabok A, Andreasson K, Nikberg M. Low risk of complications in patients with first-time acute uncomplicated diverticulitis. Int J Color Dis. 2017;32(12):1699–702.
99. Bolkenstein HE, van de Wall BJM, Consten ECJ, Broeders IAMJ, Draaisma WA. Risk factors for complicated diverticulitis: systematic review and meta-analysis. Int J Color Dis. 2017;32(10):1375–83.
100. Jaung R, Kularatna M, Robertson JP, Vather R, Rowbotham D, Maccormick AD, et al. Uncomplicated acute diverticulitis: identifying risk factors for severe outcomes. World J Surg. 2017;41(9):2258–65.
101. Biondo S, Parés D, Martí Ragué J, Kreisler E, Fraccalvieri D, Jaurrieta E. Acute colonic diverticulitis in patients under 50 years of age. Br J Surg. 2002;89(9):1137–41.
102. Vogels S, Frouws M, Morks AN, Roos D, van den Bremer J, Koch SMP, et al. Treating acute colonic diverticulitis with extraluminal pericolic air: an acute care surgery in the Netherlands (ACCSENT) multicenter retrospective cohort study. Surgery. 2021;169(5):1182–7.

Treatment for Complicated Acute Diverticulitis

23

Tomica Milosavljević and László Herszènyi

Clinically, diverticulitis is defined as a severe episode of lower abdominal pain that is usually left-sided, accompanied by low-grade fever, leukocytosis, and change in bowel movements [1–3]. Complicated diverticulitis occurs when inflammation leads to abscess, perforation and/or peritonitis, obstruction, and/or fistula. Approximately 12% of patients with diverticulitis present with complicated disease.

Risk factors for complicated diverticulitis include immunosuppression (e.g., corticosteroids and other immunosuppressive medications, chemotherapy, organ transplantation, and chronic renal failure). Nonsteroidal anti-inflammatory drug (NSAID) use is strongly associated with complicated diverticulitis including perforation. Another medication associated with complicated diverticulitis includes opiate analgesics. The risk of complicated diverticulitis is usually the highest during the first episode and decreases with subsequent episodes.

Guidelines classify diverticulitis as complicated and uncomplicated, based on computed tomography (CT) images.

Many associations strongly recommend an initial examination consisting of a specific history of the presenting complaint, physical examination, complete blood count, and urinalysis [4, 5]. Commencing treatment without imaging is reasonable in symptomatic patients with a previous history of diverticulitis, after completing a detailed history and physical examination. Yet, despite improved clinical scoring systems, misdiagnosis is common for patients presenting with the first episode of diverticulitis, due to the many differential diagnostic possibilities: irritable bowel syndrome, appendicitis, urinary tract infections, kidney stones, neoplasia, and

T. Milosavljević (✉)
Clinical Centre of Serbia, University of Belgrade, Belgrade, Serbia
e-mail: tommilos@hotmail.com

L. Herszènyi
Second Department of Medicine, Semmelweis University, Budapest, Hungary
e-mail: hersz@bel2.sote.hu

© The Author(s), under exclusive license to Springer Nature Switzerland AG 2022
A. Tursi et al. (eds.), *Colonic Diverticular Disease*,
https://doi.org/10.1007/978-3-030-93761-4_23

bowel obstruction. Clinical evaluation alone is often insufficient in the first diagnosis of diverticulitis and can lead to misdiagnosis. A radiological evidence of inflammation is needed for a definitive diagnosis of diverticulitis.

23.1 Biochemical Tests

All guidelines recommend that clinical diagnosis should consider the presenting complaint, physical examination, and biochemistry [3]. However, there is a controversy on whether biochemical tests can confirm diagnosis. All guidelines recognize that biochemistry alone is insufficient. CRP is recognized as the most powerful independent factor in the differentiation of diverticulitis from other abdominal conditions, but it only has diagnostic power if considered in combination with other factors, including white blood cell count. Other guidelines do not discuss the biochemical markers of diverticulitis. The negative predictive value of CRP below 50 mg/L is 79% for perforation in acute sigmoid diverticulitis.

In summary, biochemical markers are recommended in a routine evaluation. A high CRP and a high white blood cell count may help determine the severity of disease. Biochemical tests, however, do not confirm diagnosis.

Computed tomography (CT) is considered the best imaging choice for initial evaluation of patients with suspected diverticulitis because of its high sensitivity and specificity (94 and 99%, respectively) and its ability to detect other causes of left lower quadrant pain. CT confirms the diagnosis of diverticulitis, evaluates the severity and extent of the disease, guides management plans for the treatment of abscesses, and detects other causes of abdominal pain [1].

All major guidelines agree on its high predictive accuracy in diagnosing diverticulitis [3]. CT is not indicated routinely as a means to assess resolution of diverticulitis. However, when an outpatient's symptoms are not improving or have worsened after 5 days, a repeat CT would be recommended to ensure that the disease has not progressed. There is generally a lack of consensus regarding the use of a contrast in CT. Some guidelines and studies classify CT using oral, intravenous, or colonic contrasts as optimal. Other guidelines do not offer discussions or recommend contrast-enhanced CT over unenhanced CT. In the past, barium enema was the first-line imaging examination for diverticulitis. It is now surpassed by CT, mostly due to evidence showing superior diagnostic accuracy with CT. Barium enema is now discouraged following case studies reporting diverticular perforations. Nevertheless, water-soluble iodinated contrast enema is still used in some centers to evaluate suspected perforation.

In summary, CT has replaced barium enema as the primary imaging choice.

Ultrasound: High-resolution transabdominal ultrasound is considered an alternative imaging modality for suspected diverticulitis. The reported summary sensitivity is 92% and specificity is 90%. The guidelines from the Association of Coloproctology of Great Britain and Ireland (ACPGBI) recommend that CT or ultrasound should be used depending on local expertise. This was agreed upon by expert physicians from six countries at the 3rd International Symposium on Diverticular Disease of the Colon in 2019 [2]. Contrast-enhanced computer tomography (CE-CT) should be considered as the first-line colonic examination since it offers a more comprehensive evaluation of both uncomplicated and complicated forms; CE-CT can also be used to guide therapeutic interventions. Ultrasound has slightly lower sensitivity and specificity compared to those of CT in the assessment of acute diverticulitis, and its use as a first-line diagnostic procedure—followed by a CT scan in the case of inconclusive sonographic findings—may spare the use of CT in more than 50% of cases. Most guidelines also recognize that ultrasound may be useful in patients in whom CT scanning is contraindicated (e.g., pregnancy, contrast allergy, renal insufficiency). Ultrasound coupled with i.v. contrast agents (CEUS) differentiates between peri-intestinal phlegmon and abscess and demonstrates the actual extension of the abscess in acute diverticulitis. Two European guidelines recommend a conditional CT scan after a negative or inconclusive ultrasound [6, 7]. Ultrasound has acknowledged limitations compared with CT. It is highly operator-dependent and requires sonographer expertise. It is also dependent on body habitus as it cannot penetrate the extensive soft tissue or air-filled structures, resulting in poor image quality in obese patients or in those with overlying gas. In addition, probing may cause discomfort in patients with abdominal tenderness. In summary, ultrasound can be used to diagnose diverticulitis if carried out by an expert sonographer and is preferred in select patients where CT scanning is contraindicated. Ultrasound is useful in monitoring patients after acute diverticulitis and in particular the lesions treated conservatively.

23.2 Magnetic Resonance Imaging

The use of magnetic resonance imaging (MRI) in the diagnosis of diverticulitis is an area of controversy. Preliminary data show potential for MRI in assessing diverticulitis, with one of its major advantages being its lack of ionizing radiation. Moreover, it is less operator-dependent than ultrasound. Two small studies also suggest that MRI provides a better image to distinguish colonic carcinoma from inflammation; however, these preliminary data require confirmation by larger studies. The sensitivity and specificity of MRI are reported to be as high as 94 and 92%, respectively. The ASCRS recommends MRI as a useful alternative to CT to limit the patient's radiation exposure. The American College of Radiology, ACPGBI, NSS, and DSS acknowledge the potential of MRI, but fall short of recommendation due to lack of systematic analysis and consensual data. The clinical applicability in Australia is further questioned, as Medicare rebates do not apply to MRI scans for this indication. In summary, MRI use is not currently widely recommended for diagnosis of diverticulitis.

23.3 Colonoscopy

Whether patients should have a colonoscopy after an episode of diverticulitis depends on the patient's history, most recent colonoscopy, disease severity, and course. Colonoscopy is advised after an episode of complicated diverticulitis and after a first episode of uncomplicated diverticulitis, but can be deferred if a recent high-quality colonoscopy (within 1 year) was performed [1]. After an acute episode of diverticulitis, colonoscopy should be delayed by 6–8 weeks or until complete resolution of the acute symptoms, whichever is longer. Colonoscopy should be considered sooner if alarming symptoms are present [8].

Perforated colon cancer mimics both clinical evaluation and CT findings of diverticulitis. Owing to this, in the past, all major guidelines recommended a routine colonoscopy after CT-diagnosed diverticulitis to avoid misdiagnosis of a colonic neoplasm. However, systematic reviews of the literature have now specified that the evidence base supports routine colonoscopy only for cases of complicated diverticulitis. There are insufficient data to support the recommendation of routine colonoscopy for uncomplicated diverticulitis; its value has been further rebuked by large studies showing that the incidence of colorectal cancers after uncomplicated diverticulitis was not different to that observed in the general population. A systematic review and meta-analysis reported that routine colonoscopy in this group of patients yielded the same cancer incidence (around 0.7%) as that of the general population undergoing asymptomatic screening. Nonetheless, colonoscopy is still indicated for some uncomplicated diverticulitis cases, such as patients in whom a CT scan has identified short segments of disease with several diverticula (suggesting a more malign pathology) and patients who would otherwise fulfill the criteria for routine national screening. In Australia, the need for colonoscopy is based on the results of fecal occult blood testing, age, and other risk factors, including family history, set out in the National Bowel Cancer Screening Program. Similar recommendations are shared by the American Gastroenterological Association [9], which adds that colonoscopy should only be performed if a high-quality colonoscopy has not been performed recently (within 12 months). This decision is based on the timing and quality of previous colonoscopy, comorbidities, persistent symptoms, and patient preference. For complicated cases of diverticulitis, a follow-up colonoscopy is still warranted to rule out a colonic neoplasm. Even when colonoscopy is indicated, the NSS does not recommend it in the acute phase, as air insufflation and scope manipulation may cause a full perforation. A 6-week waiting period after diagnosis is recommended by several guidelines, to allow time for resolution of inflammation. In summary, colonoscopy is recommended for all cases of complicated diverticulitis 6 weeks after CT-diagnosed inflammation and in uncomplicated diverticulitis where there are concerning findings on CT or where the patient otherwise meets the national screening criteria.

23.4 Management of Complicated Diverticulitis

All guidelines currently recommend the use of intravenous broad-spectrum antibiotics and bowel rest for patients with complicated diverticulitis [2, 3, 7, 9–13].

Due to the lack of quality trials to provide evidence of the optimal treatment strategy, there is no universal practice for the management of complicated diverticulitis [14, 15].

According to the widely used modified Hinchey classification based on CT findings, patients with stage 0 and stage Ia diverticulitis have uncomplicated diverticulitis, whereas patients with stages Ib, II, III, and IV disease have complicated diverticulitis. The management of patients with stage Ib disease depends on the size of the abscess and the severity of presentation. It is generally agreed that bowel rest and intravenous antibiotics are sufficient for small abscesses of less than 3 cm. Patients with stage II (distant and larger abscesses of 3–5 cm) require antibiotics and generally percutaneous drainage as a bridge to elective surgical resection. Patients with stages III and IV disease (purulent and feculent peritonitis, respectively) require urgent surgical management [16].

Inpatient nonoperative treatment, including broad-spectrum antibiotics, bowel rest, and percutaneous drainage (followed by oral antibiotics and liquids or a low-residue diet in outpatients) are successful in 91% of all patients with complicated diverticulitis and in 95% of patients deemed appropriate for nonoperative treatment (i.e., perforation with or without abscess without peritonitis).

There is no recommended method for drainage [6, 12, 13, 17, 18]. In summary, smaller pericolic abscesses can be conservatively managed with bowel rest and antibiotics; larger abscesses of 3–5 cm should be percutaneously drained. Patients with peritonitis and sepsis should receive fluid resuscitation, rapid antibiotic administration, and urgent surgery.

Inpatient intravenous antibiotic treatment of mild-to-moderate complicated diverticulitis includes as single agents moxifloxacin and amoxicillin–clavulanic acid and cephalosporin, ciprofloxacin, and levofloxacin each in combination with metronidazole as multiple agents, whereas inpatient treatment of severe complicated diverticulitis, peritonitis, includes imipenem–cilastatin, meropenem, and piperacillin–tazobactam as single agents and cephalosporin, ciprofloxacin, and levofloxacin each in combination with metronidazole as multiple agents.

With up to 20% of patients with acute diverticulitis failing nonoperative management, it is important to understand the main criteria that warrant surgical intervention [18, 19]. In general, patients who require emergency or urgent surgery for diverticulitis in the acute setting fall into three main categories: (1) signs of diffuse peritonitis and/or free perforation; (2) suspicion of underlying malignancy; and (3) inadequate response to nonoperative measures (antibiotics, bowel rest, percutaneous abscess drainage) after 72 h as demonstrated by persistent symptoms and lack of normalization of objective findings (fever, tachycardia, leukocytosis). The presence of complicated diverticulitis (abscess, fistulae, stricture) by itself generally does not mandate an emergency/urgent surgical intervention [20–22].

References

1. Kaiser AM, Jiang JK, Lake JP, Ault G, Artinyan A, Gonzalez-Ruiz C, Essani R, Beart RW. The management of complicated diverticulitis and the role of computed tomography. Am J Gastroenterol. 2005;100(4):910–7. https://doi.org/10.1111/j.1572-0241.2005.41154.x.
2. Tursi A, Brandimarte G, Di Mario F, et al. International consensus on diverticulosis and diverticular disease. Statements from the 3rd international symposium on diverticular disease. J Gastrointestin Liver Dis. 2019;28(4):57–65.
3. You H, Sweeny A, Michelle L, Cooper ML, et al. The management of diverticulitis: a review of the guidelines. MJAFI. 2019;211(9):421–7.
4. Hanna MH, Kaiser AM. Update on the management of sigmoid diverticulitis. World J Gastroenterol. 2021;27(9):760–81.
5. Lambrichts DPV, Birindelli A, Tonini V, Cirocchi R, Cervellera M, Lange JF, Bemelman WA, Di Saverio S. The multidisciplinary management of acute complicated diverticulitis. Inflamm Intest Dis. 2018;3(2):80–90.
6. Gregersen R, Mortensen LQ, Burcharth J, Pommergaarg H-C, Rosenberg J. Treatment of patients with acute colonic diverticulitis complicated by abscess formation: a systematic review and meta-analysis. Int J Surg. 2016. https://doi.org/10.1016/j.ijsu.2016.10.006.
7. Schultz JK, Azhar N, Binda GA, et al. European Society of Coloproctology: guidelines for the management of diverticular disease of the colon. Color Dis. 2020. https://doi.org/10.1111/codi.15140.
8. Rottier SJ, van Dijk ST, van Geloven AA, et al. Meta-analysis of the role of colonoscopy after an episode of left-sided acute diverticulitis. BJS. 2019;106:988–97.
9. Peery AF, Shaukat A, Strate LL. AGA clinical practice update on medical management of colonic diverticulitis. Exp Rev Gastroenterol. 2021;160:906–11.
10. Binda GA, Cuomo R, Laghi A, et al. Practice parameters for the treatment of colonic diverticular disease: Italian Society of Colon and Rectal Surgery (SICCR) guidelines. Tech Coloproctol. 2015;19:615–26.
11. Francis NK, Sylla P, Abou-Khalil M, et al. EAES and SAGES 2018 consensus conference on acute diverticulitis management: evidence-based recommendations for clinical practice. Surg Endosc. 2019;33:2726–41.
12. Hall J, Hardiman K, Lee S, et al. The American Society of Colon and rectal surgeons clinical practice guidelines for the treatment of left-sided colonic diverticulitis. Dis Colon Rectum. 2020;63:728–47.
13. Sartelli M, Weber DG, Kluger Y, et al. 2020 update of the WSES guidelines for the management of acute colonic diverticulitis in the emergency setting. World J Emerg Surg. 2020;15:32. https://doi.org/10.1186/S13017-020-00313-4.
14. Strate LL, Morris AM. Epidemiology, pathophysiology, and treatment of diverticulitis. Gastroenterology. 2019;156(5):1282–98.
15. Young-Fadok TM. Diverticulitis. N Engl J Med. 2018;379:1635–42. https://doi.org/10.1056/NEJMcp1800468.
16. Sher ME, Agachan F, Bortul M, Nogueras JJ, Weiss EG, Wexner SD. Laparoscopic surgery for diverticulitis. Surg Endosc. 1997;11(3):264–7. https://doi.org/10.1007/s004649900340.
17. Hinchey EJ, Schaal PG, Richards GK. Treatment of perforated diverticular disease of the colon. Adv Surg. 1978;12:85–109.
18. Lee YF, Tang DD, Patel SH, Battaglia MA, Shanker BA, Cleary RK. Recurrence of acute right colon diverticulitis following nonoperative management: a systematic review and meta-analysis. Dis Colon Rectum. 2020;63(10):1466–73.
19. Fowler H, Gachabayov M, Vimalachandran D, Clifford R, Orangio GR, Bergamaschi R. Failure of nonoperative management in patients with acute diverticulitis complicated by abscess: a systematic review. Int J Color Dis. 2021. https://doi.org/10.1007/s00384-021-03899-6.
20. Swanson S, Strate LL. Acute colonic diverticulitis. Ann Intern Med. 2018;168:65–80.

21. Tursi A, Scarpignato C, Strate LL, et al. Colonic diverticular diseases. Nat Rev Dis Primers. 2020;6(1):20. https://doi.org/10.1038/s41572-020-0153-5.
22. van Dijk ST, Bos K, de Boer MG, Draaisma WA, van Enst WA, Felt RJ, Klarenbeek BR, Otte JA, Puylaert JB, van Geloven AA, Boermeester MA. A systematic review and meta-analysis of outpatient treatment for acute diverticulitis. Int J Color Dis. 2018;33(5):505–12.

Part VII

Surgical Treatment

Open Treatment of Acute Diverticulitis 24

Roberto Persiani, Roberto Pezzuto, and Cristina Marmorale

24.1 Introduction

Acute diverticulitis is a heterogeneous pathological process that varies from mild uncomplicated inflammation to complicated disease, including abdominal abscesses or free perforation with purulent or fecal peritonitis [1]. The severity of complicated diverticulitis is commonly classified into four stages by the CT-based Hinchey score [2].

In Western countries, acute diverticulitis represents a significant socioeconomic burden on patients and health-care systems. Indeed, the prevalence of hospitalization for diverticulitis is reported to be as high as 70–160 per 100,000 population per year [3, 4]. Furthermore, it is estimated that 8–38% of patients with acute diverticulitis present a complicated disease [5, 6].

The management of acute diverticulitis has evolved over time. In recent years, the improvement of antibiotics and the development of percutaneous techniques have allowed a successful nonsurgical management in 80% of patients with acute diverticulitis [7]. In particular, uncomplicated disease and diverticulitis with a localized abscess (stages I–II) are generally approached with conservative treatment. Surgical treatment is considered the standard therapy for severe diverticulitis with

R. Persiani (✉) · R. Pezzuto
Department of Surgical Sciences, First General Surgery Unit, "A. Gemelli" IRCCS Foundation, School of Medicine, Catholic University of the Sacred Heart, Rome, Italy
e-mail: roberto.persiani@unicatt.it; robertopezzuto@gmail.com

C. Marmorale
Department of Experimental and Clinical Medicine, School of Medicine and Surgery, Politechnical University of Marche, Ancona, Italy
e-mail: c.marmorale@univpm.it

© The Author(s), under exclusive license to Springer Nature Switzerland AG 2022
A. Tursi et al. (eds.), *Colonic Diverticular Disease*,
https://doi.org/10.1007/978-3-030-93761-4_24

perforation and generalized peritonitis (stages III–IV) or if conservative treatment fails [7, 8].

Optimal surgical treatment of diverticulitis remains poorly defined with regard to patient selection, timing, and technical approach in both elective and acute settings. Based on high-quality evidence, laparoscopic resection with primary anastomosis (PRA) is considered the preferred approach to elective colectomy if adequate expertise is available [9, 10]. In emergent and urgent settings, the role and outcomes of the type of operations, such as PRA or Hartmann's procedure (HP), as well as the approach, laparoscopic or open, have not been well studied and data are limited to low-quality randomized controlled trials and retrospective and nonrandomized studies. Based on a common context, general peritonitis, in hemodynamically unstable patients, is considered a contraindication for primary anastomosis and laparoscopic approach, especially when fecal. In this setting, laparotomy and Hartmann's procedure are still the most commonly used procedures [11]. The surgical treatment of acute complicated diverticulitis in stable patients is still a matter of intense debate. The treatment goals in this setting are different: resolution of the sepsis and symptoms and low complication rate maintaining intestinal continuity. Current guidelines and systematic reviews state that laparoscopy in an urgent setting should be restricted to selected cases in high-volume centers [10, 12]. Unquestionably, advanced skills in emergency minimally invasive colorectal surgery are crucial for successful laparoscopic treatment. However, in an acute setting, the presence of an experienced colorectal surgeon is not always realistic and open surgery still represents a valid choice.

The open surgical treatment of acute diverticulitis was first described by Mayo in 1907 [13]. It consisted of a three-stage approach: first, peritoneal lavage and creation of a proximal loop colostomy, followed by resection of the diseased colonic segment with anastomosis, and finally colostomy closure.

During the 1980s, HP became the standard therapy because resection of the source of sepsis at the time of index procedure was shown to improve postoperative morbidity and mortality [14]. The Hartmann's procedure consists of a sigmoid resection without reconstruction, burying the rectal stump, and performing a terminal colostomy. At the second stage, the colostomy is reversed. However, Hartmann's reversal may be a complex and time-consuming procedure associated with high surgical risk, particularly in older patients with many comorbidities [15]. As a result, up to 50% of patients remain with an ostomy [16, 17]. For this reason, during the 1990s, some authors [18] reported the role of resection and primary anastomosis (PRA) in the treatment of acute diverticulitis even in case of diffuse purulent or fecal peritonitis.

Based on the current evidences, the surgical strategy for diverticular disease remains challenging, with the needs to be tailored and individualized based on the severity and stage of disease, patient's comorbidities, surgeon's skills, and hospital resources. Despite the development of minimally invasive surgery, open surgery continues to play an important role in the treatment of diverticulitis. The indications for the open approach vary according to the clinical setting: emergent, urgent, or elective.

24.2 The Role of Open Surgery in Acute Settings

24.2.1 Urgent Surgery

Surgical strategy in perforated diverticulitis with diffuse purulent or fecal peritonitis in hemodynamically stable patients remains controversial. The goal is a balance between the increased risk of anastomotic failure and the consideration that end colostomies created under these circumstances are often permanent [16].

The open Hartmann's procedure has been the standard of care for perforated diverticulitis [12] and remains a safe approach for sigmoidectomy in diverticular peritonitis, especially in elderly patients and in patients with multiple comorbidities.

Hartmann's procedure is still the most commonly performed operation in an acute setting, with rates remaining relatively constant over the past decade [7]. Moreover, the open approach remains the most widely used [7], and although in highly selected and fit patients and in expert hands, laparoscopic sigmoidectomy for perforated diverticulitis is feasible, this approach cannot be extended unconditionally to the routine practice.

Computed tomography image of perforated diverticulitis with free air and fluids

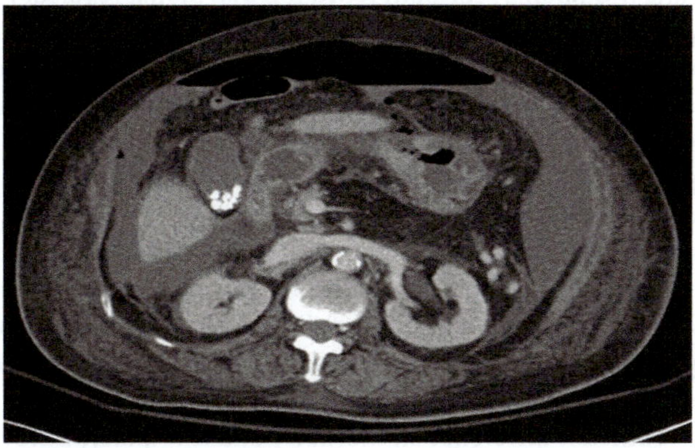

ED management of an eczematous flare

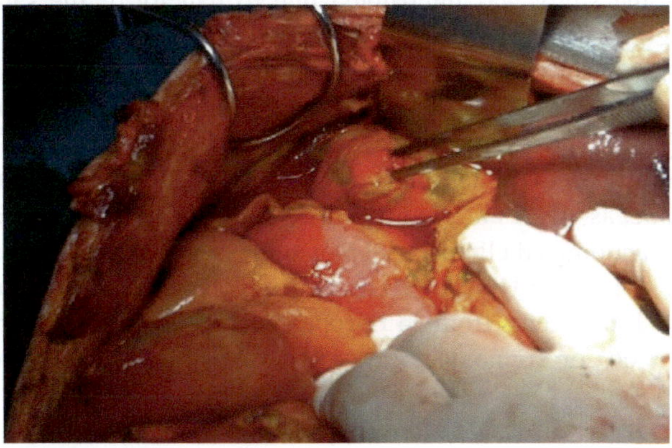

International guidelines recommend open resection without a clear preference for restoring bowel continuity: the decision should take into account patient factors, intraoperative findings, and surgeon preference [10, 12].

Some authors reported the role of primary resection and anastomosis with or without a diverting stoma. Temporary loop ileostomy has the major benefit of avoiding end colostomy and significant risks, in terms of morbidity and mortality, associated with Hartmann's procedure reversal [17]. Most of the evidences relating to the safety of primary anastomosis in this setting are obtained from retrospective case series, with their limitations and selection bias [19, 20]. Few randomized trials have been published.

A randomized clinical trial comparing Hartmann's procedure (HP) and resection with primary anastomosis (PRA) and diverting ileostomy in the treatment of Hinchey III and IV was published in 2012. Oberkofler et al. [21] compared patients from four different centers with colonic perforation and purulent or fecal peritonitis who underwent nonrestorative resection ($n = 30$) or resection with primary anastomosis and defunctioning ileostomy ($n = 32$). In both groups, the stoma reversal operation was planned after 3 months. The study was prematurely interrupted due to a low accrual rate and safety reasons. An interim analysis was carried out and showed a significant difference in relevant secondary outcomes. The overall complication rate (primary outcome) for both resection and stoma reversal operations was similar (80 vs 84%, respectively, $P = 0.813$). Although the outcome after the initial colon resection did not show any significant differences in mortality and morbidity, the stoma reversal rate after PRA with diverting ileostomy was higher (90 vs 57%, respectively, $P = 0.005$), and serious complications (Clavien–Dindo IIIb–IV: 0 vs 20%, $P = 0.046$), operating time, hospital stay, and in-hospital costs were significantly reduced in the PRA group.

Another randomized trial, by Binda et al. [22], was conducted to compare Hartmann's operation and resection with primary anastomosis in terms of adverse events, defined as mortality and morbidity following PRA or HP and stoma reversal, as the primary end point. During a 9-year period, 90 patients from 14 centers in 8 countries were randomly assigned to undergo PRA (34 patients) or HP (56 patients). There was no significant difference in mortality and morbidity, following PRA and HP. Despite a similar stoma reversal rate, adverse event rates following stoma reversal were significantly lower after PRA than HP (4.5 vs 23.5%; $P = 0.0589$). Unfortunately, the study was interrupted due to paucity of the sample size and authors reported it as inconclusive.

In 2017, Bridoux et al. [23] provided additional evidence in favor of resection with primary anastomosis. They demonstrated a significantly higher rate of definitive colostomy (stoma reversal rate at 18 months: 96% PA vs 65% HP; $p = 0.0001$) after Hartmann's procedure, despite a comparable rate of mortality, which was the primary outcome, as well as morbidity and a severe complication rate.

The largest randomized clinical trial that addressed the issue is the DIVA arm of the LADIES trail [24] for Hinchey III and IV, which analyses the 12-month stoma-free survival in 130 patients from 34 European centers who underwent Hartmann's procedure ($n = 66$) or sigmoidectomy with primary anastomosis ($n = 64$). This particular outcome describes both the risk of mortality and the likelihood of stoma reversal. Lambrichts et al. reported a significantly better 12-month stoma-free survival in patients with primary anastomosis, both for Hinchey III (79.8% HP vs 95.3 PRA; $p = 0.00025$) and IV (51.9% HP vs 92.2% PA; $p = 0.0016$). This result suggests not only a higher rate of stomal reversal after primary anastomosis but also describes a group of patients without defunctioning ileostomy. This innovative feature introduced in the LADIES trial highlights another important advantage, which is obviously impossible to achieve in Hartmann's procedure: the possibility to avoid a stoma. Moreover, despite no significant differences in short-term morbidity and mortality after the index procedures, lower overall morbidity (30% HP vs 8% PRA; $p = 0.023$) after stoma reversal in PRA is reported.

Based on these findings supporting resection with primary anastomosis as a safe and beneficial alternative to Hartmann's procedure, especially in terms of the stoma reversal rate, in 2014, the American Society of Colon and Rectal Surgeons (ASCRS) included it as an option for perforated diverticulitis in hemodynamically stable patients [25]. Despite these, in the clinical practice, its adoption is still limited.

In 2017, Cauley et al. [11] published a national retrospective cohort study. They showed that although the rate of primary anastomosis with diverting ileostomy increased from 30 to 60 per 1000 operative diverticulitis cases in a period from 1998 to 2011, the overall use remained low, with more than 90% of patients undergoing end colostomy. Moreover, they observed a higher rate of mortality and complications in patients undergoing primary anastomosis versus those receiving nonrestorative operations.

This evidence may be explained taking into account that randomized studies supporting primary anastomosis were conducted in large-volume referral centers by surgeons with colorectal board certification and thus may not reflect what really happens in a general practice. Some surgeons have expressed concerns over performing these more complex operations in the middle of the night with support staff who are unfamiliar with the equipment needed for a primary colorectal anastomosis [26, 27].

Goldstone et al. [28], in their state-wide retrospective cohort study, underlined that utilization of primary anastomosis with proximal diversion was greater among colorectal surgeons with significantly reduced postoperative mortality, but the vast majority of emergent surgeries for perforated diverticulitis (94%) are not performed by colorectal surgeons.

Limited data are available for studying the role of laparoscopic resection in patients with diffuse peritonitis due to perforated diverticulitis. However, laparoscopic resection may be feasible in stable patients even in the presence of purulent and fecal diverticular peritonitis [29].

The WSES (World Society of Emergency Surgery) guidelines [12] and the EASES (European Association of Endoscopic Surgery) and SAGES (Society of American Gastrointestinal and Endoscopic Surgery) 2018 consensus conference [10] suggest performing a laparoscopic sigmoidectomy for perforated diverticulitis only in an appropriate clinical setting, with proper equipment and technical skills. These guidelines are based on low-quality evidence because no randomized controlled trial has been published about this topic.

In 2016, Vennix et al. [30] performed a systematic review of 4 case series and 1 cohort study in which a total of 104 patients underwent emergency laparoscopic resection for perforated diverticulitis (84 Hartmann and 20 primary anastomosis without defunctioning ileostomy). No anastomotic leak was observed, surgical reintervention was necessary in two patients, the conversion rate varied from 0 to 19%, and three patients died postoperatively. A recent meta-analysis [29], including more than 400 patients from 4 prospective studies, has revealed significant advantages associated with a laparoscopic over the open approach to emergency sigmoidectomy in acute diverticulitis in terms of postoperative complication rates. Despite these excellent results, high-quality prospective or randomized studies are needed to demonstrate the benefits of emergency laparoscopic sigmoidectomy compared to those of open sigmoidectomy for perforated diverticulitis.

24.2.2 Emergent Surgery

Severe diffuse peritonitis in hemodynamically unstable patients with an overwhelming systemic inflammatory response is a life-threatening condition characterized by high mortality and morbidity rates [31, 32]. An immediate surgical intervention for source control is the cornerstone of treatment, besides adequate antimicrobial therapy, restoration of fluid and electrolyte imbalances, and physiological support of organ systems.

In this scenario, the goal is to save life and time is a luxury. These kinds of patients are not excellent candidates for complex or long procedures. Common sense suggests that surgery should be fast and lean and thus the open approach, limited resection with a complete multiquadrant peritoneal toilet, avoiding anastomosis, is preferred.

Despite low-quality evidence proving or disproving these concerns, Hartmann's procedure is strongly recommended in critically ill patients by the WSES guidelines [12] and by the EASES and SAGES 2018 consensus conference [10].

Moreover, the WSES guidelines [12] and the EASES and SAGES 2018 consensus conference [10] suggest considering a "damage control strategy" (DCS), with staged laparotomies, for unstable patients with perforated diverticulitis, to improve outcomes and to reduce the rate of end colostomies. In a DCS, patients are initially managed with peritoneal lavage, limited resection of the involved bowel, and suture of blind colonic stumps, with temporary abdominal closure. After stabilization in the intensive care unit, a second-look surgery is performed to restore intestinal continuity.

In 2010, Kafka-Ritsch et al. [33] published a prospective observational study including 51 patients with perforated diverticulitis Hinchey III or Hinchey IV. Patients were initially managed with limited resection, lavage, and temporary abdominal closure, followed by reconstructive operation 24–48 h later. Bowel continuity was restored in 84% patients. The overall mortality rate was 9.8%, anastomotic leak rate was 13%, and fascial closure was achieved in all patients.

In 2016, Sohn et al. [34] performed a case–control study comparing traditional strategy with damage control. They found no differences in morbidity and mortality, but the stoma rate was significantly reduced in the damage control group.

In 2020, Cirocchi et al. [35] published a meta-analysis on the role of damage control surgery in the treatment of perforated colonic diverticulitis. They reported about 62.1% of restoring intestinal continuity following the DCS approach, with a major leak rate of 4.7% and an overall mortality rate of 9.2%.

Limitations related to significant heterogeneity of the inclusion criteria, in particular the low rate of patients with septic shock, might suggest considering these results with extreme caution. Guidelines limit this strategy only in extremely ill patients who cannot withstand major surgery [12].

24.3 The Role of Open Surgery in Elective Settings

Determining the optimal management for patients with diverticular disease after recovery from complicated and uncomplicated diverticulitis involves a balance of the morbidity, mortality, risk of recurrence, and quality of life expected. The indications for elective colectomy following uncomplicated and complicated diverticulitis remain unclear. In general, guidelines [10, 12] favor individualized treatment decisions and a more selective use of elective colectomy. It has been estimated that 4–35% of successfully nonoperatively managed patients will undergo elective surgery [8].

The role of the open approach in elective surgery is limited and decreases over time. In 2016, Papageorge et al. [36] published a retrospective cohort study of a prospectively maintained National Surgical Quality Improvement Program (NSQIP) database, including patients undergoing nonemergent surgery for diverticulitis from 2005 to 2013. The use of laparoscopy increased significantly from 48% in 2005/2006 to 70% in 2013 ($p < 0.001$), and the absolute risk of any postoperative complication decreased by 5.8% over the study period, driven primarily by a reduction in infectious complications. In 2021, Napolitano et al. [37] published a retrospective review of the prospectively maintained Veterans Affairs Surgical Quality Improvement Program (VASQIP) database, including patients undergoing elective surgery for diverticular disease from 2004 to 2018. The 15-year time period of the study was then divided into 3-year increments to assess changes in approaches and outcomes over time. The rates of open surgery decreased from 81.7 to 46.9% ($p < 0.001$), whereas use of laparoscopy increased from 18.3 to 47.8% ($p < 0.001$) during the study period. Increased utilization of laparoscopy coincided with fewer complications and a shorter length of stay.

Since 2005, a Cochrane review [38] of short-term outcomes among 3526 patients from 25 randomized trials including surgeries for benign or malignant colorectal diseases has showed clinically relevant advantages of laparoscopic resections over the open approach in terms of surgical morbidities, length of postoperative hospital stay, and postoperative pain.

Laparoscopic surgery for elective resection for diverticular disease and its complications is strongly recommended over open surgery in several international guidelines [9, 10]. It seems important to underline that these recommendations are limited to surgeons with wide laparoscopic experience and in referral centers. High-volume surgeons and hospitals are significantly more likely to perform laparoscopic surgery for diverticular disease compared with low-volume surgeons and hospitals [39]. If this expertise is not available, or other technical concerns render minimally invasive surgery unsafe, then traditional open techniques should be used to perform the safest possible operation with optimal outcomes for the patient. However, caution is needed in complex cases, such as patients with complicated intestinal fistula. Although the laparoscopic approach for fistulized diverticulitis has shown to be feasible and safe, conversion rates as high as 18–61% have been reported for left colectomies for colovesical fistula [40, 41].

Despite the approach, laparoscopic or open, there are some technical cornerstones in elective surgical treatment for diverticulitis. Complete sigmoid colonic resection is mandatory, with distal transection at or below the rectosigmoid junction, to avoid the risk of recurrent disease. The proximal margin should be on the descending colon, in an area free from inflammation or thickening. Contrary to the principle of colorectal oncological surgery, high ligation of the inferior mesentery artery (IMA) is not imperative; its preservation should be considered to guarantee an optimal vascular supply for any anastomosis. Although routine mobilization of the splenic flexure is not supported by evidence, the descending colon should be fully mobilized to provide sufficient colonic length to form a tension-free anastomosis [10].

24.4 Conclusions

Surgery for diverticular disease and its complications may be difficult and challenging even in an elective setting. Multidisciplinary evaluation and careful selection of patients is necessary to achieve good results.

There seems to be a lack of a universal approach that can be considered the gold standard in case of diverticular disease and its complications. The best therapeutic option is definitely a customized evaluation based on the severity of disease and its symptoms, the quality of life expected for patients undergoing surgery, and its potential risks, taking into account the surgeon's expertise and hospital resources.

In the era of minimally invasive colorectal surgery, the open approach seems to be dated and antique but still represents a valid and safe choice especially in acute settings, in technically complex cases and in critically ill patients.

References

1. Hawkins AT, Wise PE, Chan T, et al. Diverticulitis: an update from the age old paradigm. Curr Probl Surg. 2020;57(10):100862. https://doi.org/10.1016/j.cpsurg.2020.100862.
2. Hinchey EJ, Schaal PG, Richards GK. Treatment of perforated diverticular disease of the colon. Adv Surg. 1978;12:85–109.
3. Jeyarajah S, Faiz O, Bottle A, Aylin P, Bjarnason I, Tekkis PP, Papagrigoriadis S. Diverticular disease hospital admissions are increasing, with poor outcomes in the elderly and emer-

gency admissions. Aliment Pharmacol Ther. 2009;30(11-12):1171–82. https://doi.org/10.1111/j.1365-2036.2009.04098.x.
4. Strate LL, Liu YL, Syngal S, Aldoori WH, Giovannucci EL. Nut, corn, and popcorn consumption and the incidence of diverticular disease. JAMA. 2008;300(8):907–14. https://doi.org/10.1001/jama.300.8.907.
5. Komen N, Morsink MC, Beiboer S, Miggelbrink A, Willemsen P, van der Harst E, Lange JF, van Leeuwen WB. Detection of colon flora in peritoneal drain fluid after colorectal surgery: can RT-PCR play a role in diagnosing anastomotic leakage? J Microbiol Methods. 2009;79(1):67–70. https://doi.org/10.1016/j.mimet.2009.08.004.
6. Biondo S, Ramos E, Deiros M, Ragué JM, De Oca J, Moreno P, Farran L, Jaurrieta E. Prognostic factors for mortality in left colonic peritonitis: a new scoring system. J Am Coll Surg. 2000;191(6):635–42. https://doi.org/10.1016/s1072-7515(00)00758-4.
7. Li D, Baxter NN, McLeod RS, Moineddin R, Wilton AS, Nathens AB. Evolving practice patterns in the management of acute colonic diverticulitis: a population-based analysis. Dis Colon Rectum. 2014;57(12):1397–405. https://doi.org/10.1097/DCR.0000000000000224.
8. Li D, Baxter NN, McLeod RS, Moineddin R, Nathens AB. The decline of elective colectomy following diverticulitis: a population-based analysis. Dis Colon Rectum. 2016;59(4):332–9. https://doi.org/10.1097/DCR.0000000000000561.
9. Hall J, Hardiman K, Lee S, Lightner A, Stocchi L, Paquette IM, Steele SR, Feingold DL. The American Society of Colon and Rectal Surgeons clinical practice guidelines for the treatment of left-sided colonic diverticulitis. Dis Colon Rectum. 2020;63(6):728–47. https://doi.org/10.1097/DCR.0000000000001679.
10. Francis NK, Sylla P, Abou-Khalil M, et al. EAES and SAGES 2018 consensus conference on acute diverticulitis management: evidence-based recommendations for clinical practice. Surg Endosc. 2019;33(9):2726–41. https://doi.org/10.1007/s00464-019-06882-z.
11. Cauley CE, Patel R, Bordeianou L. Use of primary anastomosis with diverting ileostomy in patients with acute diverticulitis requiring urgent operative intervention. Dis Colon Rectum. 2018;61(5):586–92. https://doi.org/10.1097/DCR.0000000000001080.
12. Sartelli M, Weber DG, Kluger Y, et al. 2020 update of the WSES guidelines for the management of acute colonic diverticulitis in the emergency setting. World J Emerg Surg. 2020;15(1):32. https://doi.org/10.1186/s13017-020-00313-4.
13. Mayo Wilson LB, Griffin HZWJ. Acquired diverticulitis of the large intestine. Surg Gynecol Obstet. 1907;5:8–15.
14. Krukowski ZH, Matheson NA. Emergency surgery for diverticular disease complicated by generalized and faecal peritonitis: a review. Br J Surg. 1984;71(12):921–7. https://doi.org/10.1002/bjs.1800711202.
15. Aydin HN, Remzi FH, Tekkis PP, Fazio VW. Hartmann's reversal is associated with high postoperative adverse events. Dis Colon Rectum. 2005;48(11):2117–26. https://doi.org/10.1007/s10350-005-0168-8.
16. Vermeulen J, Coene PP, Van Hout NM, van der Harst E, Gosselink MP, Mannaerts GH, Weidema WF, Lange JF. Restoration of bowel continuity after surgery for acute perforated diverticulitis: should Hartmann's procedure be considered a one-stage procedure? Color Dis. 2009;11(6):619–24. https://doi.org/10.1111/j.1463-1318.2008.01667.x.
17. Breitenstein S, Kraus A, Hahnloser D, Decurtins M, Clavien PA, Demartines N. Emergency left colon resection for acute perforation: primary anastomosis or Hartmann's procedure? A case-matched control study. World J Surg. 2007;31(11):2117–24. https://doi.org/10.1007/s00268-007-9199-8.
18. Cirocchi R, Afshar S, Di Saverio S, Popivanov G, De Sol A, Gubbiotti F, Tugnoli G, Sartelli M, Catena F, Cavaliere D, Taboła R, Fingerhut A, Binda GA. A historical review of surgery for peritonitis secondary to acute colonic diverticulitis: from Lockhart-Mummery to evidence-based medicine. World J Emerg Surg. 2017;12:14. https://doi.org/10.1186/s13017-017-0120-y.
19. Salem L, Flum DR. Primary anastomosis or Hartmann's procedure for patients with diverticular peritonitis? A systematic review. Dis Colon Rectum. 2004;47(11):1953–64. https://doi.org/10.1007/s10350-004-0701-1.

20. Constantinides VA, Tekkis PP, Athanasiou T, Aziz O, Purkayastha S, Remzi FH, Fazio VW, Aydin N, Darzi A, Senapati A. Primary resection with anastomosis vs. Hartmann's procedure in nonelective surgery for acute colonic diverticulitis: a systematic review. Dis Colon Rectum. 2006;49(7):966–81. https://doi.org/10.1007/s10350-006-0547-9.
21. Oberkofler CE, Rickenbacher A, Raptis DA, Lehmann K, Villiger P, Buchli C, Grieder F, Gelpke H, Decurtins M, Tempia-Caliera AA, Demartines N, Hahnloser D, Clavien PA, Breitenstein S. A multicenter randomized clinical trial of primary anastomosis or Hartmann's procedure for perforated left colonic diverticulitis with purulent or fecal peritonitis. Ann Surg. 2012;256(5):819–26. https://doi.org/10.1097/SLA.0b013e31827324ba.
22. Binda GA, Karas JR, Serventi A, Sokmen S, Amato A, Hydo L, Bergamaschi R. Primary anastomosis vs nonrestorative resection for perforated diverticulitis with peritonitis: a prematurely terminated randomized controlled trial. Color Dis. 2012;11:1403–10. https://doi.org/10.1111/j.1463-1318.2012.03117.x.
23. Bridoux V, Regimbeau JM, Ouaissi M, Mathonnet M, Mauvais F, Houivet E, Schwarz L, Mege D, Sielezneff I, Sabbagh C, Tuech JJ. Hartmann's procedure or primary anastomosis for generalized peritonitis due to perforated diverticulitis: a prospective multicenter randomized trial (DIVERTI). J Am Coll Surg. 2017;225(6):798–805. https://doi.org/10.1016/j.jamcollsurg.2017.09.004.
24. Lambrichts DPV, Vennix S, Musters GD, et al. Hartmann's procedure versus sigmoidectomy with primary anastomosis for perforated diverticulitis with purulent or faecal peritonitis (LADIES): a multicentre, parallel-group, randomised, open-label, superiority trial. Lancet Gastroenterol Hepatol. 2019;4(8):599–610. https://doi.org/10.1016/S2468-1253(19)30174-8.
25. Feingold D, Steele SR, Lee S, Kaiser A, Boushey R, Buie WD, Rafferty JF. Practice parameters for the treatment of sigmoid diverticulitis. Dis Colon Rectum. 2014;57(3):284–94. https://doi.org/10.1097/DCR.0000000000000075.
26. Schilling MK, Maurer CA, Kollmar O, Büchler MW. Primary vs. secondary anastomosis after sigmoid colon resection for perforated diverticulitis (Hinchey stage III and IV): a prospective outcome and cost analysis. Dis Colon Rectum. 2001;44(5):699–703. https://doi.org/10.1007/BF02234569.
27. Constantinides VA, Heriot A, Remzi F, Darzi A, Senapati A, Fazio VW, Tekkis PP. Operative strategies for diverticular peritonitis: a decision analysis between primary resection and anastomosis versus Hartmann's procedures. Ann Surg. 2007;245(1):94–103. https://doi.org/10.1097/01.sla.0000225357.82218.ce.
28. Goldstone RN, Cauley CE, Chang DC, Kunitake H, Ricciardi R, Bordeianou L. The effect of surgical training and operative approach on outcomes in acute diverticulitis: should guidelines be revised? Dis Colon Rectum. 2019;62(1):71–8. https://doi.org/10.1097/DCR.0000000000001240.
29. Cirocchi R, Fearnhead N, Vettoretto N, Cassini D, Popivanov G, Henry BM, Tomaszewski K, D'Andrea V, Davies J, Di Saverio S. The role of emergency laparoscopic colectomy for complicated sigmoid diverticulits: a systematic review and meta-analysis. Surgeon. 2019;17(6):360–9. https://doi.org/10.1016/j.surge.2018.08.010.
30. Vennix S, Boersema GS, Buskens CJ, Menon AG, Tanis PJ, Lange JF, Bemelman WA. Emergency laparoscopic sigmoidectomy for perforated diverticulitis with generalised peritonitis: a systematic review. Dig Surg. 2016;33(1):1–7. https://doi.org/10.1159/000441150.
31. van Ruler O, Boermeester MA. Surgical treatment of secondary peritonitis: a continuing problem. Chirurg. 2017;88(Suppl 1):1–6. https://doi.org/10.1007/s00104-015-0121-x.
32. Sartelli M, Catena F, Di Saverio S, et al. Current concept of abdominal sepsis: WSES position paper. World J Emerg Surg. 2014;9(1):22. https://doi.org/10.1186/1749-7922-9-22.
33. Kafka-Ritsch R, Birkfellner F, Perathoner A, et al. Damage control surgery with abdominal vacuum and delayed bowel reconstruction in patients with perforated diverticulitis Hinchey III/IV. J Gastrointest Surg. 2012;16(10):1915–22. https://doi.org/10.1007/s11605-012-1977-4.
34. Sohn M, Agha A, Heitland W, Gundling F, Steiner P, Iesalnieks I. Damage control strategy for the treatment of perforated diverticulitis with generalized peritonitis. Tech Coloproctol. 2016;20(8):577–83. https://doi.org/10.1007/s10151-016-1506-7.

35. Cirocchi R, Popivanov G, Konaktchieva M, et al. The role of damage control surgery in the treatment of perforated colonic diverticulitis: a systematic review and meta-analysis. Int J Color Dis. 2021;36(5):867–79. https://doi.org/10.1007/s00384-020-03784-8.
36. Papageorge CM, Kennedy GD, Carchman EH. National trends in short-term outcomes following non-emergent surgery for diverticular disease. J Gastrointest Surg. 2016;20(7):1376–87. https://doi.org/10.1007/s11605-016-3150-y.
37. Napolitano MA, Sparks AD, Randall JA, Brody FJ, Duncan JE. Elective surgery for diverticular disease in U.S. veterans: a VASQIP study of national trends and outcomes from 2004 to 2018. Am J Surg. 2021;221(5):1042–9. https://doi.org/10.1016/j.amjsurg.2020.08.050.
38. Schwenk W, Haase O, Neudecker J, Müller JM. Short term benefits for laparoscopic colorectal resection. Cochrane Database Syst Rev. 2005;3:CD003145. https://doi.org/10.1002/14651858.CD003145.pub2.
39. Weber WP, Guller U, Jain NB, Pietrobon R, Oertli D. Impact of surgeon and hospital caseload on the likelihood of performing laparoscopic vs open sigmoid resection for diverticular disease: a study based on 55,949 patients. Arch Surg. 2007;142(3):253–9. https://doi.org/10.1001/archsurg.142.3.253.
40. Vargas HD, Ramirez RT, Hoffman GC, Hubbard GW, Gould RJ, Wohlgemuth SD, Ruffin WK, Hatter JE, Kolm P. Defining the role of laparoscopic-assisted sigmoid colectomy for diverticulitis. Dis Colon Rectum. 2000;43(12):1726–31. https://doi.org/10.1007/BF02236858.
41. Laurent SR, Detroz B, Detry O, Degauque C, Honoré P, Meurisse M. Laparoscopic sigmoidectomy for fistulized diverticulitis. Dis Colon Rectum. 2005;48(1):148–52. https://doi.org/10.1007/s10350-004-0745-2.

Laparoscopic Treatment of Acute Diverticulitis

25

Savvas Papagrigoriadis and Valerio Papa

Nowadays, acute diverticulitis is a condition that is treated primarily medically, and surgery is kept as a reserve when medical treatment fails. This is in spite of a known higher recurrence with medical treatment versus surgical resection. The data are not from comparative studies; however, a systematic review showed that medical treatment has a threefold risk of recurrence of diverticulitis than surgical resection (18 v. 6%) [1]. The reason that guidance has become more conservative is that elective surgery for diverticulitis carries considerable operative risks with an overall risk of complications of 50% [2].

The current guidance [3] has moved away from considering the number of acute episodes as an indication for elective surgery, and the recommendation of several national guidelines is to make an individualized decision regarding resection which is individualised, based on patient condition and circumstances. There is no justification in surgery in the absence of evidence of inflammation (either ongoing or in documented prior attacks) [4]. However, this concerns the decision for elective surgery, in view of recurrent episodes or to treat chronic symptoms and in some cases to eliminate the risk of recurrence. Elective surgery for diverticular disease is described in another chapter of this book.

Emergency surgery in diverticulitis is often performed as an "open" laparotomy, and this topic is also described in another chapter.

The question this chapter examines is: is there a place for laparoscopic surgery for acute diverticulitis and its complications?

S. Papagrigoriadis (✉)
Department of Colorectal Surgery, King's College Hospital, London, UK
e-mail: lapasurgeon@gmail.com

V. Papa
Department of Digestive Surgery, "A. Gemelli" IRCCS Foundation, School of Medicine, Catholic University of the Sacred Heart, Rome, Italy
e-mail: valeriopapa@msn.com

© The Author(s), under exclusive license to Springer Nature Switzerland AG 2022
A. Tursi et al. (eds.), *Colonic Diverticular Disease*,
https://doi.org/10.1007/978-3-030-93761-4_25

Laparoscopic abdominal surgery is already three decades old, so it should not be considered novel any longer. Following the initial reports, laparoscopic colectomy for cancer has been affirmed by randomized trials [5] and systematic reviews [6] for more than 20 years now.

However, the acute abdomen presents many technical challenges and is also often accompanied by systemic illness, sepsis, and its consequences. The systemic condition of the patient should always be taken into consideration when the surgical approach is chosen. This is because, for all its advantages, laparoscopic surgery also has some occasional disadvantages such as the potential for a longer operating time, which may be undesirable in unstable patients.

Laparoscopic surgery has been tried and has succeeded in all kinds of abdominal emergencies in the hands of appropriately trained surgeons [7]. Acute diverticulitis can occasionally present as one of the more severe abdominal emergencies, both in terms of anatomy (adhesions, abscesses, fistulas) and in terms of septic unstable patients.

Nonelective surgery for acute diverticulitis and its complications can be *emergency* (in free perforation), *urgent* (within days due to failure of medical treatment), or *expedited* (within weeks of the attack). In case of expedited surgery, this is usually for the type of condition recently described as "*smouldering diverticulitis*" [8], i.e., inflammation that does not settle completely and flares up once again a few days or weeks after discharge and interruption of antibiotics. Typically, those patients have a "cluster" of symptomatic episodes, clinical attendances, or readmissions within a short period of a few months. Many of those patients are consistent with the description provided by Ambrosetti et al. [9] who showed that the formation of abscess and extracolonic contrast or gas predicts the failure of medical treatment and the development of complications, hence indicating a need for surgery.

Surgery for Hinchey III and IV peritonitis would be expected to take place as emergency, whereas Hinchey I and II would comprise the great majority of surgery that is performed as urgent or expedited.

25.1 Technical Considerations

From the technical point of view, laparoscopic pneumoperitoneum is safe and fast to perform. In the presence of abdominal distension caused by peritonitis, the open Hasson trocar technique can minimize the risk of injuring the bowel. After the initial camera port, the remaining ports can be placed safely under direct vision. It will then be immediately obvious whether there is fecal material or free pus in the abdomen and thus a decision on how to proceed can be made. In contemporary Western hospitals, almost all surgeons are trained in laparoscopy and this initial diagnostic step can be performed by the average on-call general surgeon and not just by the specialist. If the patient is not overtly septic and the circulation is stable, there is no harm in performing a diagnostic laparoscopy in almost all patients.

The amount of adhesions in the abdomen can be highly variable, and thus substantial surgical skills may be required for safe adhesiolysis. A full small bowel adhesiolysis may be necessary to completely visualize the left colon, which is the site of diverticulitis in the vast majority of cases in the Western hemisphere. In the rare event of right-sided diverticulitis, this is usually associated with solitary diverticula, which are easier to locate and manage surgically.

In the presence of Hinchey I peritonitis, a thickened inflamed sigmoid is identified and a sigmoid colectomy can be performed in a standard manner as for any other colonic pathology. There has been some debate as to whether the preservation of the inferior mesenteric artery or the superior rectal artery should be practiced for the theoretical purposes of maintaining better vascular supply of the distal stump and thus also theoretically decreasing the risk of anastomotic leak. A study by Lehmann et al. [10] looked into that dilemma and their conclusion was that the preservation of those vessels does not offer any advantage in terms of anastomotic leak. From the technical point of view, dissection—mobilization of the sigmoid colon alongside the same planes as for colorectal cancer with high ligation of the inferior mesenteric artery—is easier for most surgeons both because they are familiar with it and also because the increased inflammation and edema of the mesocolon is likely to cause bleeding and delay. The "lateral-to-medial" approach is also easier in left colectomy for diverticulitis because of the thickness of the mesocolon.

In the presence of Hinchey II peritonitis, the abscess must be located and it must be ensured that there is no formation of any fistula with other organs. The sigmoid colon may have to be fully mobilized for that purpose if the abscess is posterior. The mobilization of the splenic flexure is believed to be protective of the anastomosis and it is generally preferred by many colorectal surgeons but it cannot be considered mandatory. Nevertheless, there are supporting studies although they are not randomized supporting splenic flexure mobilisation in case of short left colon [11]. It has to be noted that laparoscopy offers the advantage of full views of the splenic flexure and the spleen and thus has a technical advantage over the open approach.

The left ureter can be at risk of being entangled in the inflammatory tissues and great caution should be exercised for its recognition. The preoperative CT scan of the patient should have been examined for any warning signs such as subtle hydronephrosis or the presence of an inflammatory mass in the anatomical proximity of the left ureter. In case of any concerns, the safest practice is to perform a cystoscopy prior to the laparoscopy and place pigtail catheters in the ureters. Even though there are no comparative trial results yet to support this recommendation, it is a precaution increasingly taken by many surgeons [12].

Once inside the abdomen, the decision as to which operation to perform is critical. Laparoscopic peritoneal lavage has been shown to provide relief from symptoms of diverticulitis in the short term even in Hinchey III peritonitis [13]; however, there are concerns that there can be more recurrences and eventually a need for colectomy. Lavage is discussed in another chapter; however, it should be noted that for successful lavage, sufficient laparoscopic adhesiolysis and visualization of all abdominal quadrants has to be performed.

The point of transection of the colon can be difficult to decide on occasion. In most of the cases, acute diverticulitis is a condition localized in the sigmoid colon, which is separated by the descending colon with a gradual demarcation zone of receding inflammation. In those cases, it is relatively easy to decide to place a stapler for transection in a reasonably healthy area of the descending colon. In many cases, there are more diverticula on the descending colon and even in the whole colon. It is not advisable to attempt eliminating all diverticula if they are not inflamed. Reports on extended left colectomies or subtotal colectomies for diverticulitis have not shown any benefit and can occasionally cause long-term disability from chronic diarrhea. However, there can be occasions where active diverticulitis involves or extends up to the descending colon. In those cases, it is an error to leave inflamed diverticulitis behind. If that is the case a full mobilization of the left colon and an extended left hemicolectomy has to be performed. In those cases, there may be surgical wisdom in trying to preserve the left branch of the middle colic artery if the anatomy allows sufficient mobilization, although we have no data to confirm that yet.

Following complete mobilization with recognition and preservation of both ureters and also mobilization of the spleen, laparoscopic colectomy is performed using intracorporeal transection with an endoscopic linear stapler. Anastomosis is performed using a circular stapler. A tire leak test is recommended in general for checking the anastomosis. If the tire test is negative then an ileostomy is not necessary. The specimen can be extracted via either a Pfannenstiel hypogastric incision or a 6 cm umbilical incision. Although specimen extraction through the anus has been described in elective diverticular resection, it is not likely that an edematous inflamed colon will be suitable for that extraction route. The decision for the extraction incision depends on the anatomy and body habitus of the patient, and there is no difference in either postoperative pain or incisional hernias, irrespective of the choice.

At that point, there comes the decision as to anastomose or not. Hartmann's sigmoidectomy with an end colostomy used to be a common choice in the past.

In Hinchey I, II, and III peritonitis, the evidence supports primary anastomosis [14]. An ileostomy is not mandatory, and it is not recommended as the standard practice. In fact, complications of the ileostomy formation and also the ileostomy reversal are added to the overall morbidity and should be avoided if possible.

Abundant evidence has accumulated in recent years suggesting that Hartmann's has more disadvantages than benefits: it requires a complex major reversal operation and if the patient is not fit or willing to undergo that then they are left with a permanent colostomy. Most reasonable surgeons would choose Hartmann's only in case of a septic unstable patient on the table; in all other cases, there is sufficient evidence that even in the presence of Hinchey IV fecal peritonitis anastomosis with a defunctioning ileostomy can be equally safe. Several randomized trials have shown that in Hinchey III and even in Hinchey IV fecal peritonitis, a primary anastomosis with a diverting stoma has not only equally good outcomes with Hartmann's but in fact better [15–18].

It is believed that if no sigmoid colon is left distally and anastomosis is performed on the rectum, then there may be less long-term recurrence of diverticulitis, but the data available is not of high quality [19].

25.2 Safety of Laparoscopic Surgery for Diverticulitis

As in medicine and surgery, the wisdom is "primum non nocere"; we can make an overall statement that many studies have shown that laparoscopic surgery for diverticulitis is safe.

In many studies in the last 20 years, elective laparoscopic surgery for diverticular disease has been shown to be safe and noninferior, and in some aspects superior, to open surgery [20]. However, most of those cases described in the literature are "cold" without the surgery taking place in the middle of inflammatory episodes. How does active inflammation affect the outcome? To answer this question, a study by Rotholtz et al. [21] compared the outcomes of laparoscopic surgery between a group (G1) of 72 patients who had laparoscopic colectomy for diverticular complications (abscess, perforation, fistula, or stenosis) and a group (G2) of 188 patients who had surgery for recurrent diverticulitis. The G1 patients had a higher conversion rate (18 vs. 3.2%) and longer hospital stay by 1 day. However, there were no differences in either complications or mortality, which shows that complications should not be a deterrent for the laparoscopic approach for skilled laparoscopic surgeons.

It is important to distinguish between the earlier stages of peritonitis, i.e., Hinchey I to Hinchey III on one hand and Hinchey IV fecal peritonitis on the other. Unfortunately, not all published studies present an analysis of the mixture of their cases, which weakens the conclusions of the systematic reviews.

25.2.1 Laparoscopic Surgery for Hinchey Peritonitis I–III

Katsuno et al. [14] published a series of laparoscopic resection of 58 patients with Hinchey I–II diverticulitis. They found that complications were significantly lower in the laparoscopic group (16.7 vs. 43.8%) and that the group also had a shorter hospital stay. There were no stomas or anastomotic leaks in either group.

El Zarrok Elgazwi et al. [22] published a series of 260 sigmoid colectomies for diverticulitis with a conversion rate of 5.7%, complication rate of 11.5%, 5 anastomotic leaks, and 2 deaths. Most of the patients in this series (230/260) had Hinchey stage I diverticulitis, but it is interesting that there were even 23/260 patients with Hinchey III perforated diverticulitis. This report shows that in the hands of experienced laparoscopic surgeons, perforations and even fistulas or stenosis are not a contraindication for laparoscopy. There is extremely low mortality, which cannot be avoided in any large series of those difficult cases.

Levack et al. [23] found in a nonrandomized comparison that laparoscopic sigmoid colectomy for diverticulitis had a much lower risk of anastomotic leak than in open surgery (2.4 vs. 8.2%); however, it is unclear whether this was due to group differences, for example, the laparoscopic group had a higher rate of splenic flexure mobilization.

The Sigma trial [24] included patients with Hinchey I or Hinchey IIb symptomatic diverticulitis. Patients were operated 3 months after the last attack of diverticulitis. Therefore, this trial should be considered as examining the "expedited" group of operations and not those performed as part of an emergency admission or shortly after that. They found that laparoscopic surgery had lower complications (9.6 vs. 25%), involved less pain, and had earlier discharge.

A systematic review by Biondo et al. [25] examined 92 studies of which 10 were randomized controlled trials. The review identified that laparoscopic lavage can be successful in many perforated patients and also that careful selection of patients allowed the performance of colectomy with primary anastomosis.

In terms of technical difficulties, it has been shown that increasing the number of attacks increases the conversion rate in laparoscopic diverticulitis surgery [26]. Three prior attacks raised the conversion rate to 25%.

Le Moine et al. [27] showed that the nonconverted patients maintained significant advantages of laparoscopy than did the converted patients: overall operating time, the need for nasogastric suction, bowel mobilization, resumption of eating, the need for analgesics, intensive care stay, and general hospital stay were all of lesser incidence in the cases completed laparoscopically. However, there was no difference in the incidence of postoperative complications.

A Cochrane systematic review by Abraha et al. [28] examined 635 publications and selected 3 trials comparing open surgery with laparoscopic surgery for sigmoid diverticulitis. The included trials were the Sigma trial [29] by Gervaz et al. [30, 31] and by Raue et al. [32] and the total number of reviewed patients was 360. All patients were of Hinchey peritonitis stages I–III. The main results were as follows:

The length of stay was not different between open and laparoscopic surgeries. The 30-day postoperative mortality was lower in the laparoscopic group (0%) than in the open group (1.7%). This was the same even for late mortality. The rate of overall surgical complications was lower in the laparoscopic group (RR 0.84, 95% CI). There was no difference in the rate of overall major complications between the open and laparoscopic groups (RR 0.74, 95% CI 0.43–1.25). The same was true for minor complications.

Laparoscopic surgery was associated with a longer operating time than open surgery. The Sigma trial examined whether this longer time was associated with more intraoperative blood loss and found that it was not.

With regard to postoperative pain, all 360 participants filled questionnaires of pain scales and quality of life and there was only a small difference around the fourth postoperative day. Both groups had similar results with regard to postoperative feeding and bowel mobilization. There was no difference in the reoperations and other major complications. The meta-analysis did not find evidence in favor of either the laparoscopic or the open surgery for acute diverticulitis.

Another systematic review by Ahmed et al. [33] of randomized trials comparing laparoscopic with open surgery for diverticulitis and its complications found no difference between the groups regarding overall postoperative morbidity, no difference regarding mortality, and no difference regarding the occurrence of incisional hernia.

The DILALA trial [34] compared laparoscopic lavage with resection as treatment for perforated diverticulitis. Patients with laparoscopic lavage had a 45% reduction of risk to undergo colectomy and colostomy at 2 years. There was no other difference.

A US study found that in a database of 1314 patients [35] who underwent emergency surgery for diverticulitis, a total of 991 patients (75.4%) were managed with HP, 285 (21.7%) had a colectomy with PA, and 38 (2.9%) had colectomy with PA and proximal diverting colostomy or ileostomy. It was also found that laparoscopic surgery was performed in only 83 patients of whom 43 had primary anastomosis, 32 had Hartmann's, and 2 had primary anastomosis with a stoma. The PA group (13.3%) was more likely to have a laparoscopic procedure compared with HP (4.3%) and PAPD (5.3%). The multiple regression analysis did not find any difference in any of the surgical techniques in terms of mortality, complications, surgical wound infections, or thrombotic events.

Hand-assisted laparoscopic surgery (HALS) is a variation of the technique applied in cases of inflamed colon or extensive pelvic adhesions. Pendlimari et al. [36] analyzed 361 patients of whom 136 had complicated diverticulitis and compared laparoscopic surgery with HALS, which showed both techniques to be equivalent and also safe and effective.

A mathematical model analysis of the optimal operative strategy for Hinchey III sigmoid diverticulitis by Dossa et al. [37] concluded that primary resection and anastomosis is the optimal approach yielding higher quality-adjusted life years.

25.2.2 Laparoscopic Surgery for Hinchey III and IV Peritonitis

Lee et al. [38] published a study on the database of the American College of Surgeons in which 3299 open operations of perforated diverticular peritonitis were compared with 282 laparoscopic-completed cases. There were also 175 cases of conversion to open. The laparoscopic-completed approach had better outcomes than did the open surgery, i.e., fewer complications, less unplanned intubation, and acute renal failure. The advantages of laparoscopy remained even if the case had to be converted to open.

Cassini et al. [39] examined 60 patients with Hinchey III and IV diffuse diverticular peritonitis, who had undergone either laparoscopic [34] or open [23] surgery. Laparoscopic patients had around half the incidence of complications of the open one while the mortality was high in both groups, around 16%. As this was not a randomized trial, it cannot serve as guidance, and it is likely that the sicker patients may have gotten open surgery.

A particular case of complicated diverticulitis is when it involves colovesical fistulas, which are a technically challenging variance. A systematic review by Cirocchi et al. [40] examined 25 studies and 202 patients with laparoscopic resection and primary anastomosis of colovesical fistulas. There was zero mortality and only one anastomotic leak. The authors concluded that laparoscopic surgery was feasible even for those complex cases.

Table 25.1 List of studies supporting the safety and efficacy of laparoscopic surgery in diverticulitis

Clinical studies		
	Type	*N* = patients
Le Moine (2003)	Prospective series	168
Killingback (2004)	Prospective series	206
Klarenbeek (2009)	Randomized controlled trial	104
Cole (2009)	Retrospective	216
El Zarrok Elgazwi (2010)	Retrospective	260
Gervaz (2010)	Randomized trial	113
Katsuno (2011)	Retrospective	58
Masoomi (2011)	Database analysis	124,734
Levack (2011)	Retrospective	249
Raue (2011)	Randomized trial	143
Rotholtz (2016)	Retrospective	236
Systematic reviews		
Biondo (2012)	Systematic review	92 studies
Abraha (2017)	Systematic review of randomized trials	3 studies
Ahmed (2018)	Systematic review and meta-analysis of randomized trials	5 studies

25.3 Conclusions

There is now abundant evidence that laparoscopic surgery can be safely performed for all stages and forms of diverticulitis. The quality of evidence is not adequate to prove superiority of either laparoscopic or open surgery. Considering that laparoscopy has already become the new gold standard in colorectal surgery and all surgeons of the latest generations are trained in the method, laparoscopic surgery is not likely to be researched against open surgery for much longer. Most current trials are designed to compare laparoscopy against robotic or natural orifice surgery. This real-life situation has been recognized in the recent guidelines of both the UK NICE and the European Society of Coloproctology, both of which state that in the absence of evidence of superiority of either technique, surgeons prefer practicing laparoscopy.

References

1. Peppas G, Bliziotis IA, Oikonomaki D, Falagas ME. Outcomes after medical and surgical treatment of diverticulitis: a systematic review of the available evidence. J Gastroenterol Hepatol. 2007;22(9):1360–8. https://doi.org/10.1111/j.1440-1746.2007.05118.x.
2. Killingback M, Barron PE, Dent OF. Elective surgery for diverticular disease: an audit of surgical pathology and treatment. ANZ J Surg. 2004;74(7):530–6. https://doi.org/10.1111/j.1445-2197.2004.03071.x.
3. Hall J, Hardiman K, Lee S, Lightner A, Stocchi L, Paquette IM, Steele SR, Feingold DL. The American Society of Colon and rectal surgeons clinical practice guidelines for the treat-

ment of left-sided colonic diverticulitis. Dis Colon Rectum. 2020;63(6):728–47. https://doi.org/10.1097/DCR.0000000000001679.
4. Schultz JK, Azhar N, Binda GA, Barbara G, Biondo S, Boermeester MA, Chabok A, Consten ECJ, van Dijk ST, Johanssen A, Kruis W, Lambrichts D, Post S, Ris F, Rockall TA, Samuelsson A, Di Saverio S, Tartaglia D, Thorisson A, Winter DC, Bemelman W, Angenete E. European Society of Coloproctology: guidelines for the management of diverticular disease of the colon. Color Dis. 2020;22(Suppl 2):5–28. https://doi.org/10.1111/codi.15140.
5. COLOR Study Group. COLOR: a randomized clinical trial comparing laparoscopic and open resection for colon cancer. Dig Surg. 2000;17(6):617–22. https://doi.org/10.1159/000051971.
6. Kuhry E, Schwenk WF, Gaupset R, Romild U, Bonjer HJ. Long-term results of laparoscopic colorectal cancer resection. Cochrane Database Syst Rev. 2008;2:CD003432. https://doi.org/10.1002/14651858.CD003432.pub2.
7. Jimenez Rodriguez RM, Segura-Sampedro JJ, Flores-Cortés M, López-Bernal F, Martín C, Diaz VP, Ciuro FP, Ruiz JP. Laparoscopic approach in gastrointestinal emergencies. World J Gastroenterol. 2016;22(9):2701–10. https://doi.org/10.3748/wjg.v22.i9.2701.
8. Rink AD, Nousinanou ME, Hahn J, Dikermann M, Paul C, Vestweber KH. Smoldering diverticultis - still a type of chronic recurrent diverticulitis with good indication for surgery? - Surgery for smoldering diverticulitis. Z Gastroenterol. 2019;57(10):1200–8. https://doi.org/10.1055/a-0991-0700.
9. Ambrosetti P, Becker C, Terrier F. Colonic diverticulitis: impact of imaging on surgical management - a prospective study of 542 patients. Eur Radiol. 2002;12(5):1145–9. https://doi.org/10.1007/s00330-001-1143-y.
10. Lehmann RK, Brounts LR, Johnson EK, Rizzo JA, Steele SR. Does sacrifice of the inferior mesenteric artery or superior rectal artery affect anastomotic leak following sigmoidectomy for diverticulitis? A retrospective review. Am J Surg. 2011;201(5):623–7. https://doi.org/10.1016/j.amjsurg.2011.01.011.
11. Schlussel AT, Wiseman JT, Kelly JF, Davids JS, Maykel JA, Sturrock PR, Sweeney WB, Alavi K. Location is everything: the role of splenic flexure mobilization during colon resection for diverticulitis. Int J Surg. 2017;40:124–9. https://doi.org/10.1016/j.ijsu.2017.02.094.
12. Chiu AS, Jean RA, Gorecka J, Davis KA, Pei KY. Trends of ureteral stent usage in surgery for diverticulitis. J Surg Res. 2018;222:203–11. https://doi.org/10.1016/j.jss.2017.09.050.
13. Scarpinata R, Papagrigoriadis S. A systematic review of the role of laparoscopic peritoneal lavage in Hinchey III peritonitis. World J Colorect Surg. 2014;4:1.
14. Katsuno G, Fukunaga M, Nagakari K, Yoshikawa S. Laparoscopic one-stage resection of right and left colon complicated diverticulitis equivalent to Hinchey stage I-II. Surg Today. 2011;41(5):647–54. https://doi.org/10.1007/s00595-010-4349-2.
15. Binda GA, Karas JR, Serventi A, et al. Primary anastomosis vs nonrestorative resection for perforated diverticulitis with peritonitis: a prematurely terminated randomized controlled trial. Color Dis. 2012;14:1403–10.
16. Oberkofler CE, Rickenbacher A, Raptis DA, Lehmann K, Villiger P, Buchli C, Grieder F, Gelpke H, Decurtins M, Tempia-Caliera AA, Demartines N, Hahnloser D, Clavien PA, Breitenstein S. A multicenter randomized clinical trial of primary anastomosis or Hartmann's procedure for perforated left colonic diverticulitis with purulent or fecal peritonitis. Ann Surg. 2012;256(5):819–26. https://doi.org/10.1097/SLA.0b013e31827324ba.
17. Sohn M, Iesalnieks I, Agha A, Steiner P, Hochrein A, Pratschke J, Ritschl P, Aigner F. Perforated diverticulitis with generalized peritonitis: low stoma rate using a "damage control strategy". World J Surg. 2018;42(10):3189–95. https://doi.org/10.1007/s00268-018-4585-y.
18. Cauley CE, Patel R, Bordeianou L. Use of primary anastomosis with diverting ileostomy in patients with acute diverticulitis requiring urgent operative intervention. Dis Colon Rectum. 2018;61(5):586–92. https://doi.org/10.1097/DCR.0000000000001080.
19. Benn PL, Wolff BG, Ilstrup DM. Level of anastomosis and recurrent colonic diverticulitis. Am J Surg. 1986;151(2):269–71. https://doi.org/10.1016/0002-9610(86)90085-1.

20. Masoomi H, Buchberg B, Nguyen B, Tung V, Stamos MJ, Mills S. Outcomes of laparoscopic versus open colectomy in elective surgery for diverticulitis. World J Surg. 2011;35(9):2143–8. https://doi.org/10.1007/s00268-011-1117-4.
21. Rotholtz NA, Canelas AG, Bun ME, et al. Laparoscopic approach in complicated diverticular disease. World J Gastrointest Surg. 2016;8(4):308–14. https://doi.org/10.4240/wjgs.v8.i4.308.
22. El Zarrok EK, Baca I, Grzybowski L, Jaacks A. Laparoscopic sigmoidectomy for diverticulitis: a prospective study. JSLS. 2010;14(4):469–75. https://doi.org/10.4293/108680810X12924466008088.
23. Levack M, Berger D, Sylla P, Rattner D, Bordeianou L. Laparoscopy decreases anastomotic leak rate in sigmoid colectomy for diverticulitis. Arch Surg. 2011;146(2):207–10. https://doi.org/10.1001/archsurg.2010.325.
24. Klarenbeek BR, Veenhof AA, Bergamaschi R, van der Peet DL, van den Broek WT, de Lange ES, Bemelman WA, Heres P, Lacy AM, Engel AF, Cuesta MA. Laparoscopic sigmoid resection for diverticulitis decreases major morbidity rates: a randomized control trial: short-term results of the Sigma Trial. Ann Surg. 2009;249(1):39–44. https://doi.org/10.1097/SLA.0b013e31818e416a.
25. Biondo S, Lopez Borao J, Millan M, Kreisler E, Jaurrieta E. Current status of the treatment of acute colonic diverticulitis: a systematic review. Color Dis. 2012;14(1):1–11. https://doi.org/10.1111/j.1463-1318.2011.02766.x.
26. Cole K, Fassler S, Suryadevara S, Zebley DM. Increasing the number of attacks increases the conversion rate in laparoscopic diverticulitis surgery. Surg Endosc. 2009;23(5):1088–92. https://doi.org/10.1007/s00464-008-9975-z.
27. Le Moine MC, Fabre JM, Vacher C, Navarro F, Picot MC, Domergue J. Factors and consequences of conversion in laparoscopic sigmoidectomy for diverticular disease. Br J Surg. 2003;90(2):232–6. https://doi.org/10.1002/bjs.4035.
28. Abraha I, Binda GA, Montedori A, Arezzo A, Cirocchi R. Laparoscopic versus open resection for sigmoid diverticulitis. Cochrane Database Syst Rev. 2017;11:CD009277. https://doi.org/10.1002/14651858.CD009277.pub2.
29. Klarenbeek BR, Bergamaschi R, Veenhof AA, van der Peet DL, van den Broek WT, de Lange ES, et al. Laparoscopic versus open sigmoid resection for diverticular disease: follow-up assessment of the randomized control Sigma trial. Surg Endosc. 2011;25:1121–6.
30. Gervaz P, Inan I, Perneger T, SchiMer E, Morel P. A prospective, randomized, single-blind comparison of laparoscopic versus open sigmoid colectomy for diverticulitis. Ann Surg. 2011;252(1):3–8.
31. Gervaz P, Mugnier-Konrad B, Morel P, Huber O, Inan I. Laparoscopic versus open sigmoid resection for diverticulitis: long-term results of a prospective, randomized trial. Surg Endosc. 2011;25(10):3373–8.
32. Raue W, Paolucci V, Asperger W, Albrecht R, Büchler MW, Schwenk W, et al. Laparoscopic sigmoid resection for diverticular disease has no advantages over open approach: midterm results of a randomized controlled trial. Langenbeck's Arch Surg. 2011;396:973–80.
33. Ahmed AM, Moahammed AT, Mattar OM, Mohamed EM, Faraag EA, AlSafadi AM, Huy NT. Surgical treatment of diverticulitis and its complications: a systematic review and meta-analysis of randomized control trials. Surgeon. 2018. https://doi.org/10.1016/j.surge.2018.03.011.
34. Kohl A, Rosenberg J, Bock D, Bisgaard T, Skullman S, Thornell A, Gehrman J, Angenete E, Haglind E. Two-year results of the randomized clinical trial DILALA comparing laparoscopic lavage with resection as treatment for perforated diverticulitis. Br J Surg. 2018;105(9):1128–34. https://doi.org/10.1002/bjs.10839.
35. Tadlock MD, Karamanos E, Skiada D, Inaba K, Talving P, Senagore A, Demetriades D. Emergency surgery for acute diverticulitis: which operation? A National Surgical Quality Improvement Program study. J Trauma Acute Care Surg. 2013;74(6):1385–91. https://doi.org/10.1097/TA.0b013e3182924a82.

36. Pendlimari R, Touzios JG, Azodo IA, Chua HK, Dozois EJ, Cima RR, Larson DW. Short-term outcomes after elective minimally invasive colectomy for diverticulitis. Br J Surg. 2011;98(3):431–5. https://doi.org/10.1002/bjs.7345.
37. Dossa F, Acuna SA, Baxter NN, Bayoumi AM. Optimal operative strategy for Hinchey III sigmoid diverticulitis: a decision analysis. Dis Colon Rectum. 2020;63(8):1108–17. https://doi.org/10.1097/DCR.0000000000001648.
38. Lee YF, Brown RF, Battaglia M, Cleary RK. Laparoscopic versus open emergent sigmoid resection for perforated diverticulitis. J Gastrointest Surg. 2020;24(5):1173–82. https://doi.org/10.1007/s11605-019-04490-9.
39. Cassini D, Miccini M, Manoochehri F, Gregori M, Baldazzi G. Emergency Hartmann's procedure and its reversal: a totally laparoscopic 2-step surgery for the treatment of Hinchey III and IV diverticulitis. Surg Innov. 2017;24(6):557–65. https://doi.org/10.1177/1553350617722226.
40. Cirocchi R, Cochetti G, Randolph J, Listorti C, Castellani E, Renzi C, Mearini E, Fingerhut A. Laparoscopic treatment of colovesical fistulas due to complicated colonic diverticular disease: a systematic review. Tech Coloproctol. 2014;18(10):873–85. https://doi.org/10.1007/s10151-014-1157-5.

Endoluminal Treatment for Diverticular Disease: Therapeutic Endoscopy and Endo-Surgery Approaches

26

Silvio De Melo, Chihiro Kosugi, and Keiji Koda

26.1 Introduction

The prevalence of diverticular disease increases with age [1, 2] and so does the medical complexity of patients. Complicated diverticulosis includes diverticular bleeding, diverticular perforation with abscess formation, diverticular perforation with fistula formation to adjacent organs (such as the bladder, small bowel, etc.), large bowel obstruction due to severe stenosis from acute or chronic diverticulitis, and segmental colitis associated with diverticulosis (SCAD) [1, 3]. Traditionally, these complications were considered surgical indications; however, due to recent advancements in minimally invasive endoscopic, surgical, and interventional radiological techniques, these indications are starting to be challenged [4]. As medical comorbidity increases, there is a parallel increase in surgical risks and complications; therefore, ideally, we would like to have a minimally invasive technique that could render similar outcomes compared to surgery but without the associated negative effects on patients in terms of intrasurgical and postoperative risks. In this chapter, we will discuss the endoscopic options for the management of diverticular disease-associated strictures and diverticular disease-associated abscesses (SCAD is covered in another chapter), to determine which one could be applied to select patients in the appropriate clinical scenario.

S. De Melo
Department of Medicine, Oregon Health and Science University, Portland, OR, USA
e-mail: demelo@ohsu.edu

C. Kosugi · K. Koda (✉)
Department of Surgery, Teikyo University Chiba Medical Center, Ichihara City, Chiba, Japan
e-mail: ckosugi0126@yahoo.co.jp; k-koda@med.teikyo-u.ac.jp

© The Author(s), under exclusive license to Springer Nature Switzerland AG 2022
A. Tursi et al. (eds.), *Colonic Diverticular Disease*,
https://doi.org/10.1007/978-3-030-93761-4_26

26.2 Endoscopic Therapy for Colonic Strictures Associated with Diverticular Disease

There are several types of colonic strictures such as those associated with diverticular disease, postoperative strictures, colonic strictures from inflammatory bowel disease, particularly Crohn's disease, strictures from ischemic colitis, post-endoscopic resection strictures, and malignant strictures, both luminal malignancy (most frequently adenocarcinoma of the colon) and extrinsic compression of the colon from extracolonic malignancies, such as gastric cancer, ovarian cancer, etc. [5–7]. Each stricture type has its own pathophysiological mechanism and response to different therapeutic options. Endoscopic interventions for the management of luminal strictures include endoscopic dilation, needle knife stricturoplasty, placement of a self-expandable metal stent (SEMS), and endoscopic bypass of the stenosed segment if feasible. The last modality is not common in the lower gastrointestinal tract.

Endoscopic dilation consists of utilizing a dilation balloon, which can be passed through the scope until it reaches the area of interest. Fluoroscopy may be needed to aid in stricture characterization, such as length, diameter, and complexity of the area. Often a large, 15–20 mm biliary balloon catheter is used to probe the area of interest. Subsequently, the dilation balloon is advanced through the narrowed area and then inflated to a predetermined size. The major complication with balloon dilation is perforation; therefore, it is recommended that the dilation be gradual and sequential 1 mm at a time starting from the diameter of the untreated segment. The balloon in kept inflated for a period of time, approximately 1 min, and then deflated and removed; the area is carefully inspected to assess the response to the dilation and for complications, mainly uncontrolled bleeding and perforation. Short, less than 1 cm postoperative strictures can respond extremely well to endoscopic dilation [8].

Endoscopic stricturoplasty is used for the treatment of strictures associated with inflammatory bowel disease, post-endoscopic resection strictures, and postoperative strictures. It is often used in combination with endoscopic dilation. In this technique, a needle knife is used to cut through the fibrotic, scarred segment, providing a scaffold to control the area of "tear" from the balloon dilation. It has been highly effective in the therapy of densely fibrotic, short (1–2 cm) segments [9].

Diverticular disease-associated colonic strictures are believed to occur due to recurrent episodes of acute diverticulitis causing fibrosis of a segment of the colon, most commonly the sigmoid colon. These diverticulitis episodes can be clinical or subclinical [10]. They do not respond to endoscopic dilation nor are they poised for therapeutic success by endoscopic stricturoplasty [11]. Therefore, the treatment option is the placement of self-expandable metal stents (SEMSs). These are often used as a "bridge to surgery" and, rarely, as a destination therapy. SEMSs are composed of a metal alloy compressed into a delivery catheter, which is then advanced through a wire-guided method across the strictured segment with or without fluoroscopy (although fluoroscopy is recommended), where it is deployed. The metal alloy can be covered by a material to prevent tissue ingrowth through the mesh, which then renders the SEMS classification of uncovered (bare metal alloy), partially covered, and fully covered (metal alloy completely surrounded by an anti-ingrowth substance, often silicone). Most colonic stents are uncovered metal stents.

26.2.1 Self-Expandable Metal Stent (SEMS) Deployment Technique

SEMSs are used for symptomatic large bowel obstruction. There is no role for prophylactic SEMS placement. The area of interest was previously identified by a computed tomography examination. The minimal information needed is location of the obstruction, length, and evidence of perforation or impending perforation (cecal size and pneumatosis coli). If the length of the stenosis is not available, one could use the previously described technique of utilizing a large biliary stone extraction balloon (15–20 mm) to inject a contrast and measure the length. There should be at least 2 cm of unaffected area proximal and distal to the stent. For instance, utilizing the balloon technique, we measured the stenotic segment to be approximately 5 cm; we would select a stent of at least 9 cm in length to account for the needed 2 cm of unaffected bowel, proximally and distally. The stent should be at least 24 mm in diameter. Pre- or post-dilation of the stenosis is not recommended due to an increased risk of perforation. Enemas should be performed to facilitate visualization. After appropriate lower bowel cleansing with enemas (tap water enemas usually suffice), the endoscopic instrument is advanced to the area of interest; one could use a therapeutic gastroscope, a colonoscope, or a pediatric colonoscope. Our personal preference is the therapeutic gastroscope, which provides better fine tip control. A 15–20 mm balloon catheter preloaded with a long, 450 cm, 0.035 inch biliary wire is advanced through the working channel of the instrument. Under fluoroscopic guidance, the wire is negotiated proximal to the stricture. The balloon is inflated to 20 mm and the contrast is injected to obtain a colography. The balloon is pulled back until it is met with resistance. The area from the balloon to the tip of the instrument is measured. The stent selected should be at least 4 cm longer than the area of interest (2 cm proximally and distally). The balloon is removed, maintaining the wire in place. The stent delivery catheter is advanced through the wire past the stricture. The stent is deployed under both endoscopic and fluoroscopic monitoring. After deployment, the endoscopic instrument is withdrawn (Fig. 26.1) [5, 6, 12].

26.2.2 Efficacy of Self-Expandable Metal Stents in Diverticular Disease-Associated Strictures

The traditional approach for patients with diverticular disease-associated strictures is surgical [13, 14]. In an acute setting, it is often a two-stage operation consisting of a diverting colostomy creation, followed by another intervention for colostomy take down, resection of the strictures, and reanastomosis. However, diverticulosis is more frequent in the elderly and increases with age; those patients often have an increased number of comorbidities. Therefore, a therapeutic option, which can

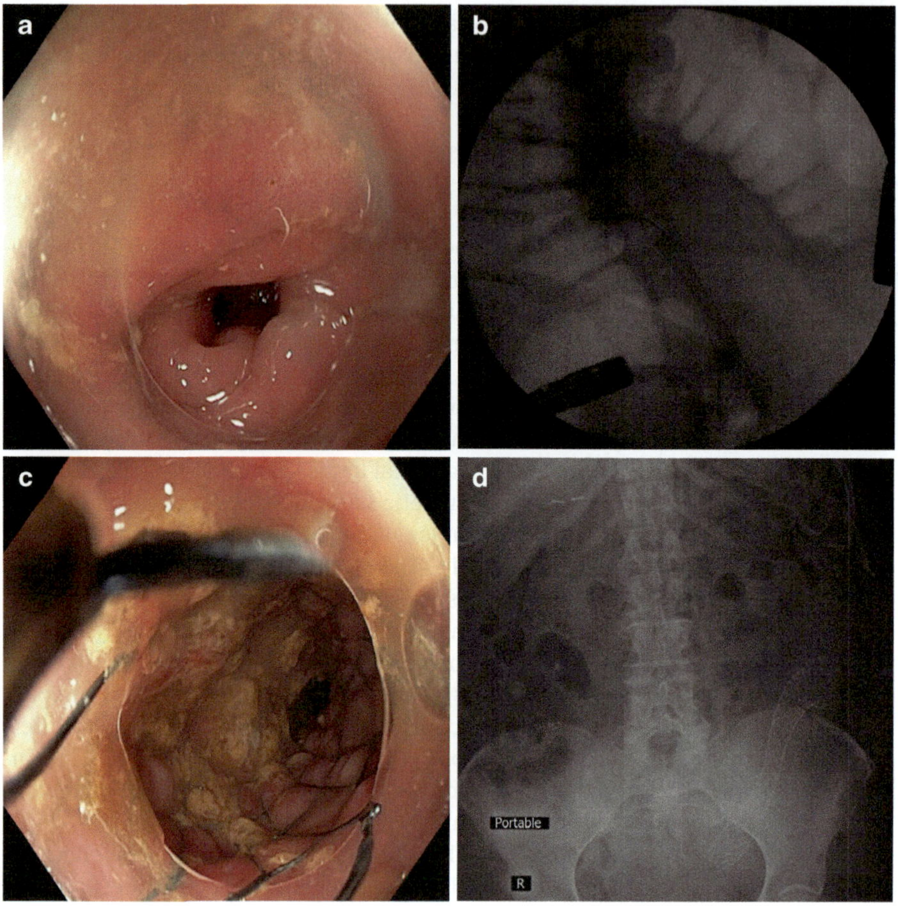

Fig. 26.1 Use of an uncovered metal stent to treat diverticular colonic strictures. (**a**) Diverticular colonic strictures. (**b**) Fluoroscopic image of colonic stent deployment. (**c**). Endoscopic image of the colonic stent after deployment. (**d**) Final fluoroscopic image of the colonic stent after deployment (Source: World J Gastrointest Endosc 2020 February 16;12(2):53–82)

transform the surgical intervention from a two-stage into a one-stage, a strategy also known as a "bridge to surgery", has the potential to minimize long-term complications in this patient population. There is no randomized trial comparing SEMSs as a bridge to surgery versus the traditional two-stage surgical approach in the management of diverticulosis-associated colonic strictures. All the information is obtained from a single-center case series and systematic reviews. With that in mind, the clinical efficacy is as follows. The overall efficacy, defined as the successful decompression of the colon, allowing for a full colonic decompression and a one-stage surgical intervention, has been reported to be 43–95% [10, 15–21]. A recent review has recommended against the routine use of SEMSs in the treatment of diverticular disease-associated colonic strictures, but it can be used in select patients with planned surgical intervention within 1 month [16].

26.2.3 Complications of Self-Expandable Metal Stents

SEMSs have several complications. They can be divided into early (less than 30 days) or late (more than 30 days). The main early adverse events include perforation, stent failure after a successful technical placement, stent migration, reobstruction, pain, and bleeding. Late complications include reobstruction, tenesmus (if low in the rectum), incontinence, fistula, migration, and perforation. Stent-related perforations can occur through several mechanisms: guidewire or catheter malposition, dilation of the strictures before or after placement, stent-induced direct perforation, or proximal perforation from barotrauma [22]. The 30-day stent-related mortality is less than 4% [5]. The median stent patency in a palliative setting ranges from 55 to 343 days [5]. Complications differ when we evaluate SEMSs in a malignant versus benign situation, particularly the use of SEMSs in the treatment of diverticular disease-associated colonic strictures. A systematic review on the use of SEMSs in the management of benign colonic obstruction, in which diverticulosis was 54% of the cause, reported a rate of perforation of 17%, reobstruction of 14%, stent migration of 20%, 61% in the bridge-to-surgery scenario, median time to operation of 14 days, and stoma avoidance of 43% with overall complications of 52% [15]. This is much higher than the reported complications for malignant obstruction with perforation of around 4%, migration rate of around 10–11%, and stent occlusion of approximately 7–12% [23, 24]. A recent review article on SEMSs for diverticular strictures has reported an overall complication rate ranging from 6 to 43% [16].

26.3 Endoscopic Therapy for Diverticular Abscess

The treatment strategy for diverticulitis has been determined based on both patient's pathophysiological symptoms, including laboratory data, and diagnostic images, including CT or ultrasound scan. When diverticulitis is accompanied by abscess formation, and if it is persistent after the administration of antibiotics, percutaneous drainage would be the most frequently attempted intervention to treat the locoregional inflammation. However, percutaneous drainage is technically not always an easy maneuver depending on the location or the size of the abscess. In particular, when the abscess is located in the area surrounded by the small intestine, or regions close to the vessels or ureters, percutaneous abscess drainage has a risk of injuring the intestine, vessels, or ureters. Here, we describe a novel method of intraluminal abscess drainage and lavage using endoscopy.

26.3.1 Indication

Localized abscess caused by diverticulitis would be the candidate for intraluminal abscess drainage (Fig. 26.2). Disseminated abscess with peritonitis is not suitable for this technique. Patients with a life-threatening condition may not be indicative of this maneuver. The appropriate timing for this procedure would be

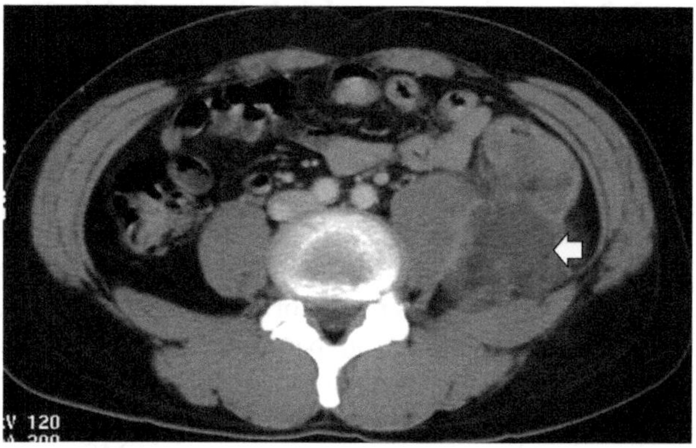

Fig. 26.2 Localized retroperitoneal abscess that was treated with intraluminal abscess drainage (arrow)

a few days after conservative antibiotic therapy, since this procedure may expand the abscess cavity by the pressure of washing water before the cavity wall becomes firm enough.

26.3.2 Description of the Procedure

26.3.2.1 Pre-Procedure Preparation

Usually, bowel preparation is not necessary since the majority of patients indicative of this technique are under fasting conditions for several days; small amounts of enema may be applied for preparation. Mild sedation may be necessary when there is a possibility of causing abdominal pain during the procedure.

26.3.2.2 Localization of the Culprit Diverticulum

The location of the diverticulum responsible for causing the abscess should be estimated using either CT or ultrasound before performing the procedure (Fig. 26.3). During endoscopy, the inflamed diverticulum is examined. Usually, the diverticulum responsible for causing the abscess can be identified as it is highly inflamed, sometimes filled and packed with purulent exudate. It is often lifted by the abscess located outside the colon (Fig. 26.4).

26.3.2.3 Puncture of the Diverticulum and Access to the Abscess Cavity

The diverticulum responsible for the abscess formation is then punctured using either endoscopic forceps or a catheter (Fig. 26.5). We usually divert the ERCP catheter for this purpose. When we access the proper abscess cavity by this puncture, purulent exudate comes out of the punctured hole (Fig. 26.6). Thereafter, the abscess cavity is investigated under fluoroscopy with a contrast agent to assess whether the cavity is localized and has not expanded to a wide area of the abdominal cavity.

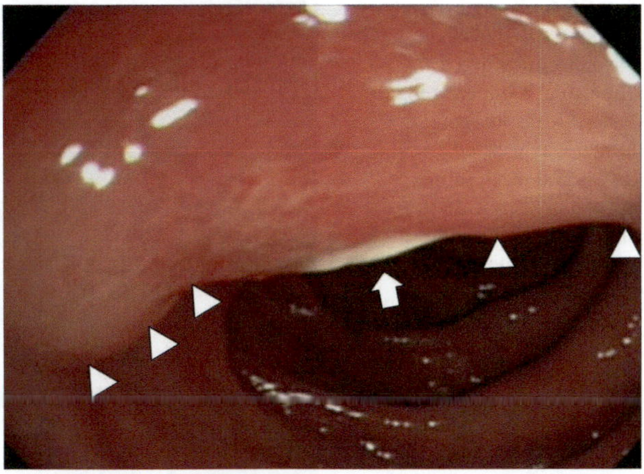

Fig. 26.3 Diverticulum that is believed to be the origin of the abscess (Fig. 26.2, arrow). It is packed with purulent exudate, located on the dome-like lifting toward the colonic lumen (arrow head)

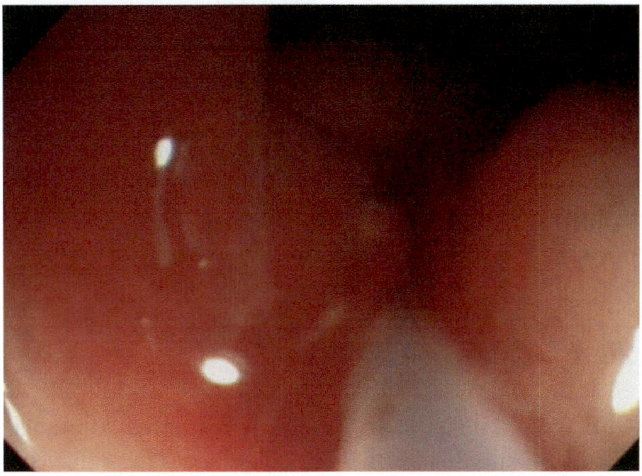

Fig. 26.4 Access to the diverticulum and puncture with a catheter

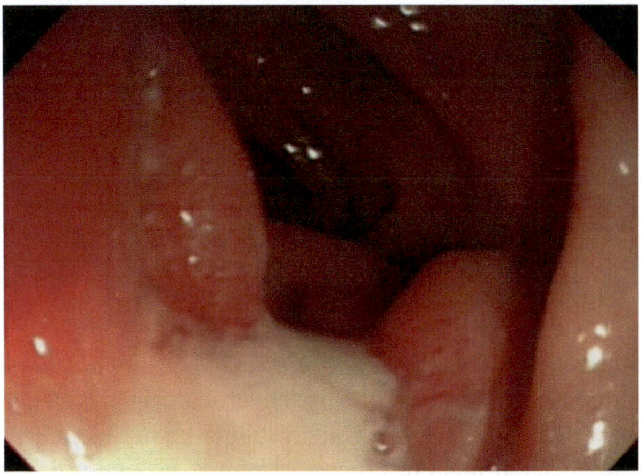

Fig. 26.5 Pus discharge from the punctured diverticulum

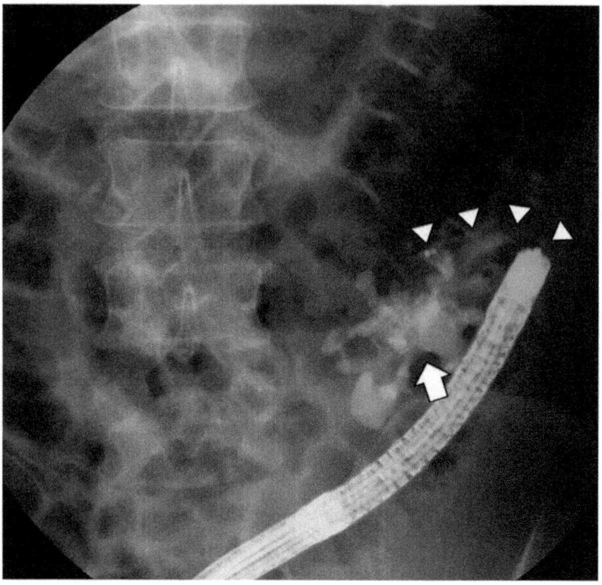

Fig. 26.6 X-ray image to measure the size of the abscess cavity and to confirm it is a localized lesion. After imaging, the lumen was washed thoroughly with saline. Arrow, abscess cavity; arrow heads, the catheter inside the lumen

26.3.2.4 Lavage of the Abscess Cavity

Following the fluoroscopic evaluation, the abscess cavity is washed thoroughly with saline thorough the inserted catheter. Usually, we use more than 500 ml of saline until the draining water becomes completely clear.

26.4 Outcomes

Until now, we have performed intraluminal drainage in 14 cases with localized abscess formation in the last 13 years. The indication of this technique has been expanded in recent years since we observed that this technique is safe to perform. Drainage failed in two cases in whom we could not access their abscess cavities. It was successful in the remaining 12 cases. No adverse effects were noted in these 14 cases. The 12 cases in whom this technique was successful were discharged from the hospital 3–17 days after the procedure (median 6 days). In the two cases in whom this technique was unsuccessful, conservative therapy for 12 and 30 days after the procedure was necessary before discharge. There is no recurrent diverticulitis among these cases.

26.5 Final Remarks

Our patients live longer and with an increasing number of medical problems increasing their medical complexity. Diverticulosis prevalence increases with age, and the best treatment for each patient should be individualized by involving the patient in the decision-making process. There is no one-size-fits-all treatment plan when it comes to the increasingly more complex care of diverticular disease. We should recognize that, based on the best available evidence, the use of SEMSs to treat diverticular disease-associated colonic stenosis carries a higher complication rate compared to its use in malignant colonic obstruction; however, it can allow a successful one-stage surgical intervention in up to 75% of patients, which can minimize risks for the patients and be more cost-effective. It is clear that it is time for a multicenter, randomized clinical study to assess the role of SEMSs as a bridge to surgery in the treatment algorithm of diverticulosis-associated colonic strictures.

For the treatment of diverticulitis with abscess formation, the conservative therapy including antibiotic administration is first considered, and the majority of small abscesses are reported to be cured without further interventions [25]. Whether abscess drainage is necessary is still a controversial issue [26]; however, percutaneous abscess drainage (PAD) has been a major approach for nonoperative treatment of complicated diverticulitis [27]. In this chapter, we introduced an alternative approach to PAD, that is, intraluminal drainage under colonoscopy. Although not many cases have been examined, intraluminal drainage using endoscopy for localized abscess of the colonic diverticulum was safe to perform. In addition, once it is performed successfully, the outcomes in patients have been satisfactory [28]. When a localized abscess remains unhealed after conservative therapy with antibiotics, intraluminal abscess drainage may as well be tried before performing PAD or a surgical maneuver.

Conflicts of Interest None.

References

1. Strate LL, et al. Diverticular disease as a chronic illness: evolving epidemiologic and clinical insights. Am J Gastroenterol. 2012;107(10):1486–93.
2. Kang J-Y, Melville D, Maxwell JD. Epidemiology and management of diverticular disease of the colon. Drugs Aging. 2004;21(4):211–28.
3. Mendez-Pastor A, Garcia-Henriquez N. Complicated diverticulitis. Dis Colon Rectum. 2020;63(1):26–8.
4. You H, et al. The management of diverticulitis: a review of the guidelines. Med J Aust. 2019;211(9):421–7.
5. van Hooft JE, et al. Self-expandable metal stents for obstructing colonic and extracolonic cancer: European Society of Gastrointestinal Endoscopy (ESGE) clinical guideline. Gastrointest Endosc. 2014;80(5):747–61. e1–75
6. Committee, A.S.o.P, et al. The role of endoscopy in the management of patients with known and suspected colonic obstruction and pseudo-obstruction. Gastrointest Endosc. 2010;71(4):669–79.
7. Hunt RH, et al. Colonoscopy in management of colonic strictures. Br Med J. 1975;3(5979):360–1.
8. Kwon YH, Jeon SW, Lee YK. Endoscopic management of refractory benign colorectal strictures. Clinical Endosc. 2013;46(5):472–5.
9. Sinh P, Shen B. Endoscopic evaluation of surgically altered bowel in patients with inflammatory bowel diseases. Inflamm Bowel Dis. 2015;21(6):1459–71.

10. Fejleh MP, Tabibian JH. Colonoscopic management of diverticular disease. World J Gastrointestinal Endos. 2020;12(2):53–9.
11. Graham DY, et al. Evaluation of the effectiveness of through-the-scope balloons as dilators of benign and malignant gastrointestinal strictures. Gastrointest Endosc. 1987;33(6):432–5.
12. Gargallo CJ, et al. Short- and long-term clinical outcomes of self-expandable metal stents inserted for colorectal obstruction and efficacy of different insertion techniques. Gastroenterologia y hepatologia. 2019;42(3):157–63.
13. Venara A, et al. Sigmoid stricture associated with diverticular disease should be an indication for elective surgery with lymph node clearance. J Visc Surg. 2015;152(4):211–5.
14. Sawai RS. Management of colonic obstruction: a review. Clin Colon Rectal Surg. 2012;25(4):200–3.
15. Currie A, et al. Systematic review of self-expanding stents in the management of benign colorectal obstruction. Colorectal Dis. 2014;16(4):239–45.
16. Venezia L, et al. Feasibility and safety of self-expandable metal stent in nonmalignant disease of the lower gastrointestinal tract. World J Gastrointest Endosc. 2020;12(2):60–71.
17. Keranen I, et al. Outcome of patients after endoluminal stent placement for benign colorectal obstruction. Scand J Gastroenterol. 2010;45(6):725–31.
18. Small AJ, Young-Fadok TM, Baron TH. Expandable metal stent placement for benign colorectal obstruction: outcomes for 23 cases. Surg Endosc. 2008;22(2):454–62.
19. Forshaw MJ, et al. Self-expanding metallic stents in the treatment of benign colorectal disease: indications and outcomes. Colorectal Dis. 2006;8(2):102–11.
20. Tamim WZ, et al. Experience with endoluminal colonic wall stents for the management of large bowel obstruction for benign and malignant disease. Arch Surg (Chicago, Ill. 1960). 2000;135(4):434–8.
21. Davidson R, Sweeney WB. Endoluminal stenting for benign colonic obstruction. Surg Endosc. 1998;12(4):353–4.
22. Baron TH, Song LMWK, Repici A. Role of self-expandable stents for patients with colon cancer (with videos). Gastrointest Endosc. 2012;75(3):653–62.
23. Watt AM, et al. Self-expanding metallic stents for relieving malignant colorectal obstruction: a systematic review. Ann Surg. 2007;246(1):24–30.
24. Khot UP, et al. Systematic review of the efficacy and safety of colorectal stents. Br J Surg. 2002;89(9):1096–102.
25. Gregersen R, et al. Treatment of patients with acute colonic diverticulitis complicated by abscess formation: a systematic review. Int J Surg. 2016;35:201–8.
26. Lambrichts DPV, et al. Multicentre study of non-surgical management of diverticulitis with abscess formation. Br J Surg. 2019;106(4):458–66.
27. Lamb MN, Kaiser AM. Elective resection versus observation after nonoperative management of complicated diverticulitis with abscess: a systematic review and meta-analysis. Dis Colon Rectum. 2014;57(12):1430–40.
28. Kosugi C, et al. Endoscopic transluminal abscess drainage for Hinchey II colonic diverticulitis. Int J Color Dis. 2012;27(9):1239–40.

Peritoneal Lavage for Perforated Diverticulitis

27

Ricardo Escalante, Enio Chaves de Oliveira, Leonardo Bustamante-Lopez, and Narimantas Evaldas Samalavicius

27.1 Introduction

Diverticular diseases are frequently considered a twentieth century development, which is not strictly correct, but supports the circumstance that the advances in diagnosis and treatment of this now common condition have been predominantly evolving in the past century [1]. This disease was common only in Western countries; however, underdeveloped nations have now acquired the wrong habits and passive lifestyle of developed countries, and the incidence of diverticular diseases has increased in other urban areas of the world. Diseases in the ascending colon are almost exclusively found in Asian populations, particularly genetic diseases [2].

Diverticular disease of the colon is a medical condition that is highly related to the aging of the population in Western countries. It is estimated that at the age of 40 years, diverticulosis affects approximately 10% of the population, whereas, at the age of 85 years, its prevalence increases to more than two-thirds of the population [3, 4].

R. Escalante (✉)
Universidad Central de Venezuela, Loira Medical Center, Caracas, Venezuela
e-mail: r_escalanteg@hotmail.com

E. C. de Oliveira
Department of Surgery, Universidade Federal de Goiás, School of Medicine, Goiânia, Brazil
e-mail: eco1.br@gmail.com

L. Bustamante-Lopez
Department of Diverticular Disease, Hospital das Clinicas da Universidade de São Paulo, Saõ Paulo, Brazil
e-mail: leonardoabustmante@yahoo.com

N. E. Samalavicius
Department of Surgery, Klaipėda University Hospital, Klaipėda, Lithuania
e-mail: narimantas.samalavicius@nvi.lt

© The Author(s), under exclusive license to Springer Nature Switzerland AG 2022

A. Tursi et al. (eds.), *Colonic Diverticular Disease*,
https://doi.org/10.1007/978-3-030-93761-4_27

Diverticular disease accounts for approximately 300,000 hospitalizations per year in the United States, resulting in 1.5 million days of inpatient care. In addition, roughly 1.5 million outpatient visits each year are due to diverticular disease.

Over the past several years, research describing the natural biology of diverticulitis has been incorporated into the management recommendations for this challenging disease [2].

Diverticular disease is not a new concept, and the presence of diverticula within the colon was documented as early as 1700 by the French surgeon Alexis Littre [5]. This author said that a diverticulum could be formed when a part of the intestinal wall enters the hernial sac, and, therefore, only one side of the intestine is pulled out and finally becomes a longer canal.

27.2 Historical Aspects

The first in-depth description of the disease process of inflammation of the diverticula with resultant benign fistulas to the bladder was presented by Cruveilhier in 1849 [6]. In 1899, 50 years later, Graser [7] introduced the term "peridiverticulitis," suggesting that herniation of the mucosa through areas of penetration of the vasa recta was the pathogenesis for the development of diverticula; this is now a well-established concept. In 1904, Beer [8] proposed that the mechanism of the development of diverticulitis was impaction of feces in the neck of the diverticulum, causing inflammation and subsequent abscess with possible fistula formation. In 1908, Telling [9] reported 80 cases of diverticulitis of the sigmoid and proposed that the illness may be more predominant than previously assumed. In 1907, William Mayo presented the first report of surgical treatment for diverticulitis. He operated on a case of internal fecal fistula into the bladder and later resected the colon [10]. Two years earlier, Humphry Rolleston [11], an English surgeon, had published in *The Lancet* a case with an intraperitoneal abscess circumscribed around the sigmoid. At that time, he called it pericolitis sinistra with abscess formation. Now we are aware that it was perforated diverticulitis. He performed the treatment in the same manner as we do in some patients today: "evacuated the pus, washed out the cavity and inserted a drainage tube" [11].

The first surgical technique, known as the "three-stage procedure", was developed in the Mayo Clinic from where the first experience with the classic three-stage operation was reported in 1924 [12]. The technique consists of a colostomy at the level of the transverse colon and the positioning of drainage, resection of the diseased colon after a period of 3–6 months, and stoma closure after a further 3–6 months. This technique had a high mortality rate. Antibiotics were not available. This three-stage procedure was mainly used in perforation, obstruction, and fistula formation.

The second method, the "two-stage" or Hartmann's procedure, was used for the first time by Henry Hartmann in 1921 [13] to perform sigmoid resection for the treatment of neoplastic disease. It consists of a segmental resection of the diseased colon without a primary anastomosis but with an end colostomy; intestinal continuity can be restored during the second operation. Widely used since the 1950s, the

Hartmann procedure became the standard of care in the 1980s but has a significant complication rate, and mortality rates range from 5 to 14%. The restoration of bowel continuity was not possible in around 25–80% of patients at the time.

Over the years, many papers have reported a controversy between three-stage and two-stage procedures. In 2000, the American Society of Colon and Rectal Surgeons (ASCRS) pointed out that the "Three-stage operative approach strategy (nonresectional surgery) was no longer recommended for most patients." Thereafter, Hartmann's procedure was considered the gold standard for complicated acute diverticulitis [2].

The advantages of Hartman's procedure over resection with primary anastomosis with or without ileostomy were controversial. Many studies were conducted, but no significant differences were found between primary resection with anastomosis and Hartmann's procedure with respect to mortality, morbidity, sepsis, wound complications, and duration of these procedures. The key has been in cost issues. With the goal to reduce the mortality and morbidity associated with an emergency surgery, two methods have been used: percutaneous drainage by ultrasound or computed tomography and peritoneal lavage with drainage [14].

27.3 Classification Systems

Different classification systems have been proposed over the years to assess the severity of acute diverticulitis, the most commonly used of which is the Hinchey classification [12], which classifies complicated diverticulitis. The Hinchey classification, modified by Wasvary [15] in 1999, is the most frequently used nowadays, but other classification systems remain in use as well, notably the Ambrosetti classification [16], the Hansen–Stock classification [17], and, more recently, the modified Neff classification [18].

Traditionally, the Hinchey classification (1978) was used to define the severity of acute diverticulitis based on clinical and operative findings [19]. However, this system lacks details on intermediate severities, which are recognized by modern imaging [20]. The CT-based classification by Ambrosetti et al. [16] distinguishes between mild and severe (complicated) acute diverticulitis, but the system insufficiently distinguishes the different grades of complicated diverticulitis, thus limiting its usefulness in decision-making and in tracking disease progression for outcome analysis. The modified (1999) and further adapted (2005) Hinchey classification system added subgroups for both milder and complicated forms of acute diverticulitis and categories for chronic complications (obstruction, fistula) with the goal to define criteria for management decisions [15, 21].

Computed tomography imaging represents the standard for classifying the severity of diverticulitis (Figs. 27.1 and 27.2) and allows opening alternatives for treatment strategies [22]. Over the past few decades, management has evolved with an emphasis on tailoring surgical intervention on the basis of the Hinchey stage [22]. A combination of clinical judgment and analysis of the CT findings is quintessential for sound decision-making.

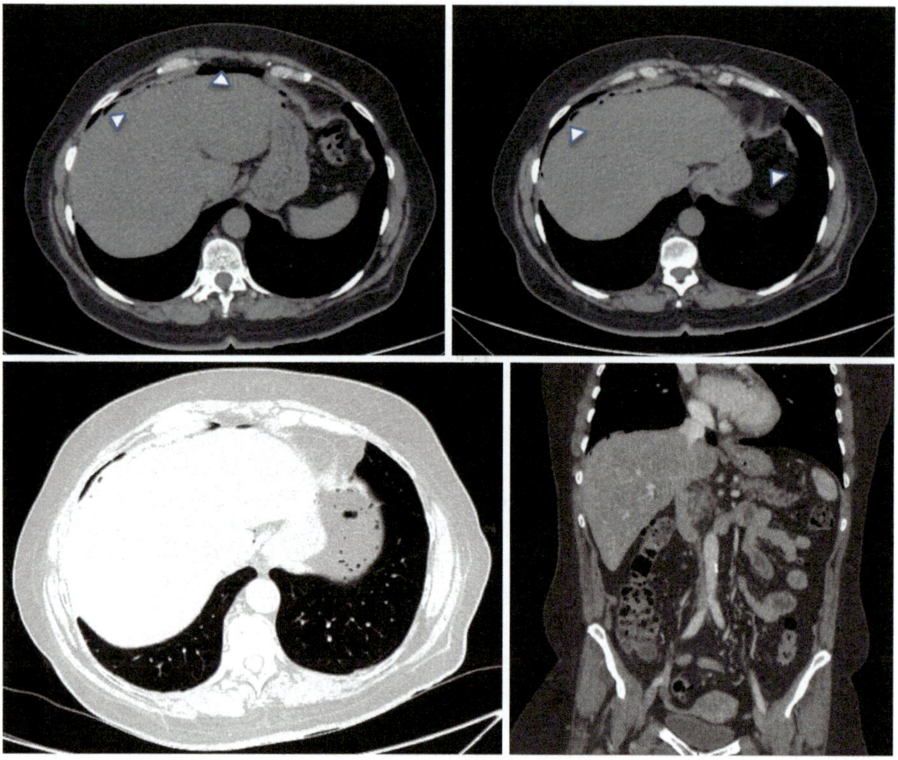

Fig. 27.1 Abdominal CT scan: pneumoperitoneum (arrow heads)

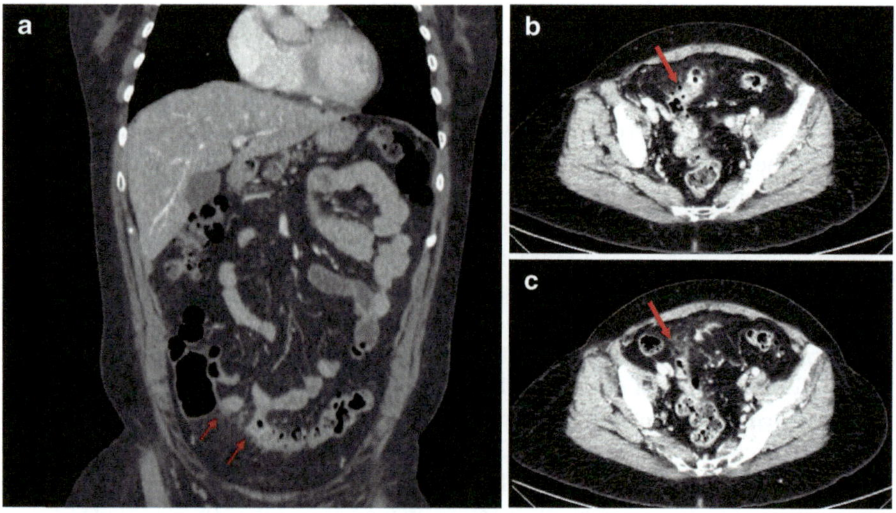

Fig. 27.2 Abdominal CT scan: coronal view showing sigmoide colon diverticulitis blocked by the small bowel (**a**) and axial view showing inflammatory process with fat tissue involvement (arrows) (**b**, **c**)

27.4 Surgical Alternatives

Operative management in the emergency situation should be reserved for the treatment of those patients who do not respond for conservative treatment.

Traditionally, management of complicated diverticular disease has involved open damage control operations with large definitive resections and colostomies. Studies are now showing that in a subset of patients who would typically have undergone an open Hartmann's procedure for Hinchey III/IV diverticulitis, a laparoscopic approach is equally safe and has better outcomes. Laparoscopic sigmoidectomy is superior to open sigmoidectomy for treating perforated diverticulitis with regard to fewer short-term and long-term complications, decreased pain, improvement in length of stay, and maintenance of better cost effectiveness than open resections [23, 24]. Lin et al. conducted a search in MEDLINE, EMBASE, Science Citation Index Expanded, and the Cochrane database until November 2019 and reviewed 14 articles. This meta-analysis concluded that laparoscopic surgery does not show significant advantages over open surgery in postoperative complications for the emergency treatment of complicated diverticulitis [25].

The choice of operation for these patients has been the subject of debate and will remain controversial without large-scale, prospective studies. The current techniques include: (1) resection with primary colorectal anastomosis with or without additional loop ileostomy; (2) end colostomy (Hartmann's procedure); (3) damage control strategy [26, 27]; (4) and laparoscopic lavage and placement of a drainage.

Laparoscopic peritoneal lavage is an alternative to sigmoid resection in Hinchey III diverticulitis (generalized purulent peritonitis). Lavage is not appropriate in the setting of fecal contamination or overt colonic perforation. When patients require an emergency intervention for unrelenting diverticulitis with abscess formation or with diffuse peritonitis, laparoscopic lavage and drainage has emerged as a potential alternative to resection and for a while gained some popularity, primarily in European centers [28, 29].

The technique of lavage and drainage regained popularity during the 1990s. This procedure can also be performed laparoscopically with the advantage of faster recovery and shorter hospital stay. This strategy allows resectional surgery to be postponed or avoided altogether in many patients; and higher rates of primary resection and anastomosis can be achieved avoiding the need for a stoma [30, 31]. The concept of this approach is that on some occasions, perforations have already sealed at the time of the surgery and the only intervention that seems necessary is to lavage the abdominal cavity to remove the pus.

27.5 Randomized Controlled Trials

There have been multiple early reports with encouraging results; they were small [32] and uncontrolled series, with a high risk of selection bias [28, 33–36].

Three prospective randomized controlled multicenter trials (LADIES trial, DILALA trial, and SCANDIV trial) on laparoscopic peritoneal lavage were launched and resulted in high-quality evidence [22].

The LADIES trial was conducted from 2010 to 2013 in Belgium, Italy, and The Netherlands and consisted of two subarms: comparing the Hartmann vs primary anastomosis and laparoscopic lavage vs sigmoidectomy [37]. The laparoscopic lavage arm of the trial, however, was terminated early upon governmental oversight pressure due to a significantly increased rate of perioperative morbidity, mortality, and need for surgical interventions compared to the resection groups.

The DILALA trial included patients with only Hinchey III peritonitis diagnosed by laparoscopy and with a 1-year reoperation rate as the primary outcome. The preliminary analysis of the short-term results (12 weeks) in 76 patients reported no statistically significant differences regarding morbidity and mortality, statistically significant longer periods of abdominal drainage but shorter hospital stay in the LPL group compared to the HP group [38].

The Scandinavian diverticulitis (SCANDIV) trial encompassed 101 laparoscopic lavage vs 98 resection patients in 21 centers in Norway and Sweden from 2010 to 2014 [39]. In contrast to the LADIES trial, the SCANDIV trial was continued to completion. The authors reported a nonstatistically significant higher incidence of the primary outcome in the laparoscopic peritoneal lavage group and comparable mortality. However, there were statistically significantly higher rates of abscesses, secondary peritonitis, and reoperations in the peritoneal lavage group along with missed malignancy in four cases. However, the study has several limitations such as inclusion of patients with Hinchey I and II and participation of more experienced surgeons in the resection group, which might be a source of significant bias [40].

The actual technique of laparoscopic lavage used in those three randomized controlled trials studying this approach was not uniform and the trials were designed differently and examined different end points. The volume of saline irrigation, number of drains used, and management of intraoperative adhesions around the area of presumed diverticular perforation varied across the studies.

27.6 Surgical Technique

The patient is placed in a modified lithotomy position, with shoulder pads and leg pads.

The surgeon and his assistant stand to the right of the patient. A 10–12 mm umbilical trocar is placed at the introduction of the 0° optics, plus two or three 5 mm ports according to the surgeon's needs.

The surgery begins with the inspection of the sigmoid colon from medial to lateral. The omentum, intestine, pelvic structures, cecal appendix, and the entire colon should be search of collections that could pass unnoticed. The debridement of these should be performed carefully, avoiding unnecessary bleeding [41].

Aspiration of the purulent content is carried out (Fig. 27.3), collecting samples for culture and irrigation of all four quadrants of the abdomen with saline (3L or more).

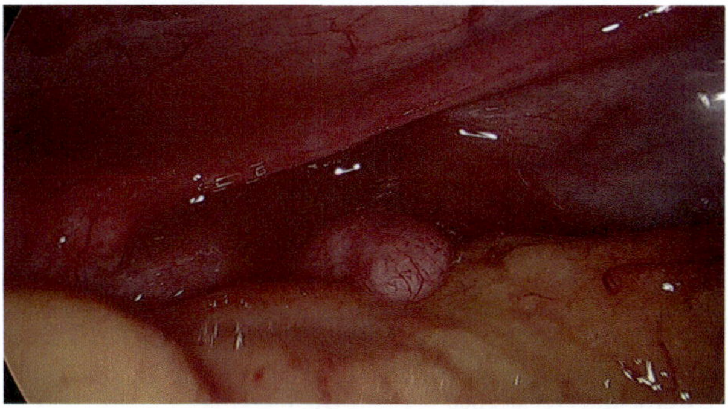

Fig. 27.3 Laparoscopy view showing purulent peritonitis

Once a completely clear liquid is obtained in aspiration, continuous suction drains are placed in Douglas cul-de-sac, in the left parieto-colic groove and others according to the surgeon's criteria.

The adhesions that exist in the septate area should not be released and routine gas-leak testing should be considered at laparoscopy through transanal carbon dioxide or air insufflation of the sigmoid colon to avoid missing a breach in the colonic wall [42]. The findings of fecal peritonitis or an overt colon perforation should prompt the surgeon to perform a resection. Patients deemed to be candidates for LL need to be advised on the possibility of a resurgery if they fail to respond to the LL or if a sigmoid carcinoma is subsequently found. They also need to be advised on the likely need for a delayed elective sigmoid resection [31].

27.7 Discussion

The most obvious advantage advocated by the supporters of this technique consists of the avoidance of a large laparotomy and derivative procedures, thus reducing their consequent complications. The advantages of laparoscopic lavage include shorter operative times, reduction of postoperative pain, a lowering of surgical site infections, reduced cardiac complications, a potential reduction of the rate of incisional hernias and stoma formation, and shorter length of hospital stay; based on the results of some trials, reduced costs and an amelioration in postoperative disability should be considered [43–47]. However, laparoscopic lavage is associated with significantly increased risks of intra-abdominal abscess, peritonitis. Future emergency reoperation and long-term diverticulitis recurrence with reintervention and readmission after laparoscopic lavage is high [48]. The major criticism of the nonresectional laparoscopic lavage technique is the continued presence of the perforated colon as a septic focus and the column of feces remaining in the colon proximal to the perforation as a potential ongoing source of contamination [49].

The future of lavage as a treatment for perforated diverticulitis remains unclear (see Table 27.1). Recently, three different societies have published their guidelines. The Clinical Practice Guidelines of the American Society of Colon and Rectal Surgeons set practice parameters in 2020 and concluded that the safety of lavage for

Table 27.1 Outcomes of laparoscopic lavage vs sigmoid resection

	Laparoscopic lavage	Sigmoid resection
Acute reintervention rate	High	Low
Elective reinterventions	Similar	Similar
Indication	Young and stable patients	Critically ill patients
Readmission to ICU	Similar	Similar
Stoma frequency	Low	High
Stoma reversal	Low	High
Severe complications	Similar	Similar
Hospital stay	Similar	Similar
Diverticulitis recurrence	High	Low
Cost	Little cheaper	More expensive

purulent or feculent peritonitis was unclear and it was not recommended as an appropriate alternative to colectomy, and thus colectomy should typically be performed in this situation. Moreover, these guidelines pointed out that in patients with purulent peritonitis, colectomy is preferred over laparoscopic lavage, considering that studies are needed to better identify the selection criteria for patients who might benefit from laparoscopic lavage and to standardize the operative technique [50]. The European Society of Coloproctology considers that laparoscopic lavage is cheaper than Hartmann's procedure and reduces the risk of colostomy at 1- and 2-year follow-up but may in the short term result in intra-abdominal abscesses and overlooked free perforations or tumor perforations requiring reintervention (drainage or reoperation). It concluded that laparoscopic lavage is feasible in selected patients with Hinchey III peritonitis. Alternatively, resection is recommended [51]. Finally, the World Society of Emergency Surgery (WSES) updated its guidelines for management of acute left-sided colonic diverticulitis, according to the most recent available literature, and suggests performing laparoscopic peritoneal lavage and drainage only in highly selective patients with generalized peritonitis and not be considered as the first-line treatment in patients with peritonitis from acute colonic diverticulitis [52].

27.8 Conclusions

Laparoscopic peritoneal lavage may be considered an effective and safe option for the treatment of patients with sigmoid diverticulitis with Hinchey stage III peritonitis and can be performed as a "bridge" procedure with the intention to avoid the Hartmann procedure.

This technique should be considered suitable to patients without systemic toxicity, no comorbidities, and only in centers experienced in minimally invasive surgeries.

In comparison to sigmoid resections, laparoscopic peritoneal lavage results in higher rates of postoperative abscess formation, requiring more percutaneous drainage interventions without any difference in perioperative mortality and serious morbidity.

Patient selection is of paramount importance. Studies are needed to better identify the selection criteria for patients who might benefit from laparoscopic lavage and to standardize the operative technique. Surgeons utilizing laparoscopic lavage should be aware of the clinical outcomes and risks of unresolved septic foci associated with this approach and should be prepared to offer secondary interventions, as needed.

Several controversies remain about laparoscopic lavage and drainage. Further evidence from randomized clinical trials is needed to define the role of laparoscopic peritoneal lavage and drainage in the treatment of patients with complicated Hinchey III diverticulitis.

References

1. Heise CP. Epidemiology and pathogenesis of diverticular disease. J Gastrointest Surg. 2008;12:1309–11.
2. Feingold D, Steele SR, Lee S, et al. Practice parameters for the treatment of sigmoid diverticulitis. Dis Colon Rectum. 2014;57:284–94.
3. De Sousa L, Chacín B, Escalante R, Do Nascimiento J, Simoes M. Colon dicerticulosis: autopsies findings. Gene. 1997;51(3):184–9.
4. Roberts P, Abel M, Rosen L, Cirocco W, Fleshman J, Leff E. Practice parameters for sigmoid diverticulitis. The standards task force American society of colon and rectal surgeons. Dis Colon Rectum. 1995;38(2):125–32.
5. Littre A. Diverticulitis and its surgical treatment. Proc Interstate Post-Grad Med Assembly N Am. 1928;55:57–65.
6. Cruveilhier J. Traite d'anatomie pathologique generale, vol. 1. Paris: Bailliere; 1849.
7. Graser E. The wrong bowel diverticulum. Arch Klin Chir. 1899;59:63–7.
8. Beer E. Some pathological and clinical aspects of acquired (false) diverticula of the intestine. Am J Med Sci. 1904;128:135–45.
9. Telling WH. Acquired diverticula of the sigmoid flexure, considered especially in relation to secondary pathological processes and their clinical symptoms. Lancet. 1908;1:843–50.
10. Mayo WJ, Wilson LB, Gfffin HZ. Acquired diverticulitis of the large intestine. Surg Gynecol Obstet. 1907;5:8–15.
11. Rolleston HD. Pericolitis sinistra. Lancet. 1905;854:860.
12. Painter NS, Burkitt DP. Diverticular disease of the colon, a 20th century problem. Clin Gastroenterol. 1975;4:3–21.
13. Hartmann H. Chirurgie du rectum. Travaux de Chirurgie, No. 8, Chap XIV. Cancer du rectum. Masson, Paris. 1931.
14. Stabile BE, Puccio E, Van Sonnenberg E, et al. Preoperative percutaneous drainage of diverticular abscesses. Am J Surg. 1990;159:99–105.
15. Wasvary H, Turfah F, Kadro O, Beauregard W. Same hospitalization resection for acute diverticulitis. Am Surg. 1999;65:632–5.
16. Ambrosetti P, Becker C, Terrier F. Colonic diverticulitis: impact of imaging on surgical management – a prospective study of 542 patients. Eur Radiol. 2002;12:1145–9.
17. Hansen O, Graupe F, Stock W. Prognostic factors in perforating diverticulitis of the large intestine. Chirurg. 1998;69:443–9.
18. Mora Lopez L, Serra Pla S, Serra-Aracil X, Ballesteros E, Navarro S. Application of a modified Neff classification to patients with uncomplicated diverticulitis. Color Dis. 2013;15(11):1442–7.
19. Hinchey EJ, Schaal PG, Richards GK. Treatment of perforated diverticular disease of the colon. Adv Surg. 1978;12:85–109.

20. Kaiser AM, Jiang JK, Lake JP, Ault G, Artinyan A, Gonzalez-Ruiz C, Essani R, Beart RW Jr. The management of complicated diverticulitis and the role of computed tomography. Am J Gastroenterol. 2005;100:910–7.
21. Broderick-Villa G, Burchette RJ, Collins JC, Abbas MA, Haigh PI. Hospitalization for acute diverticulitis does not mandate routine elective colectomy. Arch Surg. 2005;140:576–81.
22. Hanna M, Kaiser A. Update on the management of sigmoid diverticulitis. World J Gastroenterol. 2021;27:760–81.
23. Madiedo A, Jason H. Minimally invasive management of diverticular disease. Clin Colon Rectal Surg. 2021;34:113–20.
24. Abraha I, Binda GA, Montedori A, Arezzo A, Cirocchi R. Cochrane Database Syst Rev. 2017;11:CD009277.
25. Lin H, Zhuang Z, Huang X, Li Y. The role of emergency laparoscopic surgery for complicated diverticular disease. Medicine. 2020;99:e22421.
26. Sohn M, Agha A, Heitland W, Gundling F, Steiner P, Iesalnieks I. Damage control strategy for the treatment of perforated diverticulitis with generalized peritonitis. Tech Coloproctol. 2016;20:577–83.
27. Cirocchi R, Popivanov G, Konaktchieva M, Chipeva S, Tellan G, Mingoli A, Zago M, Chiarugi M, Binda GA, Kafka R, Anania G, Donini A, Nascimbeni R, Edilbe M, Afshar S. The role of damage control surgery in the treatment of perforated colonic diverticulitis: a systematic review and meta-analysis. Int J Color Dis. 2021;36:867–79.
28. Bretagnol F, Pautrat K, Mor C, Benchellal Z, Huten N, de Calan L. Emergency laparoscopic management of perforated sigmoid diverticulitis: a promising alternative to more radical procedures. J Am Coll Surg. 2008;206:654–7.
29. Radé F, Bretagnol F, Auguste M, Di Guisto C, Huten N, de Calan L. Determinants of outcome following laparoscopic peritoneal lavage for perforated diverticulitis. Br J Surg. 2014;101:1602–6.
30. Cirocchi R, Afshar S, Di Saverio S, Georgi Popivanov G, De Sol A, Gubbiotti F, Tugnoli G, Sartelli M, Fausto Catena F, Cavaliere D, Taboła R, Fingerhut A, Binda GA. A historical review of surgery for peritonitis secondary to acute colonic diverticulitis: from Lockhart-Mummery to evidence-based medicine. World J Emerg Surg. 2017;12:14.
31. Theodoropoulos D. Current options for the emergency management of diverticular disease and options to reduce the need for colostomy. Clin Colon Rectal Surg. 2018;31:229–35.
32. Escalante R, Bustamante-Lopez L, Lizcano A, Acosta B. Peritoneal lavage in complicated acute diverticulitis. Back to the future. J Clin Gastroenterol. 2016;50:83–5.
33. O'Sullivan GC, Murphy D, O'Brien MG, Ireland A. Laparoscopic management of generalized peritonitis due to perforated colonic diverticula. Am J Surg. 1996;171:432–4.
34. White SI, Frenkiel B, Martin PJ. A ten-year audit of perforated sigmoid diverticulitis: highlighting the outcomes of laparoscopic lavage. Dis Colon Rectum. 2010;53(11):1537–41.
35. Karoui M, Champault A, Pautrat K, Valleur P, Cherqui D, Champault G. Laparoscopic peritoneal lavage or primary anastomosis with defunctioning stoma for Hinchey 3 complicated diverticulitis: results of a comparative study. Dis Colon Rectum. 2009;52(04):609–15.
36. Rossi GL, Mentz R, Bertone S, et al. Laparoscopic peritoneal lavage for Hinchey III diverticulitis: is it as effective as it is applicable? Dis Colon Rectum. 2014;57:1384–90.
37. Vennix S, Musters GD, Mulder IM, Swank HA, Consten EC, Belgers EH, van Geloven AA, Gerhards MF, Govaert MJ, van Grevenstein WM, Hoofwijk AG, Kruyt PM, Nienhuijs SW, Boermeester MA, Vermeulen J, van Dieren S, Lange JF. Laparoscopic peritoneal lavage or sigmoidectomy for perforated diverticulitis with purulent peritonitis: a multicentre, parallel-group, randomised, open-label trial. Lancet. 2015;386:1269–77.
38. Angenete E, Thornell A, Burcharth J, Pommergaard HC, Skullman S, Bisgaard T, Jess P, Lackberg Z, Matthiessen P, Heath J, Roesenberg J, Haglind E. Laparoscopic lavage is feasible and safe for the treatment of perforated diverticulitis with purulent peritonitis: the first results from the randomized controlled trial DILALA. Ann Surg. 2016;263:117–22.
39. Schultz JK, Yaqub S, Wallon C, Blecic L, Forsmo HM, Folkesson J, Buchwald P, Körner H, Dahl FA, Oresland T. G Laparoscopic lavage vs primary resection for acute perforated diver-

ticulitis: the SCANDIV randomized clinica trial. JAMA. 2015;314(13):1364–75. https://doi.org/10.1001/jama.2015.12076.
40. Mandrioli M, Tugnoli G, Di Saverio S. Laparoscopic lavage vs primary resection for perforated diverticulitis. JAMA. 2016;315(10):1053. https://doi.org/10.1001/jama.2015.17864.
41. Pinedo G, Inostrosa G. Cirugía laparoscópica en la enfermedad diverticular. In: Enfermedades del colon, recto y ano, vol. 89. 3rd ed. Capitulo: Enriquez H. Amolca; 2013. p. 1731–5.
42. Zaborowski A, Des C, Winter DC. Evidence-based treatment strategies for acute diverticulitis. Int J Color Dis. 2021;36:467–75.
43. Cirocchi R, Stefano Trastulli S, Vettoretto N, Milani D, Cavaliere D, Renzi C, Adamenko O, Desiderio J, Burattini MF, Prof PA, Arezzo A, Abe FA. Laparoscopic peritoneal lavage: a definitive treatment for diverticular peritonitis or a "bridge" to elective laparoscopic sigmoidectomy? Medicine. 2015;94:334.
44. Shaikh F, Stewart P, Walsh S, Davies R. Laparoscopic peritoneal lavage or surgical resection for acute perforated sigmoid diverticulitis: a systematic review and meta-analysis. Int J Surg. 2017;38:130–7.
45. Gehrman J, Angenete E, Björholt I, Bock D, Rosenberg J, Haglind E. Health economic analysis of laparoscopic lavage versus Hartmann's procedure for diverticulitis in the randomized DILALA trial. Br J Surg. 2016;103:1539–47.
46. Angenete E, Bock D, Rosenberg J, Haglind E. Laparoscopic lavage is superior to colon resection for perforated purulent diverticulitis—a meta-analysis. Int J Color Dis. 2017;32(2):163–9.
47. Vennix S, van Dieren S, Opmeer B, Lange J, Bemelman W. Cost analysis of laparoscopic lavage compared with sigmoid resection for perforated diverticulitis in the Ladies trial. Br J Surg. 2017;104:62–8.
48. Sneiders D, Lambrichts D, Swank H, Blanken-Peeters C, Nienhuijs S, Govaert M, Gerhards M, Hoofwijk A, Bosker R, van der Bilt J, Heijnen B, ten Cate HH, Kleinrensink G, Lange J, Bemelman W. Long-term follow-up of a multicentre cohort study on laparoscopic peritoneal lavage for perforated diverticulitis. Color Dis. 2019;21(6):705–14.
49. Vermeulen J, Lange J. Treatment of perforated diverticulitis with generalized peritonitis: past, present, and future. J World J Surg. 2010;34(3):587–93.
50. Hall J, Hardiman K, Lee S, Lightner A, Stocchi L, Paquette I, Steele S, Feingold D. The American Society of Colon and Rectal Surgeons clinical practice guidelines for the treatment of left-sided colonic diverticulitis. Dis Colon Rectum. 2020;63:728–47.
51. Schultz J, Azhar N, Binda G, Barbara G, Biondo S, Boermeester M, Chabok A, Consten E, van Dijk S, Johanssen A, Kruis W, Lambrichts D, Post S, Ris F, Rockal T, Samuelsson A, Di Saverio S, Tartaglia D, Thorisson A, Winter D, Bemelman W, Angenete E. European Society of Coloproctology: guidelines for the management of diverticular disease of the colon. Color Dis. 2020;22(2):5–28. https://doi.org/10.1111/codi.15140.
52. Sartelli M, Weber DG, Kluger Y, Ansaloni L, et al. 2020 update of the WSES guidelines for the management of acute colonic diverticulitis in the emergency setting. World J Emerg Surg. 2020;15:32.

Elective Surgery 28

Gian Andrea Binda, Antonio Amato, and Johannes Schultz

In recent years, the indications for surgical treatment of diverticular disease have diminished [1, 2], especially for elective procedures.

28.1 Indications

Traditionally, the indications for elective surgery were prophylaxis of recurrence after uncomplicated or complicated episodes of diverticulitis, treatment of chronic symptoms related to diverticular disease, and treatment of chronic complications like fistula or stenosis.

In the late 1990s, the guidelines of several medical and surgical associations [3–5] agreed on the necessity of prophylactic interval sigmoidectomy after two previous episodes of acute uncomplicated diverticulitis (AUD) or after just one episode if the patient was under 50.

This policy was mainly based on outdated studies [6, 7], suggesting a higher probability of further attacks after recurrent episodes of diverticulitis. Furthermore, it was argued that the response to medical treatment would decrease and the risk of complications would increase (to as high as 60%), with a doubling of the mortality rate.

G. A. Binda (✉)
General Surgery, BioMedical Institute, Genoa, Italy
e-mail: gianbinda1@gmail.com

A. Amato
Department of General Surgery, S. Agata Hospital, Imperia, Italy
e-mail: ab.amato@libero.it

J. Schultz
Department of Gastrointestinal Surgery, Akershus University Hospital, Lørenskog, Norway
e-mail: josc@ahus.no

© The Author(s), under exclusive license to Springer Nature Switzerland AG 2022
A. Tursi et al. (eds.), *Colonic Diverticular Disease*,
https://doi.org/10.1007/978-3-030-93761-4_28

In more recent years, with the improvement of knowledge obtained on the natural history of the disease [8–10], those statements have been questioned. In fact, the long-term risk of relapse, the risk of failure of conservative treatment or poor outcome after recurrent episodes of AUD, and the long-term risk of emergency surgery (3–7%), stoma (0–4%), and death (<1%) are lower than previously anticipated. Furthermore, the risk of free perforation decreases with the number of previous episodes of AUD [11, 12], and, therefore, the protective role of surgery after a previous attack is minimal. A US Nationwide Inpatient Sample study reported a significant decline of surgical treatment for diverticulitis, in the period 1991–2005, from 17.9 to 13.7%, whereas the proportion of free perforations among patients, discharged after an admission with diverticular disease, remained unchanged (1.5%) [13]. In addition, surgery does not fully protect against relapses [14, 15].

Previous guidelines also recommended elective surgery after only one previous episode of conservatively managed complicated diverticulitis. However, recent studies evaluating a conservative approach to diverticulitis complicated by an abscess show no increased risk of complicated recurrent attacks [16, 17]. Although others [18, 19] report a higher risk of complicated recurrences, a substantial number of patients can still be treated nonoperatively, whereas the risk of recurrence requiring urgent operation following conservative management of acute complicated diverticulitis is relatively low [18, 20]. Only one small randomized trial compared elective surgery to observation in patients with extraluminal air and/or abscesses. The majority of patients in the observation group did not require elective surgery. However, health-related quality of life (HRQoL) was not evaluated in this trial [21].

To date, elective surgery for preventing complications of diverticulitis is no more indicated [22–24], regardless of the number of previous episodes of diverticulitis. In the past, a more aggressive approach was suggested for young [25] and immunocompromised patients [26]. The rationale was an assumed higher risk of frequent and serious complicated recurrences. However, there is no strong evidence of a worse prognosis after an episode of acute diverticulitis in younger patients, and, for immunocompromised patients, the risk of complications is higher both during recurrent attacks and during elective surgery. Therefore, the indications for elective surgery in young or immunocompromised patients should follow the same principles as those in other patients, i.e., not routinely recommended [27, 28].

Currently, the indications for elective surgery are tailored and surgical treatment should be recommended to patients with persisting symptoms clearly related to diverticular disease and affecting the patient's quality of life.

The first step is to connect the symptoms to DD, especially if uncomplicated, as the differential diagnosis with IBS, segmental colitis associated with diverticulosis (SCAD), or other colitis could be extremely challenging. Chronic complications of diverticulitis as fistula or stenosis, when symptomatic, are still the main indications for elective surgery. Colovesical or colovaginal fistulas may cause septic symptoms such as cystitis and vaginitis with passage of gas or feces through the ureteral or vulvar orifices, symptoms which often significantly impair HRQoL. A stenosis of the sigmoid may cause abdominal pain and/or subocclusive symptoms, usually indicating elective surgery. Other peculiar conditions could affect HRQoL, such as short time intervals between recurrent AD episodes or work commitments with the need to travel a lot, increasing the patient's motivation toward surgery.

If symptoms are clearly related to DD, their severity and impact on quality of life has to be discussed with the patient to balance operative risks and risk factors (i.e., age, body mass index, comorbidities, and specific surgical complications). The final decision has to be shared with the patient.

28.2 Technical Aspects

The technical aspects of elective surgical treatment of diverticulitis may influence the postoperative course and affect functional outcomes and the risk of recurrences. Unfortunately, this aspect is frequently not accounted for in clinical trials and a rigorous standardization of the procedure is still lacking [29]. The key points for the surgical approach are the extent of the resection, the level of vascular ligation, and the mini-invasive approach.

28.2.1 Extent of the Resection

There is a general agreement that the extent of the resection is related to the risk of recurrence. Although based on low-quality evidence, removal of the whole inflamed colon with healthy margins is recommended. The proximal resection margin should be in the nearest colonic segment without macroscopic evidence of inflammation to perform anastomosis in the soft supple tissue. There is no need to resect all proximal diverticula [30]. Almost one-third (28%) of the episodes of acute diverticulitis involve the descending colon; therefore, its distal or even a wider part frequently needs to be excised [31]. As an anastomosis to the distal sigmoid with retention of a sigmoid remnant could increase the risk of recurrence, the distal resection margin should be in the upper rectum [32, 33]. Gonzalez et al. reported that the risk of recurrence was 6.7 and 12% after colorectal versus colo-colic anastomosis, respectively [34]. Mobilization of the splenic flexure is not mandatory, and the need for this step is related to the anatomy and the extent of the resection. However, it should be performed if necessary to allow for a tension-free anastomosis, and the final decision is left to the surgeon's judgment. Retrospectively, Schlussel et al. found that splenic flexure mobilization is associated with a longer-median operative time with no significant differences in major morbidity, thus supporting a tailored choice on an individual basis [35]. Rectal mobilization can also provide additional length and sometimes it is required to overcome postinflammatory rectal strictures.

28.2.2 Vascular Ligation

In contrast to colorectal cancer, there is little consensus on the surgical principles for the management of diverticulitis. Different vascular approaches have been described. The inferior mesenteric artery (IMA) could be divided either proximally (high tie,

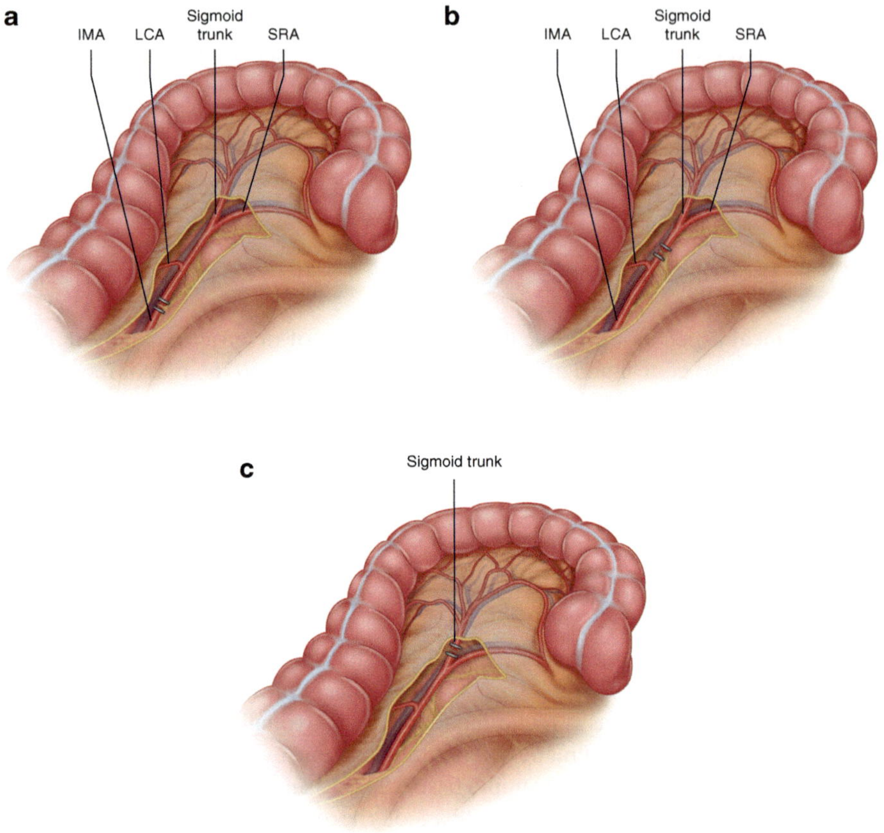

Fig. 28.1 Level of vascular ligation. (**a**) High IMA tie. (**b**) Low IMA tie. (**c**) IMA preservation

Fig. 28.1a) or distally to the origin of the left colic artery (LCA) (low tie, Fig. 28.1b) or preserved through a mid-mesocolic dissection with or without division of the left colic artery (Fig. 28.1c). After high tie, the vascular supply of the proximal colonic stump relies on the marginal artery of Drummond whose insufficiency could lead to poor perfusion of the anastomosis. A randomized study found that the rate of radiological and clinical anastomotic leakage was significantly lower after IMA preservation than that after high tie [36]. Afterward, observational studies showed conflicting results regarding the relationship between anastomotic leak and the level of section of vascular supply [37–39]. A recent meta-analysis and systematic review has failed to demonstrate any advantage for IMA preservation regarding anastomotic morbidity [40].

One randomized controlled trial found that IMA preservation in patients operated electively for diverticular disease leads to better intestinal function. The reason may be a reduced impairment of colonic innervation [41]. In cancer surgery, a series of 44 patients who were prospectively evaluated showed a significantly worse postoperative fecal continence and quality of life after ligation compared to preservation of the IMA [42]. Conversely, a prospective study in male patients undergoing elective laparoscopic sigmoidectomy for diverticular disease with IMA high tie did not observe any detrimental effects or de novo symptoms in bowel, urinary, and sexual functions. From the technical point of view, the authors focused the importance of sectioning IMA 2 cm from its origin, far from the descending sympathetic fibers lying on the aorta [43]. In summary, it seems reasonable to preserve the IMA, provided that colonic cancer requiring oncological resection can be ruled out with certainty. However, extensive postinflammatory fibrosis and adhesions could make an intramesocolic dissection complex, thus increasing the risk of ureteral lesions.

28.2.3 Mini-Invasive Approach

Since the 1990s, laparoscopic sigmoid resection has gained popularity in the elective surgery of diverticular disease. A large retrospective study extracting data from the US National Inpatient Sample database found that laparoscopy was associated with significantly lower postoperative morbidity and a shorter mean hospital stay compared to open surgery. However, 88.3% of patients underwent open surgery and selection bias cannot be ruled out [44]. Similarly, Kakarla et al., by retrospectively analyzing the ACS-NSQIP database, reported that patients treated with laparoscopic resection experienced lower overall morbidity and wound complication after risk-adjusted analysis. The operative time was significantly shorter and the length of hospital stay was significantly longer with open surgery [45]. Observational studies suggested that laparoscopic sigmoid resection is safe and feasible in the elective setting, showing advantages in short-term outcomes (earlier passage of stool, earlier return to liquid diet, less analgesic requirements, etc.). As in other fields of gastrointestinal surgery, this may translate to faster recovery [46–48]. However, laparoscopic resection may be technically challenging when dealing with a complex inflammatory process. Given the observational design of the above-mentioned trials, there is a high risk of selection bias. Randomized studies depict a variegated scenario: Raue et al. found no clear advantage of the laparoscopic over the open approach with comparable postoperative complications and mortality rate as well as early and 12-month quality of life [49]. In another single-blind trial, laparoscopic resection was associated with a significantly longer operative time and reduction of postoperative ileus and hospital stay. Both open and laparoscopic procedures achieved good long-term results in terms of gastrointestinal function, HRQoL, and patient satisfaction. The long-term benefits of laparoscopic surgery were restricted to cosmetic aspects [50, 51]. In the Sigma trial, laparoscopy was associated with a longer operative time, a 15.4% reduction of major complications, shorter hospitalization, and better HRQoL [52]. At a 6-month follow-up, a 27% reduction in the major morbidity and a decrease in HRQoL differences were observed [53]. A Cochrane review analyzing these three RTCs stated that there is uncertainty whether laparoscopic surgery has substantial advantages over open resection.

The level of evidence was low due to a high risk of bias in all included trials [54]. In the last few years, robotic surgery was introduced in the management of diverticulitis. Preliminary results suggest that the robotic approach had a lower conversion rate and significantly increased hospital charges when compared with laparoscopic surgery [55, 56]. Conversion is required in between 13.1 and 19.2% of laparoscopically treated cases and has been recognized as an independent risk factor of morbidity [52]. Factors predictive of conversion include BMI, previous abdominal surgery, the presence of stenosis/fistula, severity of diverticulitis and adhesions, bleeding, and surgical expertise [57, 58]. In a large real-world US nationwide study, high-volume surgeons were 8.80 times more likely to perform a laparoscopic sigmoid resection for diverticular disease than low-volume surgeons [59].

28.2.4 Other Technical Notes

Iatrogenic ureteral injury is a rare complication of colorectal surgery with an incidence of 0.28%. It is associated with severe morbidity and serious sequelae, and intraoperative diagnosis occurs in only 15–30% of cases [60]. After IBD and cancer surgery, procedures for diverticulitis are the third most common reason for iatrogenic ureteral lesions and the laparoscopic approach is associated with a slightly higher risk [61]. As a preventive measure, identification of the ureter should be performed during the visceral mobilization, with lateral-to-medial dissection on the colon side of the Monk's line or with medial-to-lateral dissection along the Gerota plane without entering the retroperitoneum; furthermore, especially in case of severe inflammation or fibrosis that may displace the ureter, this step should start in an unaffected area. In selected patients, prophylactic ureteric catheter placement can help in intraoperative identification even if clear selection criteria have not yet been established [62]. A US population-based study reported a longer operative time, a longer hospital length of stay, and higher cost [63]. More recently, lighted ureteric stents and intraureteral injection of indocyanine green with subsequent visualization under near-infrared fluorescence have been proposed to overcome the loss of tactile feedback during laparoscopic surgery [64, 65].

28.3 Outcomes

As mentioned earlier, the prophylactic role of surgery has expired. The main goal of elective sigmoid resections after diverticulitis is to improve patients' HRQoL. When counseling patients, surgeons need to relate the potential improvement in HRQoL to the risk of morbidity that is related to the surgical intervention. For patients with frequent recurrences of diverticulitis, the improvement of HRQoL is likely to be closely related to the prevention of new attacks.

28.3.1 Improvement in Quality of Life

Several retrospective observational studies have found an improvement in the quality of life in patients after elective sigmoid resection for recurrent diverticulitis or ongoing complaints after an episode of diverticulitis [66]. However, these studies were generally of low quality and were hampered by a probable selection bias. Recently, two randomized trials (DIRECT and LASER trials) have shown improvement of HRQoL in patients operated electively after one or more episodes of diverticulitis [67, 68]. The inclusion criteria were slightly different. Both trials included patients with frequent recurrences (>2 episodes within 2 years) or ongoing complaints (left lower quadrant pain and/or changed bowel habits for at least 3 months) after one episode of acute diverticulitis. However, in the DIRECT trial [67], confirmation of ongoing inflammation (on CT or at endoscopy) was required for patients included due to ongoing complaints. Furthermore, in the LASER trial [68], patients could be included after only one conservatively treated episode of complicated diverticulitis, regardless of the ongoing complaints.

	Direct		Laser	
	Resection *n* = 53	Conservative *n* = 56	Resection *n* = 41	Conservative *n* = 44
Inclusion criteria				
Recurrent diverticulitis (>2 episodes in 2 years)	40(36%)		66 (77%)	
	17 (32%)	23 (41%)	34(83%)	32(73%)
Ongoing complaints (> 3 months)	69(63%)		5 (6%)	
	36 (68%)	33 (59%)	2(5%)	3(7%)
Complicated diverticulitis (at least one episode)	Not an inclusion criterion		23 (27%)	
			10(24%)	13(30%)
Baseline				
Age; mean (SD)/median (IQR)	54.1 (44.6–62.1)	56.5 (48.3–63.2)	59 (51.5–63.0)	59 (50.3–62.8)
Number of episodes	3.1 (1.0)	4.1 (2.0)	4.6 (3.5)	4.0 (3.1)
GIQLI (SD)	92.6 (22.8)	92.2 (21.3)	104.8 (21.9)	99.8 (20.9)
VAS pain (SD)[a]	63.3 (21.0)	69.3 (13.6)	4.2 (2.9)	4.6 (2.6)
Results				
GIQLI 6 months (SD)	114.4 (22.3)	100.4 (22.7)	114.9(16.8)	102.0 (21.7)
GIQLI 1 year (SD)	112.8 (23.3)	101.2		
GIQLI 5 years (SD)	118.2 (21.0)	108.5(20.0)		
VAS pain 6 month (SD)[a]	23.9 (23.4)	49.8 (22.2)	1.8 (1.9)	3.3 (2.0)
Anastomotic insufficiency (6 months)	7(15%)	0	2(5%)	0

Abbreviations: *SD* Standard deviation, *IQR* Inter quartile range, *GIQLI* Gastrointestinal Quality of Life Score, *VAS* Visual analogue scale

[a] VAS 1–100 in the DIRECT trial (1 = no pain, 100 = worst imaginable pain) and VAS 1–10 in the LASER trial (1 = no pain, 10 = worst imaginable pain)

There are limitations with both trials. They were both aborted prematurely, thus limiting the conclusions that can be drawn from them, as truncated randomized controlled trails frequently overestimate the effect size of the trial intervention [69]. In the DIRECT trial there were several crossovers, especially at long-term follow-up, which further complicates the interpretation of results [70]. In addition, the inclusion of different entities (ongoing complaints and frequent recurrences) in the same trial makes it difficult to decide which of the groups would profit the most. Finally, no SHAM operation was performed in the control group for ethical reasons. Surgery is known to have a considerable placebo effect, which most certainly explains part of the effect seen in both studies [71].

It is noteworthy that both trials observed an improvement of HRQoL in both groups. The observed difference in GIQLI between the groups is just above the minimally clinical important difference at 6 months and long-term follow-up in the DIRECT trial showed a decrease in the difference over time [70]. Unfortunately, neither of the trials reported the number of patients with improved HRQoL and the number of patients with reduced HRQoL after surgery. Another interesting fact is that 68% of conservatively treated patients in the LASER trial were satisfied with the treatment 6 months after inclusion versus 78% in the surgically treated group. Pain was improved after surgery in both groups but there were still patients with daily or constant pain 6 months after surgery in the LASER trial.

28.3.2 Prevention of New Attacks

Most patients with frequent recurrences of diverticulitis have recurrent attacks in the same bowel segment. To prevent further recurrences, it is important to resect the colon from the affected bowel segment down to the colorectal junction as the recurrence rate is higher after colosigmoid anastomosis [15, 33]. Although sigmoid resection significantly reduces the risk of recurrent attacks [67, 72], the risk is far above zero [15, 54, 73]. A possible reason for that could be, as reported in one study [74], that 35% of recurrent diverticulitis attacks occur at a different colonic location than previous attacks.

28.3.3 Morbidity

Elective surgery for diverticular disease is now mostly performed laparoscopically. Although laparoscopy in general reduces the risk of superficial wound infections and wound dehiscence, the risk of anastomotic insufficiency (AI) remains. The risk of AI is reported to be between 0 and 15% [54]. Therefore, there is always the risk of a stoma for all operated patients. In the DIRECT trial [70], one patient (2%) ended up with a permanent stoma. This proportion may be higher in older patients and in patients with fistulas or stenosis, some of whom should be counseled to undergo Hartmann's procedure in the first place. A recent national inpatient propensity score-matched cohort study has found a higher risk of major complications in patients treated with elective sigmoid resection for diverticular disease than in patients treated with the same procedure for colorectal cancer [75]. The reoperation rate was also significantly higher after resection for diverticular disease. However, the AI rate was higher in the cancer group (9.2 vs 8.3%, $p < 0.001$); it is therefore difficult to explain why the reoperation rate was higher in diverticular disease. One explanation might be that most of the operations were performed openly and that wound dehiscence might be a reason for reoperation. Another explanation might be incompleteness of records in the database. It is noteworthy that the overall mortality was as high as 2.3% after resection for diverticular disease. The explanation for the high mortality might be that some of the patients were electively operated for complications of diverticular disease.

28.3.4 Risk Benefit Assessment

When counseling the patient, the surgeon has to weigh the risks of surgery against the possible gain in HRQoL. All patients should be informed that sigmoid resection for diverticular disease is associated with considerable morbidity, risk of a permanent stoma and even mortality [75]. Patients with frequent recurrences will have a lower chance of recurrence after a sigmoid resection. The expected gain in HRQoL is relatively small and patients need to be informed that symptoms may persist even after an operation.

References

1. Biondo S. The diminishing role of surgery for acute diverticulitis. Br J Surg. 2019;106(4):308–9.
2. Li D, Baxter NN, McLeod RS, Moineddin R, Nathens AB. The decline of elective colectomy following diverticulitis: a population-based analysis. Dis Colon Rectum. 2016;59:332–9.
3. Stollman NH, Raskin JB. Diagnosis and management of diverticular disease of the colon in adults. Ad hoc practice parameters Committee of the American College of gastroenterology. Am J Gastroenterol. 1999;94:3110–21.
4. Roberts P, Abel M, Rosen L, et al. Practice parameters for sigmoid diverticulitis. The standards task force American Society of Colon and Rectal Surgeons. Dis Colon Rectum. 1995;38:125–32.
5. Kohler L, Sauerland S, Neugebauer E. Diagnosis and treatment of diverticular disease: results of a consensus development conference. The scientific Committee of the European Association for endoscopic surgery. Surg Endosc. 1999;13:430–6.
6. Parks TG. Natural history of diverticular disease of the colon. A review of 521 cases. BMJ. 1969;IV:639–42.
7. Farmakis N, Tudor RG, Keighley MRB. The 5-year natural history of complicated diverticular disease. Br J Surg. 1994;84:733–5.
8. Chapman JR, Dozois EJ, Wolff BG, Gullerud RE, Larson DR. Diverticulitis: a progressive disease? Do multiple recurrences predict less favorable outcomes? Ann Surg. 2006;243(6):876–30. https://doi.org/10.1097/01.sla.0000219682.98158.11.
9. Pittet O, Kotzampassakis N, Schmidt S, Denys A, Demartines N, Calmes JM. Recurrent left colonic diverticulitis episodes: more severe than the initial diverticulitis? World J Surg. 2009;33:547–52.

10. Janes S, Meagher A, Frizelle FA. Elective surgery after acute diverticulitis. Br J Surg. 2005;92:133–42.
11. Ritz JP, Lehmann KS, Frericks B, Stroux A, Buhr HJ, Holmer C. Outcome of patients with acute sigmoid diverticulitis: multivariate analysis of risk factors for free perforation. Surgery. 2011;149(5):606–13. https://doi.org/10.1016/j.surg.2010.10.005.
12. Humes DJ, West J. The role of acute diverticulitis in the development of complicated colonic diverticular disease and one year mortality following diagnosis in the UK: population based cohort study. Gut. 2012;61:95–100.
13. Ricciardi R, Baxter NN, Read TE, Marcello PW, Hall J, Roberts PL. Is the decline in the surgical treatment for diverticulitis associated with an increase in complicated diverticulitis? Dis Colon Rectum. 2009;52:1558–63.
14. Haglund U, Hellberg R, Johnsen C, Hulten L. Complicated diverticular disease of the sigmoid colon. An analysis of short and long term outcome in 392 patients. Ann Chir Gynaecol. 1979;68:41–6.
15. Longchamp G, Abbassi Z, Meyer J, Toso C, Buchs NC, Ris F. Surgical resection does not avoid the risk of diverticulitis recurrence-a systematic review of risk factors. Int J Color Dis. 2021;36(2):227–37.
16. Aquina CT, Becerra AZ, Xu Z, Justiniano CF, Noyes K, Monson JRT, et al. Population-based study of outcomes following an initial acute diverticular abscess. Br J Surg. 2019;106:467–76.
17. Gregersen R, Mortensen LQ, Burcharth J, Pommergaard HC, Rosenberg J. Treatment of patients with acute colonic diverticulitis complicated by abscess formation: a systematic review. Int J Surg. 2016;35:201–8.
18. Devaraj B, Liu W, Tatum J, Cologne K, Kaiser AM. Medically treated diverticular abscess associated with high risk of recurrence and disease complications. Dis Colon Rectum. 2016;59:208–15.
19. Lambrichts DPV, Bolkenstein HE, van der Does DCHE, Dieleman D, Crolla RMPH, Dekker JWT, et al. Multicentre study of non-surgical management of diverticulitis with abscess formation. Br J Surg. 2019;106:458–66.
20. Buchwald P, Dixon L, Wakeman CJ, Eglinton TW, Frizelle FA. Hinchey I and II diverticular abscesses: longterm outcome of conservative treatment. ANZ J Surg. 2017;87:1011–4.
21. You K, Bendl R, Taut C, et al. Randomized clinical trial of elective resection versus observation in diverticulitis with extraluminal air or abscess initially managed conservatively. Br J Surg. 2018;105:971–9.
22. Binda GA, Cuomo R, Laghi A, Nascimbeni R, Serventi A, Bellini D, et al. Practice parameters for the treatment of colonic diverticular disease: Italian Society of Colon and Rectal Surgery (SICCR) guidelines. Tech Coloproctol. 2015;19(10):615–26.
23. Hall J, Hardiman K, Lee S, et al. The American Society of Colon and Rectal Surgeons clinical practice guidelines for the treatment of left-sided colonic diverticulitis. Dis Colon Rectum. 2020;63(6):728–47.
24. Schultz JK, Azhar N, Binda GA, et al. European Society of Coloproctology: guidelines for the management of diverticular disease of the colon. Color Dis. 2020 Sep;22(Suppl 2):5–28. https://doi.org/10.1111/codi.15140.
25. Rafferty J, Shellito P, Hyman NH, Buie WD. Standards Committee of the American Society of colon and Rectal surgeons. Practice parameters for sigmoid diverticulitis. Dis Colon Rectum. 2006;49:939–44.
26. Pourfarziani V, Mousavi-Nayeeni SM, Ghaheri H, et al. The outcome of diverticulosis in kidney recipients with polycystic kidney disease. Transplant Proc. 2007;39:1054–6.
27. van de Wall BJ, Poerink JA, Draaisma WA, Reitsma JB, Consten EC, Broeders IA. Diverticulitis in young versus elderly patients: a meta-analysis. Scand J Gastroenterol. 2013;48:643–51.
28. Biondo S, Trenti L, Elvira J, Golda T, Kreisler E. Outcomes of colonic diverticulitis according to the reason of immunosuppression. Am J Surg. 2016;212:384–90.
29. Ambrosetti P, Gervaz P. Laparoscopic elective sigmoidectomy for diverticular disease: a plea for standardization of the procedure. Color Dis. 2014 Feb;16(2):90–4.

30. Wolff BG, Ready RL, MacCarty RL, Dozois RR, Beart RW Jr. Influence of sigmoid resection on progression of diverticular disease of the colon. Dis Colon Rectum. 1984;27:645–7.
31. Hall JF, Roberts PL, Ricciardi R, et al. Colonic diverticulitis: does age predict severity of disease on CT imaging? Dis Colon Rectum. 2010;53:121–5.
32. Thaler K, Baig MK, Berho M, et al. Determinants of recurrence after sigmoid resection for uncomplicated diverticulitis. Dis Colon Rectum. 2003;46:385–8.
33. Benn PL, Wolff BG, Ilstrup DM. Level of anastomosis and recurrent colonic diverticulitis. Am J Surg. 1986;151:269–71.
34. Gonzalez R, Smith CD, Mattar SG, Venkatesh KR, Mason E, Duncan T, Wilson R, Miller J, Ramshaw BJ. Laparoscopic vs open resection for the treatment of diverticular disease. Surg Endosc. 2004 Feb;18(2):276–80.
35. Schlussel AT, Wiseman JT, Kelly JF, et al. Location is everything: the role of splenic flexure mobilization during colon resection for diverticulitis. Int J Surg. 2017;40:124–9.
36. Tocchi A, Mazzoni G, Fornasari V, Miccini M, Daddi G, Tagliacozzo S. Preservation of the inferior mesenteric artery in colorectal resection for complicated diverticular disease. Am J Surg. 2001;182:162–7.
37. Sohn M, Schlitt HJ, Hornung M, Zülke C, Hochrein A, Moser C, Agha A. Preservation of the superior rectal artery: influence of surgical technique on anastomotic healing and postoperative morbidity in laparoscopic sigmoidectomy for diverticular disease. Int J Colorectal Dis. 2017;32(7):955–60.
38. Lehmann RK, Brounts LR, Johnson EK, Rizzo JA, Steele SR. Does sacrifice of the inferior mesenteric artery or superior rectal artery affect anastomotic leak following sigmoidectomy for diverticulitis? A retrospective review. Am J Surg. 2011 May;201(5):623–7.
39. De Nardi P, Gazzetta P. Does inferior mesenteric artery ligation affect outcome in elective colonic resection for diverticular disease? ANZ J Surg. 2018;88:E778–81.
40. Cirocchi R, Popivanov G, Binda GA, et al. Sigmoid resection for diverticular disease – to ligate or to preserve the inferior mesenteric artery? Results of a systematic review and meta-analysis. Color Dis. 2019;21:623–31.
41. Masoni L, Mari FS, Nigri G, et al. Preservation of the inferior mesenteric artery via laparoscopic sigmoid colectomy performed for diverticular disease: real benefit or technical challenge: a randomized controlled clinical trial. Surg Endosc. 2013;27:199–206.
42. Dobrowolski S, Hac S, Kobiela J, Sledzinski Z. Should we preserve the inferior mesenteric artery during sigmoid colectomy? Neurogastroenterol. 2009;21:1288–e123.
43. Jolivet M, Trilling B, Sage PY, Boussat B, Girard E, Faucheron JL. Prospective evaluation of functional outcomes after laparoscopic sigmoidectomy with high tie of the inferior mesenteric artery for diverticular disease in consecutive male patients. TIC. 2020;24(1):33–40.
44. Masoomi H, Buchberg B, Nguyen B, Tung V, Stamos MJ, Mills S. Outcomes of laparoscopic versus open colectomy in elective surgery for diverticulitis. World J Surg. 2011 Sep;35(9):2143–8.
45. Kakarla VR, Nurkin SJ, Sharma S, Ruiz DE, Tiszenkel H. Elective laparoscopic versus open colectomy for diverticulosis: an analysis of ACS-NSQIP database. Surg Endosc. 2012 Jul;26(7):1837–42.
46. Martinolich J, Croasdale DR, Bhakta AS, et al. Laparoscopic surgery for diverticular fistulas: outcomes of 111 consecutive cases at a single institution. J Gastrointest Surg. 2019;23:1015–21.
47. Keller DS, Delaney CP, Hashemi L, Haas EM. A national evaluation of clinical and economic outcomes in open versus laparoscopic colorectal surgery. Surg Endosc. 2016;30:4220–8.
48. Alves A, Panis Y, Slim K, et al. French multicentre prospective observational study of laparoscopic versus open colectomy for sigmoid diverticular disease. Br J Surg. 2005;92:1520–5.
49. Raue W, Paolucci V, Asperger W, Albrecht R, Büchler MW, Schwenk W. LAPDIV-CAMIC trial group. Laparoscopic sigmoid resection for diverticular disease has no advantages over open approach: midterm results of a randomized controlled trial. Langenbeck's Arch Surg. 2011;396(7):973–80.

50. Gervaz P, Inan I, Perneger T, Schiffer E, Morel P. A prospective, randomized, single-blind comparison of laparoscopic versus open sigmoid colectomy for diverticulitis. Ann Surg. 2010;252(1):3–8.
51. Gervaz P, Mugnier-Konrad B, Morel P, Huber O, Inan I. Laparoscopic versus open sigmoid resection for diverticulitis: long-term results of a prospective, randomized trial. Surg Endosc. 2011;25(10):3373–8.
52. Klarenbeek BR, Veenhof AA, Bergamaschi R, van der Peet DL, van den Broek WT, de Lange ES, Bemelman WA, Heres P, Lacy AM, Engel AF, Cuesta MA. Laparoscopic sigmoid resection for diverticulitis decreases major morbidity rates: a randomized control trial: short-term results of the sigma trial. Ann Surg. 2009;249(1):39–44.
53. Klarenbeek BR, Bergamaschi R, Veenhof AA, van der Peet DL, van den Broek WT, de Lange ES, Bemelman WA, Heres P, Lacy AM, Cuesta MA. Laparoscopic versus open sigmoid resection for diverticular disease: follow-up assessment of the randomized control sigma trial. Surg Endosc. 2011 Apr;25(4):1121–6.
54. Abraha I, Binda GA, Montedori A, Arezzo A, Cirocchi R. Laparoscopic versus open resection for sigmoid diverticulitis. Cochrane Database Syst Rev. 2017;11(11):CD009277.
55. Raskin ER, Keller DS, Gorrepati ML, Akiel-Fu S, Mehendale S, Cleary RK. Propensity-matched analysis of sigmoidectomies for diverticular disease. JSLS. 2019;23:23.
56. Ogilvie JW Jr, Saunders RN, Parker J, Luchtefeld MA. Sigmoidectomy for diverticulitis: a propensity-matched comparison of minimally invasive approaches. J Surg Res. 2019;243:434–9.
57. Le Moine MC, Fabre JM, Vacher C, Navarro F, Picot MC, Domergue J. Factors and consequences of conversion in laparoscopic sigmoidectomy for diverticular disease. Br J Surg. 2003;90:232–6.
58. Bastawrous AL, Landmann RG, Liu Y, Liu E, Cleary RK. Incidence, associated risk factors, and impact of conversion to laparotomy in elective minimally invasive sigmoidectomy for diverticular disease. Surg Endosc. 2020 Feb;34(2):598–609.
59. Weber WP, Guller U, Jain NB, Pietrobon R, Oertli D. Impact of surgeon and hospital caseload on the likelihood of performing laparoscopic vs open sigmoid resection for diverticular disease: a study based on 55,949 patients. Arch Surg. 2007 Mar;142(3):253–9.
60. Halabi WJ, Jafari MD, Nguyen VQ, et al. Ureteral injuries in colorectal surgery: an analysis of trends, outcomes, and risk factors over a 10-year period in the United States. Dis Colon Rectum. 2014;57(2):179–86.
61. Palaniappa NC, Telem DA, Ranasinghe NE, et al. Incidence of iatrogenic ureteral injury after laparoscopic colectomy. Arch Surg. 2012 Mar;147(3):267–71.
62. Speicher PJ, Goldsmith ZG, Nussbaum DP, Turley RS, Peterson AC, Mantyh CR. Ureteral stenting in laparoscopic colorectal surgery. J Surg Res. 2014;190(1):98–103.
63. Coakley KM, Kasten KR, Sims SM, Prasad T, Heniford BT, Davis BR. Prophylactic ureteral catheters for colectomy: a national surgical quality improvement program-based analysis. Dis Colon Rectum. 2018;61:84–8.
64. Boyan WP, Lavy D, Dinallo A, et al. Lighted ureteral stents in laparoscopic colorectal surgery; a five-year experience. Ann Transl Med. 2017;5(3):44.
65. Siddighi S, Yune JJ, Hardesty J. Indocyanine green for intraoperative localization of ureter. Am J Obstet Gynecol. 2014 Oct;211(4):436.e1–2.
66. Andeweg CS, Berg R, Staal JB, ten Broek RP, van Goor H. Patient-reported outcomes after conservative or surgical Management of Recurrent and Chronic Complaints of diverticulitis: systematic review and meta-analysis. Clin Gastroenterol Hepatol. 2016;14(2):183–90.
67. van de Wall BJM, Stam MAW, Draaisma WA, et al. Surgery versus conservative management for recurrent and ongoing left-sided diverticulitis (DIRECT trial): an open-label, multicentre, randomised controlled trial. Lancet Gastroenterol Hepatol. 2017;2(1):13–22.
68. Santos A, Mentula P, Pinta T, et al. Comparing laparoscopic elective sigmoid resection with conservative treatment in improving quality of life of patients with diverticulitis: the laparoscopic elective sigmoid resection following diverticulitis (LASER) randomized clinical trial. JAMA Surg. 2021;156(2):129–36.

69. Færden AEØ T, Wasmuth HH, Schultz JK. Bekkenreservoar ved ulcerøs kolitt. Gastroenterologen; 2019. p. 10–3.
70. Bolkenstein HE, Consten ECJ, van der Palen J, et al. Long-term outcome of surgery versus conservative Management for Recurrent and Ongoing Complaints after an episode of diverticulitis: 5-year follow-up results of a multicenter randomized controlled trial (DIRECT-trial). Ann Surg. 2019;269(4):612–20.
71. Jonas WB, Crawford C, Colloca L, et al. To what extent are surgery and invasive procedures effective beyond a placebo response? A systematic review with meta-analysis of randomised, sham controlled trials. BMJ Open. 2015;5(12):e009655.
72. Azhar N, Johanssen A, Sundström T, et al. Laparoscopic lavage vs primary resection for acute perforated diverticulitis: long-term outcomes from the Scandinavian diverticulitis (SCANDIV) randomized clinical trial. JAMA Surg. 2021;156(2):121–7.
73. Andeweg C, Peters J, Bleichrodt R, van Goor H. Incidence and risk factors of recurrence after surgery for pathology-proven diverticular disease. World J Surg. 2008;32(7):1501–6.
74. Gervaz P, Platon A, Widmer L, Ambrosetti P, Poletti PA. A clinical and radiological comparison of sigmoid diverticulitis episodes 1 and 2. Color Dis. 2012;14(4):463–8.
75. Ilyas MI, Zangbar B, Nfonsam VN, et al. Are there differences in outcome after elective sigmoidectomy for diverticular disease and for cancer? A national inpatient study. Colorectal Dis. 2017;19(3):260–5.

GPSR Compliance

The European Union's (EU) General Product Safety Regulation (GPSR) is a set of rules that requires consumer products to be safe and our obligations to ensure this.

If you have any concerns about our products, you can contact us on ProductSafety@springernature.com

In case Publisher is established outside the EU, the EU authorized representative is:

Springer Nature Customer Service Center GmbH
Europaplatz 3
69115 Heidelberg, Germany

Batch number: 10726058

Printed by Printforce, the Netherlands